# Cancer Treatment and Research

Volume 129

**Series Editor**
Steven T. Rosen, Duarte, USA

This book series provides detailed updates on the state of the art in the treatment of different forms of cancer and also covers a wide spectrum of topics of current research interest. Clinicians will benefit from expert analysis of both standard treatment options and the latest therapeutic innovations and from provision of clear guidance on the management of clinical challenges in daily practice. The research-oriented volumes focus on aspects ranging from advances in basic science through to new treatment tools and evaluation of treatment safety and efficacy. Each volume is edited and authored by leading authorities in the topic under consideration. In providing cutting-edge information on cancer treatment and research, the series will appeal to a wide and interdisciplinary readership. The series is listed in PubMed/Index Medicus.

Ravi Salgia • Prakash Kulkarni
Editors

# Immunotherapies in Solid Tumors

## A Team Medicine Approach

Springer

*Editors*
Ravi Salgia
Department of Medical Oncology
and Therapeutics Research
City of Hope National Medical Center
Duarte, CA, USA

Prakash Kulkarni
Department of Medical Oncology
and Therapeutics Research
City of Hope National Medical Center
Duarte, CA, USA

ISSN 0927-3042 ISSN 2509-8497 (electronic)
Cancer Treatment and Research
ISBN 978-3-031-97241-6 ISBN 978-3-031-97242-3 (eBook)
https://doi.org/10.1007/978-3-031-97242-3



This Springer imprint is published by the registered company Springer Nature Switzerland AG
The registered company address is: Gewerbestrasse 11, 6330 Cham, Switzerland

# Preface

Immunotherapy is a type of cancer treatment which leverages the patient's own immune system to fight cancer. By either boosting or modifying the immune system's ability to recognize and attack cancer cells, immunotherapy has revolutionized cancer therapy. It can be used alone or in combination with other cancer treatments such as chemotherapy, radiation therapy, and surgery.

Currently, several different types of cancer immunotherapies exist such as T-cell therapy, immune checkpoint inhibitors, monoclonal antibodies, and cancer vaccines, which can result in sustainable responses in patients with a wide range of metastatic diseases. Despite the promising results, however, several challenges remain, such as the almost inevitable immune resistance, drug-related toxicity, and the lack of established and reliable predictive biomarkers to predict toxicity and/or discern a patient's response to immunotherapy. Thus, we undertook this endeavor to bring out this book dedicated to immunotherapy, how we can personalize it to each patient, and how basic research scientists and clinicians can work together to embrace a Team Medicine approach to derive maximum impact of this revolutionary therapy that emboldens the patient's own immune system which is comprised by the menacing disease.

To this end, we invited our esteemed colleagues at City of Hope to share their experiences in treating patients with various solid tumors. Soon, it became obvious that it may be worth sharing our collective experience and knowledge with our colleagues worldwide. This was the genesis for putting together this compendium entitled *Immunotherapies in Solid Tumors: A Team Medicine Approach.*

The book embodies 14 chapters each of which is contributed by highly experienced and renowned physicians and scientists in their respective fields. An introductory chapter provides a brief overview of the different types of cancer immunotherapies currently available, their mechanisms of action, and the benefits and potential side effects as well as the almost inevitable issue of therapy resistance. In addition, an overview of the various combination therapies such as chemotherapy, radiation therapy, and targeted therapy, which are currently used in combination with cancer immunotherapy, is presented. Finally, the chapter highlights how a "Team Medicine" approach could enable all eligible cancer patients to receive this promising treatment to treat their respective cancer types. Chapter 2 provides a brief introduction to artificial intelligence (AI) and machine learning (ML) approaches in designing immunotherapy in cancer. Artificial intelligence (AI) and machine learning (ML) are revolutionizing cancer immunotherapy by addressing the complex interplay between cancer and the immune system. This chapter explores how AI technologies enhance immunotherapy development across multiple domains: antibody design, response prediction, biomarker identification, and T-cell target discovery.

More detailed information regarding the different immunotherapies as well as their combinations when applicable in various solid tumors including breast cancer, colon cancer, glioblastoma, head and neck cancer, lung cancer, melanoma, ovarian cancer, pancreatic cancer, prostate cancer, and renal cell carcinoma is discussed in the ensuing chapters (Chaps. 3, 4, 5, 6, 7, 8, 9, 10, 11, 12, and 13). Chapter 14, "Phenotypic Plasticity, Non-genetic Mechanisms, and Immune Drug Resistance in Cancer," which serves as the concluding chapter, summarizes the mechanisms underlying cancer immunotherapy resistance, especially the contributions of phenotypic plasticity and the underlying nongenetic mechanisms. Furthermore, recent developments in preventing relapses following treatment so that the efficacy of immunotherapy can be improved are also briefly discussed. Finally, the positive impact of an interdisciplinary "Team Medicine" approach to personalize cancer immunotherapy for each patient is highlighted.

We hope this compendium will encourage our colleagues worldwide involved both in basic and translational research, to benefit from such a collaborative effort so that more effective immunotherapies and novel treatment strategies may be designed that can help the patients. We trust the book will serve as a valuable companion not only to academic researchers working in larger medical centers but also to those working in the local communities affiliated with the major centers. We believe this book will also interest our colleagues in the pharmaceutical and biotechnology sector interested in immunotherapy, especially for solid tumors. Finally, this book should serve as a major reference for graduate students, postdoctoral scientists, and academics with an interest in cancer immunotherapy from an interdisciplinary, Team Medicine perspective.

Duarte, CA, USA Ravi Salgia
Duarte, CA, USA Prakash Kulkarni

# Acknowledgments

A major part of the reason to put this compendium together were the Medical Oncology Symposia that are held every six months in the Department of Medical Oncology at City of Hope over the past several years. There has hardly been a symposium where a session is not devoted to discussing immunotherapy. Therefore, we would like to first and foremost thank the members of our respective laboratories and clinics for their enthusiasm, tremendous efforts, and invaluable contributions to make this endeavor a reality. In addition, we thank our patients and their families for putting their trust in us to advance path-breaking cancer research and cancer care.

We would like to acknowledge Gregory Sutorius, Executive Editor, Springer Nature, Switzerland AG, for soliciting our book proposal and guiding us through the publication process, which at times felt rather overwhelming, and Nishanthini Vetrivel, Production Editor (Books), for her outstanding support and meticulous attention to detail. It was a real pleasure to work with them. Greg and Nisha were very professional and helpful in making sure we stayed the course.

And last but not least, we express our gratitude to our families for their love, encouragement, and their incredible support.

Ravi Salgia
Prakash Kulkarni

# Contents

# Contributors

**Bamidele A. Adesunloye** City of Hope, Newnan, GA, USA

**Arya Amini** Department of Medical Oncology, City of Hope National Medical Center, Duarte, CA, USA

**Gagandeep Brar** Department of Medical Oncology, City of Hope National Medical Center, Duarte, CA, USA

**Justine Yang Bruce** Carbone Cancer Center, University of Wisconsin, Madison, WI, USA
Department of Medicine, School of Medicine and Public Health, University of Wisconsin, Madison, WI, USA

**Debora Bruno** Department of Medical Oncology, City of Hope, Newnan, GA, USA

**Hannah Chang** Department of Medical Oncology and Therapeutics Research, City of Hope Comprehensive Cancer Center, Duarte, CA, USA

**Vincent Chung** Department of Medical Oncology & Therapeutics Research, City of Hope National Medical Center, Duarte, CA, USA

**Bridget Crossman** Department of Human Oncology, School of Medicine and Public Health, University of Wisconsin, Madison, WI, USA

**Bridget E. Crossman** Department of Human Oncology, University of Wisconsin, Madison, WI, USA

**Dana Do** Department of Medical Oncology, City of Hope National Medical Center, Duarte, CA, USA

**Max Duesberg** Department of Internal Medicine, Santa Clara Valley Medical Center, San Jose, CA, USA

**Pankaj Garg** Department of Chemistry, GLA University, Mathura, Uttar Pradesh, India

**Tiffany Glazer** Department of Surgery, School of Medicine and Public Health, University of Wisconsin, Madison, WI, USA
Carbone Cancer Center, University of Wisconsin, Madison, WI, USA

**Regan L. Harmon** Department of Human Oncology, University of Wisconsin, Madison, WI, USA

**Vanessa Hsu** City of Hope Comprehensive Cancer Center, Duarte, CA, USA

**Mari Iida** Department of Human Oncology, University of Wisconsin, Madison, WI, USA

**Salvador Jaime-Casas** City of Hope Comprehensive Cancer Center, Duarte, CA, USA

**Irene Kang** Department of Medical Oncology and Therapeutics Research, City of Hope Comprehensive Cancer Center, Irvine, CA, USA

**Ajaz Khan** Department of Medical Oncology, Zion, IL, USA

**Randall Kimple** Department of Human Oncology, University of Wisconsin, Madison, WI, USA
Carbone Cancer Center, University of Wisconsin, Madison, WI, USA

**Sudarsan Vishnu Kollimuttathuillam** Department of Medical Oncology, City of Hope, Irvine, CA, USA

**Prakash Kulkarni** Department of Medical Oncology and Therapeutics Research, City of Hope National Medical Center, Duarte, CA, USA
Department of Systems Biology, City of Hope National Medical Center, Duarte, CA, USA

**Colton Ladbury** Department of Medical Oncology, City of Hope National Medical Center, Duarte, CA, USA

**Benjamin Leach** Department of Medical Oncology and Therapeutics Research, City of Hope National Medical Center, Mission Hills, CA, USA

**Matthew Lee** Department of Medical Oncology and Therapeutics Research, City of Hope National Medical Center, Duarte, CA, USA

**Percy Lee** Department of Radiation Oncology, City of Hope Orange County Lennar Foundation Cancer Center, Irvine, CA, USA

**Alexis LeVee** Department of Medical Oncology and Therapeutics Research, City of Hope Comprehensive Cancer Center, Duarte, CA, USA

**Aaron Lewis** Department of Surgical Oncology, City of Hope Comprehensive Cancer Center (COH), Duarte, CA, USA

**Candie Y. Lin** Department of Human Oncology, University of Wisconsin, Madison, WI, USA

**Rimas V. Lukas** Department of Neurology, Lou & Jean Malnati Brain Tumor Institute, Northwestern University, Evanston, IL, USA

**B. Madhu Krishna** Department of Medical Oncology, Beckman Research Institute, City of Hope Comprehensive Cancer Center and National Medical Center, Duarte, CA, USA

**Laleh Melstrom** Department of Surgical Oncology, City of Hope Comprehensive Cancer Center (COH), Duarte, CA, USA

**Amartej Merla** Department of Medical Oncology, Lancaster, CA, USA

**Atish Mohanty** Department of Medical Oncology & Therapeutics Research, Beckman Research Institute of City of Hope Comprehensive Cancer Center and National Medical Center, Duarte, CA, USA

**Meera Nair** William J. Brennan High School, San Antonio, TX, USA

**Charles B. Nguyen** City of Hope Orange County, Irvine, CA, USA

**Siddhika Pareek** Department of Medical Oncology & Therapeutics Research, City of Hope National Medical Center, Duarte, CA, USA

**Krushangi Patel** City of Hope Department of Medical Oncology & Therapeutics Research, City of Hope Comprehensive Cancer Center Long Beach, Long Beach, CA, USA

**Evan P. Pisick** City of Hope Chicago, Zion, IL, USA

**Swapnil Rajurkar** City of Hope National Medical Center, Upland, CA, USA

**Sravani Ramisetty** Department of Medical Oncology, Beckman Research Institute, City of Hope Comprehensive Cancer Center and National Medical Center, Duarte, CA, USA

**Mustafa Raoof** Department of Surgical Oncology, City of Hope Comprehensive Cancer Center (COH), Duarte, CA, USA

**Amanda Reyes** Department of Medical Oncology and Therapeutics Research, City of Hope National Medical Center, Duarte, CA, USA

**Ravi Salgia** Department of Medical Oncology and Therapeutics Research, City of Hope National Medical Center, Duarte, CA, USA

**Lokesh Seth** Department of Medical Oncology, City of Hope National Medical Center, Duarte, CA, USA

**Koral Shah** City of Hope Comprehensive Cancer Center, Duarte, CA, USA

**Sagun Shrestha** City of Hope Phoenix, Goodyear, AZ, USA

**Gargi Singhal** Undergraduate Medical Sciences, S.N. Medical College Agra, Agra, Uttar Pradesh, India

**Sharad S. Singhal** Department of Medical Oncology & Therapeutics Research, Beckman Research Institute, City of Hope Comprehensive Cancer Center and National Medical Center, Duarte, CA, USA

**Marissa Tadi** Department of Medical Oncology and Therapeutics Research, City of Hope Comprehensive Cancer Center, Irvine, CA, USA

**TingTing Tan** Department of Medical Oncology, City of Hope National Medical Center, Newport Beach, CA, USA

**Farzad Teymouri** Department of Internal Medicine, Eisenhower Health, Rancho Mirage, CA, USA

**Karen Tsai** Department of Endocrinology, City of Hope Comprehensive Cancer Center, Duarte, CA, USA

**Julius Weng** Department of Radiation Oncology, City of Hope Orange County Lennar Foundation Cancer Center, Irvine, CA, USA

**Deric Wheeler** Department of Human Oncology, School of Medicine and Public Health, University of Wisconsin, Madison, WI, USA
Carbone Cancer Center, University of Wisconsin, Madison, WI, USA

**Andrew Williams** Department of Neurology, Lou & Jean Malnati Brain Tumor Institute, Northwestern University, Evanston, IL, USA

**Helena T. Wu** Data Science Institute, The University of Chicago, Chicago, IL, USA

**Yan Xing** City of Hope Comprehensive Cancer Center, Duarte, CA, USA

**Sharon Xu** Department of Pharmacy, City of Hope Comprehensive Cancer Center, Irvine, CA, USA

**Jennifer Yoon** Department of Human Oncology, University of Wisconsin, Madison, WI, USA

**Peter D. Zang** City of Hope Comprehensive Cancer Center, Duarte, CA, USA

**Miguel Zugman** City of Hope Comprehensive Cancer Center, Duarte, CA, USA

# Cancer Immunotherapy—An Overview

1

Prakash Kulkarni, Dana Do, Sagun Shrestha,
Benjamin Leach, and Ravi Salgia

## Abbreviations

| | |
|---|---|
| CAR-T | Chimeric antigen receptor T cell therapy |
| TCR therapy | Engineered T cell receptor therapy |
| TILs | Tumor-infiltrating lymphocytes |
| ICIs | Immune checkpoint inhibitors |
| PD-1 | Programmed cell death protein 1 |
| PD-L1 | Programmed cell death ligand 1 |
| TME | Tumor microenvironment |
| DLI | Donor lymphocyte infusion therapy |
| CRS | Cytokine release syndrome |
| mAbs | Monoclonal antibodies |
| IV | Intravenous |
| FDA | U.S. Food and Drug Administration |

P. Kulkarni
Department of Medical Oncology and Therapeutics Research, City of Hope National Medical Center, Duarte, CA, USA

Department of Systems Biology, City of Hope National Medical Center, Duarte, CA, USA

D. Do
Department of Medical Oncology, City of Hope National Medical Center, Duarte, CA, USA

S. Shrestha
City of Hope Phoenix, Goodyear, AZ, USA

B. Leach
Department of Medical Oncology and Therapeutics Research, City of Hope National Medical Center, Mission Hills, CA, USA

R. Salgia (✉)
Department of Medical Oncology and Therapeutics Research, City of Hope Comprehensive Cancer Center, Duarte, CA, USA
e-mail: rsalgia@coh.org



R. Salgia, P. Kulkarni (eds.), *Immunotherapies in Solid Tumors*, Cancer Treatment and Research 129, https://doi.org/10.1007/978-3-031-97242-3_1

| | |
|---|---|
| CTLA-4 | Cytotoxic T-lymphocyte-associated protein 4 |
| Tregs | Regulatory T cells |
| HIV | Human immunodeficiency virus |
| ICB | Immune checkpoint blockade |
| ACT | Adoptive cell therapy |
| NCI | National Cancer Institute |

## 1.1 Introduction

Immunotherapy has come a long way from its humble beginnings in the third century in the Qin dynasty in China [1]. Since then, the earliest known attempts to leverage a patient's immune system to cure cancer were reported by two German physicians, Fehleisen and Busch back in the late 1800s. Fehleisen and Busch independently observed significant tumor regression in patients with accidental erysipelas infections [2]. At around the same time, in 1891, an American physician, William Bradley Coley, who conducted an experiment where he injected heat-inactivated bacteria into 100 s of patients with inoperable cancers, also saw significant tumor regression in these patients [2, 3]. Since that time, the field has been burgeoning, and there has been an exponential increase in our understanding of cancer immunotherapy and the therapeutic advances for cancer. However, a historical account of this fascinating field is beyond the scope of this introductory chapter; instead, the reader is recommended to consult several excellent reviews that have appeared in the recent past (see [1, 3–6]).

In this introductory chapter we provide a brief overview of immunotherapy, the different types of immunotherapies that are approved for use in the clinic at the present time, their mechanisms of action, the associated benefits and risks, and the potential side effects. Although immunotherapy has been quite successful, the emergence of resistance to the different immunotherapeutic modalities does pose a significant impediment in treating patients. Therefore, we discuss the mechanisms of resistance to immunotherapy. We also aim to provide an overview of the various combination therapies such as immunotherapy combined with chemotherapy, radiation therapy, or targeted therapy that are currently being used in the clinic or are being explored preclinically. We conclude the chapter by highlighting how immunotherapy has revolutionized cancer treatment and point out how a "Team Medicine" approach could help ensure all eligible cancer patients can receive this promising treatment. The other chapters included in this book provide detailed information regarding the different immunotherapies as well as their combinations when applicable that are currently approved for the treatment of different types of cancers. For more recent and comprehensive reviews on cancer immunotherapy, the reader is referred to several excellent reviews that have been in the literature recently [7–11].

## 1.2 What Is Cancer Immunotherapy and How Does It Work?

Broadly speaking, immunotherapy for cancer is a type of therapeutic modality that assists the body's immune system to fight the disease. The treatment can include small molecule drugs such as immune checkpoint inhibitors, as well as biologics, recombinant proteins, antibodies, and engineered cells. The latter include adoptive cell therapy which involves isolating immune cells from the body and reinjecting them following genetic engineering, and chimeric antigen receptor or (CAR)-T cell therapy whereby genetically engineered T cells produce a protein that binds to cancer cells. Another example of adoptive cell therapy is engineered T cell receptor (TCR) therapy. In this type of therapy, a patient's T cells are genetically engineered to recognize and kill cancer cells in the body [12, 13].

In a healthy individual, the body's immune system can detect cancer cells as nonself and destroy them to curb tumor growth in many cancers. However, the body's immune system is compromised in many patients allowing the tumor to grow unabated [14]. The detection of immune cells, also known as tumor-infiltrating lymphocytes (TILs), indicates a positive response by the immune system to the tumor meaning it is mounting an immune response against the tumor. Tumors with TILs are also referred to as immunologically "hot" tumors. In fact, "hot" tumors present with a better prognosis than patients whose tumors are immunologically "cold" meaning they lack TILs [15]. The different types of immunotherapies are described in more detail below.

## 1.3 Types of Cancer Immunotherapies

Several types of immunotherapies are currently in use in the clinic to treat different cancers. They typically include:

### 1.3.1 Immune Checkpoint Inhibitors (ICIs)

Checkpoints are proteins present on T cells that help them discern healthy cells in the body and prevent the T cells from attacking the healthy cells. Cancer cells are often observed to show increased expression of checkpoints, which shield them from the immune system. Immune checkpoint inhibitors or ICIs are small molecule therapeutics that block immune checkpoints. By blocking the immune checkpoints, ICIs allow immune cells to override the checkpoints so that the immune system can respond more strongly to cancer [16, 17]. Indeed, ICI therapy has dramatically impacted positive clinical outcomes and has conferred durable clinical benefits for cancer patients [18].

Several types of ICIs are currently in use in the clinic (Table 1.1) [19–54]. They include the programmed cell death protein 1 (PD-1) inhibitors such as nivolumab (Opdivo), pembrolizumab (Keytruda), the cytotoxic T-lymphocyte-associated protein 4 (CTLA-4) inhibitor ipilimumab (Yervoy), and the programmed cell death ligand 1 (PD-L1) inhibitors, namely atezolizumab (Tecentriq), durvalumab (Imfinzi), and avelumab (Bavencio). ICIs are approved for treating several types of cancers, including lung cancer, bladder cancer, kidney cancer, melanoma, breast cancer, head and neck cancer, and colorectal cancer. Some side effects typically encountered with these ICIs include fatigue, rash, itching, diarrhea, pneumonitis, and type 1 diabetes.

**Table 1.1** Different types of immunotherapies

| Type of immunotherapy | Cancer types recommended for use of the therapy | Examples of therapy | References |
|---|---|---|---|
| Monoclonal antibodies (mAbs) | Breast, lung, melanoma, head and neck cancer, chronic lymphocytic leukemia (CLL), non-Hodgkin lymphoma, multiple myeloma, sarcoma, pediatric neuroblastoma | Trastuzumab (Herceptin), Pembrolizumab, Bevacizumab (Avastin), Cetuximab (Erbitux), Rituximab (Mabthera), Elotuzumab (Empliciti), Denosumab (Xgeva), Dinutuximab (Unituxin) | [19–29] |
| Immune checkpoint inhibitors (ICIs) | Melanoma, lung, breast, kidney, bladder, head and neck cancer, gastrointestinal cancers, cervical, liver, Hodgkin's lymphoma, mesothelioma | Anti-PD-1 therapies, anti-PD-L1 therapies, anti-CTLA-4 therapies, anti-LAG-3 therapies, small molecule inhibitors like Nivolumab (Opdivo) | [30–38] |
| Cancer vaccines | Bladder, melanoma, metastatic castration-resistant prostate cancer, cervical, breast, glioblastoma | Bacillus Calmette-Guérin (BCG) | [39–46] |
| Adoptive cell transfer | Metastatic melanoma, post-transplant lymphoma, refractory lymphoma, neuroblastoma, synovial sarcoma, glioblastoma | Tumor-infiltrating lymphocyte (TIL) therapy | [47–50] |
| Cytokines | Melanoma, renal cell carcinoma, lymphoma | IL-2, IFN-α, and TNF | [51–54] |

### 1.3.2 T Cell Transfer Therapy

T cell transfer therapy refers to an immunotherapy that enhances the natural ability of the body's T cells to fight cancer. It involves the removal of the immune cells taken from the patient's tumor. T cells that are most active against the cancer to be treated are enriched or engineered to bolster activity, grown in large batches, and systemically reinjected in the patient [55].

Several types of T cell transfer therapy are currently in practice (Table 1.1). Examples include *Chimeric Antigen Receptor (CAR) T Cell Therapy* wherein a patient's T cells are genetically engineered to express a receptor that specifically targets the patient's cancer cells. TIL therapy is another example of T cell transfer therapy whereby T cells present in the tumor microenvironment (TME) are isolated, expanded, and then infused back into the patient as a bolus to enhance the immune response [56]. Yet another type of T cell transfer therapy is the donor lymphocyte infusion (DLI) therapy. Here, T cells from a healthy donor are systemically injected to treat certain types of cancers. While the different T cell transfer therapies do offer potential benefits to the patient such as target-specific cancer cells as well as stimulate the patient's own immune system to fight cancer, they do carry some risks too. For example, the cytokine release syndrome (CRS) is a serious concern. CRS can cause a life-threatening reaction that can occur when too many T cells are released into the bloodstream. Other potential risks include neurotoxicity and infection due to immunosuppression during treatment. Besides, the therapy is expensive and may not be available in all hospitals.

### 1.3.3 Monoclonal Antibodies

Monoclonal antibodies (mAbs) are antibodies that are designed to recognize and bind to specific antigens expressed on the cancer cell surface. Numerous fully human mAbs are currently in use to treat several cancer types (Table 1.1). Some examples include Rituximab (Mabthera) that targets the CD20 antigen which is expressed on B cells as well as some cancer cells enabling the immune system to kill them, Trastuzumab (Herceptin) that is highly effective in treating some breast cancers, and Blinatumomab (Blincyto) that binds to CD19, a surface protein expressed on leukemia cells as well as CD3, an antigen that is expressed on the surface of T cells, helping the T cells kill the leukemia cells. Despite their promise however, mAbs do cause some side effects such as infusion reactions (fever, chills, nausea), allergic reactions, headache, and general fatigue.

### 1.3.4 Cancer Treatment Vaccines

Therapeutic cancer vaccines are now well recognized in treating cancer in patients who are resistant to other standard-of-care immunotherapies (Table 1.1). However, cancer vaccines have yet to realize their full potential and broaden the oncologic armamentarium. Cancer treatment vaccines are a type of immunotherapy in which biological materials such as tumor cells, proteins, or dendritic cells are injected into the patient to "educate" their immune system to detect and destroy cancer cells that contain tumor-associated antigens. The different types of cancer treatment vaccines include whole tumor vaccines, where the entire cancer cell is used to create the vaccine, antigen vaccines that use only certain antigens from cancer cells to stimulate the immune system, DNA vaccines wherein, DNA from cancer cells to improve the immune system's ability to destroy cancer cells, and personalized mRNA vaccines where the patient's RNA is used to trigger an immune response, are currently being tested in clinical trials [57, 58]. Although cancer vaccines are generally well-tolerated, they can cause side effects like fatigue, chills, fever, and headache.

### 1.3.5 Immune System Modulators

Immune system modulators may be defined as entities such as ICIs that act either by enhancing or suppressing the body's immune system [59, 60]. While some immune system modulators affect only parts of the immune system, other immune modulators act on the entire immune system (Table 1.1). Other examples of immune system modulators used to treat different cancers include immunostimulants, such as cytokines and interleukin-2, immunosuppressants, to suppress the immune system in transplant patients, and allergies, as well as certain dietary supplements such as vitamin D, zinc, and selenium, which appear to have immune-modulating effects. The side effects of immune system modulators vary and are typically minor. However, in severe cases, side effects may include inflammation of organs like the lungs, liver, or intestines due to the immune system attacking healthy tissues.

## 1.4 Who Is Eligible for Immunotherapy and How Is Immunotherapy Administered to Patients?

Generally speaking, the eligibility of patients for immunotherapy depends on a few factors including cancer type, disease stage, and the overall health of the patient. Typically, patients who are determined to be eligible and would benefit from immunotherapy would include patients who have advanced disease, have failed other treatments, and have a good immune system [61].

Immunotherapy is administered via multiple routes. While some are given intravenously (IV), they may also be administered orally. In some cases, for example, in skin cancer, immunotherapy may be applied topically. In bladder cancer patients, immunotherapy is delivered intravesical directly into the bladder. Although approved to treat many types of cancer, immunotherapy drugs have not been used as widely as some of the other medical modalities such as surgery, chemotherapy, or radiation therapy [15].

## 1.5 Combination Therapies

Notwithstanding the promise of immunotherapy over other therapeutic modalities for cancer treatment, only some patients show a clear benefit while others fail to respond. In recent years, combination therapies with existing anticancer treatments such as chemo and radiation therapy and epigenetic therapy have gained considerable attention and are being extensively investigated both in preclinical and clinical studies. Examples of such combination therapies that are U.S. Food and Drug Administration (FDA) approved include the use of pembrolizumab in combination with chemotherapy as a first-line therapy for treating patients with non-small cell lung cancer, and radiation therapy in combination with immunotherapy which act synergistically [62, 63].

Combination therapies that combine cancer immunotherapy with other state-of-the-art medical modalities tend to significantly increase tumor immunogenicity, reverse tumor immunosuppression, reduce tumor burden, and increase the immune effector response. For example, a combination of a PD-1 inhibitor and a cytotoxic T-lymphocyte-associated protein 4 (CTLA-4) inhibitor appears a promising strategy in several cancers, including mesothelioma and non-small cell lung cancer [64, 65]. Similarly, combining atezolizumab (anti-PD-L1 antibody) with bevacizumab (anti-vascular endothelial growth factor antibody) has been quite successful in liver cancer [66, 67].

Cancer immunotherapy plus radiation therapy is also a promising treatment strategy. Here, radiation damages cancer cells and thus makes them more visible to the immune system. Immunotherapy simultaneously activates the immune cells to kill the damaged tumor cells, resulting in a robust anti-tumor response than either treatment alone. This approach is being explored across various cancer types [68, 69].

## 1.6 Emergence of Resistance

Resistance to therapy, regardless of the type of therapy, is an almost inevitable problem when dealing with human diseases, especially in cancer [70, 71]. With regard to immunotherapy, resistance may be defined as the stage when cancer cells develop ways to avoid the immune system making the therapeutic treatment ineffective or less effective than expected. Furthermore, patients can be innately resistant to immunotherapy or can arise in patients who initially respond well to the treatment but later develop resistance, the so-called acquired resistance. While innate resistance is typically due to genetic abnormalities in cancer cells, acquired resistance can be due to genetic or non-genetic mechanisms such as epigenetic changes and phenotypic adaptations caused by the striking phenotypic plasticity of cancer cells [72, 73]. Additional details regarding phenotypic plasticity, non-genetic mechanisms, and immune drug resistance are discussed in Chap. 14.

Among the factors that are thought to contribute to immunotherapy resistance are certain extrinsic factors such as changes in the local TME and host-related factors, T-cell exhaustion, and the gut microbiota. Another important phenomenon that contributes significantly to immunotherapy resistance is cancer immunoediting which proceeds in three phases, namely elimination, equilibrium, and escape [74, 75].

The way in which cancer cells evolve under the pressure of the body's immunosurveillance can result in tumor subclones that are less recognizable by the immune system and ultimately render them capable of evading immunotherapy. Since the different phases of immunoediting can impact the cancer cell's antigen profile, immunoediting can determine its ability to evade immune detection.

The term elimination may be considered as the same as immunosurveillance and refers to how the body's immune system uses adaptive and innate immunity to attack and kill cancer cells, a phenomenon previously referred to as cancer immunosurveillance. Equilibrium, on the other hand, occurs in the event the immune system cannot completely eliminate the tumor. In this case, the patient's immune system tries to control the growth of the tumor, but the effect is not clinically observable. Finally, the term escape refers to that stage when the tumor cells develop resistance. By this stage, an immunosuppressive environment is established, and the tumor cells flourish unabated (Fig. 1.1).

Immunoediting in cancer cells can also lead to increased expression of immune checkpoints such as PD-L1 which further suppresses immune responses and attenuates the efficacy of ICI therapies. Additionally, an immunosuppressive TME can be augmented by immunoediting, including the presence of regulatory T cells (Tregs).

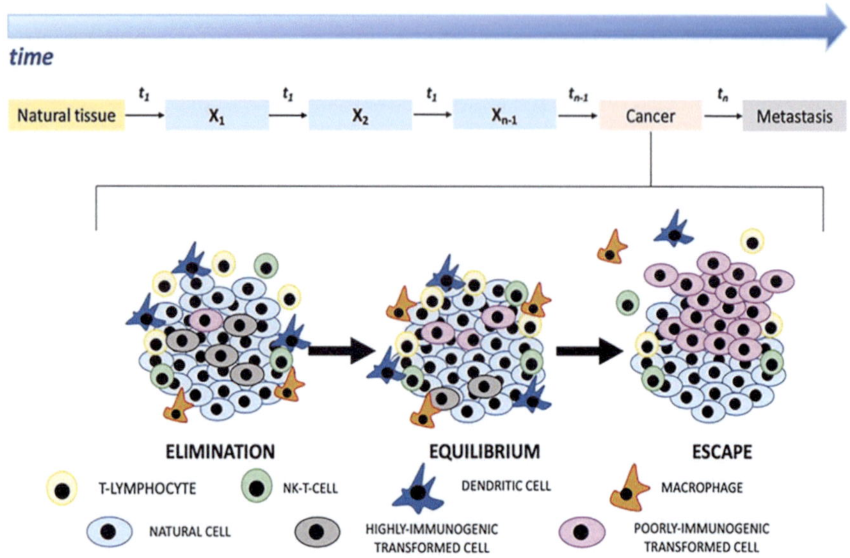


**Fig. 1.1** The cartoon shows the progression of different states (x1, x2, …, xn−1, xn) identifiable in the development of cancer from natural tissue. The exact time interval (t) between two successive states is unpredictable. Understanding how the immune system affects cancer progression still remains one of the most important topics in cancer immunology. Elimination, equilibrium, and escape represent three states that function either independently or in sequence in which a different relation between transformed cells and the immune system is established. The entire process is called "cancer immunoediting". (Taken from [76] Borroni and Grizzi (2021) with permission)

These events can hinder effector T cell infiltration and hence negatively impact immunotherapy response in patients. Therefore, understanding the mechanisms behind immunoediting is imperative for developing effective treatment strategies that can overcome immunotherapy resistance and improve treatment outcomes.

Immunoediting is a continuous process and can occur during disease progression or during the therapeutic treatment. Furthermore, it also occurs in immunosuppressed patients, such as those with human immunodeficiency virus (HIV) or the elderly. Factors that can affect cancer immunoediting include immunosuppression, tumor immunogenicity, and immunotherapy [77].

## 1.7 Team Medicine Approach

Medical centers around the world serve as critical entities of every health care system. Such centers tend to focus on clinical care, medical education, and biomedical research which is vital to the community they serve. On the other hand, community clinics/hospitals, although not engaged in medical education or research, also fill a critical need by serving as the primary sites for healthcare in these communities underscoring their complimentary role. It thus seems natural for the two healthcare providers to work together to benefit the community at large. Furthermore, new healthcare reforms and mounting economic pressures due to escalating healthcare costs, have also helped to create opportunities and incentives for the two entities to integrate and consolidate their mission and vision. Thus, most leading academic medical centers, especially in the United States have merged, acquired, or established partnerships with their community peers so that ultimately, all patients, irrespective of their proximity and accessibility to such leading institutions, can be benefited from the most recent and effective clinical advances.

While this trend is seen across most, if not all, medical specialties, it is more pronounced in medical oncology. Perhaps, one of the reasons aside from the obvious ones, is the interdisciplinary nature of the medical modalities and approaches used to treat cancer including latest breakthroughs such as robotic surgeries, machine learning, and artificial intelligence. Furthermore, many of these modalities involve highly specialized and expensive equipment, techniques, and trained and licensed personnel, adding to the difficulty in replicating such facilities in the community. Finally, new ideas and concepts adopted from the basic sciences that tend to approach the problem from a systems perspective involve an interdisciplinary team of basic research scientists that include theorists, experimentalists, and clinicians working together to better understand and treat cancer. This is also true for cancer immunotherapy given the multiple treatment options that are all based on the fundamentals of immunology. The fact that immunotherapy is administered in combination with other modalities such as radiation therapy further underscores the importance of a Team Medicine and multidisciplinary education approach where clinicians and basic research scientists with expertise in nutrition, immunobiology, and radiation biology work together to develop novel treatment strategies [78–82].

Therefore, embracing a Team Medicine approach that combines the skills, expertise, and vision of clinicians at major medical centers together with their counterparts in the community centers and hospitals they are affiliated with along those of basic research scientists are crucial to further cutting-edge translational research [83]. This will ensure that all patients regardless of whether they come from urban or suburban communities can benefit from the latest developments in science and medicine. Thus, it follows that a Team Medicine approach is not only more likely to provide more sensitive and reliable biomarkers for early diagnosis and better prognosis as well as response to therapy but is also likely to identify more safe and effective treatments against this burgeoning disease. Indeed, emerging data indicate that cancer is increasingly more prevalent in younger patients in their 40s (early onset) [84, 85]. Furthermore, on a more sobering note, according to some estimates, the number of early-onset cancer cases will rise globally by ~30% between 2019 and 2030 [86], underscoring the need for these Team Medicine to ensure that we provide young patients with effective treatment while not compromising their quality of life.

## 1.8 Conclusions and Future Directions

Immunotherapy, which harnesses the body's own immune system to fight the disease, is undoubtedly a promising therapeutic modality for treating cancer. It can be effective for a wide range of cancers. Unfortunately, however, not all patients respond to immunotherapy even if they are eligible, and there are potential side effects that need to be considered. Therefore, patients need to be made aware of the potential benefits and risks of immunotherapy by their healthcare team so that the right treatment option for each patient can be determined and personalized.

Immunotherapies like immune checkpoint blockade (ICB) and adoptive cell therapy (ACT) have transformed cancer treatment, especially for patients whose disease was thought to be incurable. Nonetheless, the emergence of primary and secondary resistance often results in treatment failure. Thus, only a minority of patients who are eligible and opt to receive immunotherapy for their specific cancer type experience long-term benefits (see [87]).

Regardless of the promise and the positive outcomes, there remain significant challenges associated with immunotherapy. Thus, currently, research in the field is focused on addressing resistance, be able to predict responses, and how to preclude or at least minimize potential side effects. Potential avenues that are being explored in the clinic to overcome resistance include testing combination therapies such as ICIs or radiation therapy plus immunotherapy. Thus, a Team Medicine approach may be the most practical way to leverage the maximum benefit of immunotherapy in cancer.

Additional information about ongoing clinical trials that involve immunotherapy can be found by visiting Find NCI-Supported Clinical Trials or calling the Cancer Information Service, National Cancer Institute's (NCI) contact center, at 1-800-4-CANCER (1-800-422-6237). NCI's list of cancer clinical trials includes all NCI-supported clinical trials that are taking place across the United States and Canada, including the National Institute of Health Clinical Center in Bethesda, MD.

## References

1. Decker WK, da Silva RF, Sanabria MH, Angelo LS, Guimarães F, Burt BM, Kheradmand F, Paust S. Cancer immunotherapy: historical perspective of a clinical revolution and emerging preclinical animal models. Front Immunol. 2017;8:829. https://doi.org/10.3389/fimmu.2017.00829. PMID: 28824608.
2. Oiseth SJ, Aziz MS. Cancer immunotherapy: a brief review of the history, possibilities, and challenges ahead. J Cancer Metastasis Treat. 2017;3:250–61.
3. Dobosz P, Dzieciątkowski T. The intriguing history of cancer immunotherapy. Front Immunol. 2019;10:2965. https://doi.org/10.3389/fimmu.2019.02965. PMID: 31921205.
4. Eno J. Immunotherapy through the years. J Adv Pract Oncol. 2017;8(7):747–53. Epub 2017 Nov 1. PMID: 30333937.
5. Abbott M, Ustoyev Y. Cancer and the immune system: the history and background of immunotherapy. Semin Oncol Nurs. 2019;35(5):150923. https://doi.org/10.1016/j.soncn.2019.08.002. Epub 2019 Sep 13. PMID: 31526550.
6. Ikeda H. Cancer immunotherapy in progress-an overview of the past 130 years. Int Immunol. 2025;2025:dxaf002. https://doi.org/10.1093/intimm/dxaf002. Epub ahead of print. PMID: 39792088.
7. Waldman AD, Fritz JM, Lenardo MJ. A guide to cancer immunotherapy: from T cell basic science to clinical practice. Nat Rev Immunol. 2020;20(11):651–68. https://doi.org/10.1038/s41577-020-0306-5. Epub 2020 May 20. PMID: 32433532; PMCID: PMC7238960.

8. Liu C, Yang M, Zhang D, Chen M, Zhu D. Clinical cancer immunotherapy: current progress and prospects. Front Immunol. 2022;13:961805. https://doi.org/10.3389/fimmu.2022.961805. PMID: 36304470; PMCID: PMC9592930.
9. Oliveira G, Wu CJ. Dynamics and specificities of T cells in cancer immunotherapy. Nat Rev Cancer. 2023;23(5):295–316. https://doi.org/10.1038/s41568-023-00560-y. Epub 2023 Apr 12. PMID: 37046001; PMCID: PMC10773171.
10. Emens LA, Romero PJ, Anderson AC, Bruno TC, Capitini CM, Collyar D, Gulley JL, Hwu P, Posey AD Jr, Silk AW, Wargo JA. Challenges and opportunities in cancer immunotherapy: a Society for Immunotherapy of Cancer (SITC) strategic vision. J Immunother Cancer. 2024;12(6):e009063. https://doi.org/10.1136/jitc-2024-009063. PMID: 38901879; PMCID: PMC11191773.
11. Hsu CY, Pallathadka H, Jasim SA, Rizaev J, Olegovich Bokov D, Hjazi A, Mahajan S, Mustafa YF, Husseen B, Jawad MA. Innovations in cancer immunotherapy: a comprehensive overview of recent breakthroughs and future directions. Crit Rev Oncol Hematol. 2025;206:104588. https://doi.org/10.1016/j.critrevonc.2024.104588. Epub 2024 Dec 10. PMID: 39667718.
12. Esfahani K, Roudaia L, Buhlaiga N, Del Rincon SV, Papneja N, Miller WH Jr. A review of cancer immunotherapy: from the past, to the present, to the future. Curr Oncol. 2020;27(Suppl 2):S87–97. https://doi.org/10.3747/co.27.5223. Epub 2020 Apr 1. PMID: 32368178; PMCID: PMC7194005.
13. Kciuk M, Yahya EB, Mohamed Ibrahim Mohamed M, Rashid S, Iqbal MO, Kontek R, Abdulsamad MA, Allaq AA. Recent advances in molecular mechanisms of cancer immunotherapy. Cancers (Basel). 2023;15(10):2721. https://doi.org/10.3390/cancers15102721. PMID: 37345057; PMCID: PMC10216302.
14. Song S, Wang C, Chen Y, Zhou X, Han Y, Zhang H. Dynamic roles of tumor-infiltrating B lymphocytes in cancer immunotherapy. Cancer Immunol Immunother. 2025;74(3):92. https://doi.org/10.1007/s00262-024-03936-7. PMID: 39891668; PMCID: PMC11787113.
15. Galon J, Bruni D. Approaches to treat immune hot, altered and cold tumours with combination immunotherapies. Nat Rev Drug Discov. 2019;18(3):197–218. https://doi.org/10.1038/s41573-018-0007-y. PMID: 30610226.
16. Bagchi S, Yuan R, Engleman EG. Immune checkpoint inhibitors for the treatment of cancer: clinical impact and mechanisms of response and resistance. Annu Rev Pathol. 2021;16:223–49. https://doi.org/10.1146/annurev-pathol-042020-042741. Epub 2020 Nov 16. PMID: 33197221.
17. Johnson DB, Nebhan CA, Moslehi JJ, Balko JM. Immune-checkpoint inhibitors: long-term implications of toxicity. Nat Rev Clin Oncol. 2022;19(4):254–67. https://doi.org/10.1038/s41571-022-00600-w. Epub 2022 Jan 26. PMID: 35082367; PMCID: PMC8790946.
18. Sharma P, Goswami S, Raychaudhuri D, Siddiqui BA, Singh P, Nagarajan A, Liu J, Subudhi SK, Poon C, Gant KL, Herbrich SM, Anandhan S, Islam S, Amit M, Anandappa G, Allison JP. Immune checkpoint therapy-current perspectives and future directions. Cell. 2023;186(8):1652–69. https://doi.org/10.1016/j.cell.2023.03.006. PMID: 37059068.
19. Ali-Thompson S, Daly GR, Dowling GP, Kilkenny C, Cox L, McGrath J, AlRawashdeh MM, Naidoo S, Power C, Hill ADK. A bibliometric analysis of HER2-positive breast cancer: 1987-2024. Front Oncol. 2024;14:1355353. https://doi.org/10.3389/fonc.2024.1355353. PMID: 38769947.
20. Johnson KCC, Ni A, Quiroga D, Pariser AC, Sudheendra PK, Williams NO, Sardesai SD, Cherian M, Stover DG, Gatti-Mays M, Ramaswamy B, Lustberg M, Jhawar S, Skoracki R, Wesolowski R. The survival benefit of adjuvant trastuzumab with or without chemotherapy in the management of small (T1mic, T1a, T1b, T1c), node negative HER2+ breast cancer. NPJ Breast Cancer. 2024;10(1):49. https://doi.org/10.1038/s41523-024-00652-4. PMID: 38898072.
21. Boutros A, Croce E, Ferrari M, Gili R, Massaro G, Marconcini R, Arecco L, Tanda ET, Spagnolo F. The treatment of advanced melanoma: current approaches and new challenges. Crit Rev Oncol Hematol. 2024;196:104276. https://doi.org/10.1016/j.critrevonc.2024.104276. Epub 2024 Jan 29. PMID: 38295889.

22. Xu J, Mu S, Wang Y, Yu S, Wang Z. Recent advances in immunotherapy and its combination therapies for advanced melanoma: a review. Front Oncol. 2024;14:1400193. https://doi.org/10.3389/fonc.2024.1400193. PMID: 39081713.
23. Mell LK, Torres-Saavedra PA, Wong SJ, Kish JA, Chang SS, Jordan RC, Liu T, Truong MT, Winquist EW, Takiar V, Wise-Draper T, Robbins JR, Rodriguez CP, Awan MJ, Beadle BM, Henson C, Narayan S, Spencer SA, Powell S, Dunlap N, Sacco AG, Hu KS, Park HS, Bauman JE, Harris J, Yom SS, Le QT. Radiotherapy with cetuximab or durvalumab for locoregionally advanced head and neck cancer in patients with a contraindication to cisplatin (NRG-HN004): an open-label, multicentre, parallel-group, randomised, phase 2/3 trial. Lancet Oncol. 2024;25(12):1576–88. https://doi.org/10.1016/S1470-2045(24)00507-2. Epub 2024 Nov 14. PMID: 39551064.
24. Knight A, Karapetyan L, Kirkwood JM. Immunotherapy in melanoma: recent advances and future directions. Cancers (Basel). 2023;15(4):1106. https://doi.org/10.3390/cancers15041106. PMID: 36831449.
25. Jain N, Wierda WG, O'Brien S. Chronic lymphocytic leukaemia. Lancet. 2024;404(10453):694–706. https://doi.org/10.1016/S0140-6736(24)00595-6.
26. Minard-Colin V, Aupérin A, Pillon M, Burke GAA, Barkauskas DA, Wheatley K, Delgado RF, Alexander S, Uyttebroeck A, Bollard CM, Zsiros J, Csoka M, Kazanowska B, Chiang AK, Miles RR, Wotherspoon A, Adamson PC, Vassal G, Patte C, Gross TG, European Intergroup for Childhood Non-Hodgkin Lymphoma, Children's Oncology Group. Rituximab for high-risk, mature B-cell non-Hodgkin's lymphoma in children. N Engl J Med. 2020;382(23):2207–19. https://doi.org/10.1056/NEJMoa1915315. PMID: 32492302.
27. Jiang H, Li L, Guo M, Li M, Wu H, Chen X, Gao M, Xu Q, Mi J, Cui C, Fu W. Efficacy of daratumumab on multiple myeloma patients with renal insufficiency: a systematic review and meta-analysis. Hematology. 2024;29(1):2399430. https://doi.org/10.1080/16078454.2024.2399430. Epub 2024 Sep 9. PMID: 39248713.
28. Wessel LE, Strike SA, Singh A, Bernthal NM, Athanasian EA. The role of denosumab in the treatment of primary tumors of bone. J Hand Surg [Am]. 2023;48(9):923–30. https://doi.org/10.1016/j.jhsa.2023.02.013. Epub 2023 Apr 7. PMID: 37032292.
29. Zheng M, Kumar A, Sharma V, Behl T, Sehgal A, Wal P, Shinde NV, Kawaduji BS, Kapoor A, Anwer MK, Gulati M, Shen B, Singla RK, Bungau SG. Revolutionizing pediatric neuroblastoma treatment: unraveling new molecular targets for precision interventions. Front Cell Dev Biol. 2024;12:1353860. https://doi.org/10.3389/fcell.2024.1353860. PMID: 38601081.
30. Wang T, Ma W, Zou Z, Zhong J, Lin X, Liu W, Sun W, Hu T, Xu Y, Chen Y. PD-1 blockade treatment in melanoma: mechanism of response and tumor-intrinsic resistance. Cancer Sci. 2025;116(2):329–37. https://doi.org/10.1111/cas.16398. Epub 2024 Nov 27. PMID: 39601129.
31. Xia Z, Hong J, Yu X, Ran Y, Xie H, Zhou Z, Zuo J, Chen T, Meng J, Yang J. Pembrolizumab versus sintilimab in patients with advanced NSCLC: a retrospective multicenter study with propensity-score matching analysis. Front Oncol. 2024;14:1422039. https://doi.org/10.3389/fonc.2024.1422039. PMID: 39703850.
32. Hossain AM. A comprehensive review of immune checkpoint inhibitors for cancer treatment. Int Immunopharmacol. 2024;143(Pt 2):113365. https://doi.org/10.1016/j.intimp.2024.113365. Epub 2024 Oct 23. PMID: 39447408.
33. Lasorsa F, di Meo NA, Rutigliano M, Milella M, Ferro M, Pandolfo SD, Crocetto F, Tataru OS, Autorino R, Battaglia M, Ditonno P, Lucarelli G. Immune checkpoint inhibitors in renal cell carcinoma: molecular basis and rationale for their use in clinical practice. Biomedicine. 2023;11(4):1071. https://doi.org/10.3390/biomedicines11041071. PMID: 37189689.
34. Struckmeier AK, Gosau M, Smeets R. Immunotherapeutic strategies beyond the PD-1/PD-L1 pathway in head and neck squamous cell carcinoma—a scoping review on current developments in agents targeting TIM-3, TIGIT, LAG-3, and VISTA. Oral Oncol. 2025;161:107145. https://doi.org/10.1016/j.oraloncology.2024.107145. Epub 2024 Dec 19. PMID: 39705929.

35. Noori M, Jafari-Raddani F, Davoodi-Moghaddam Z, Delshad M, Safiri S, Bashash D. Immune checkpoint inhibitors in gastrointestinal malignancies: an Umbrella review. Cancer Cell Int. 2024;24(1):10. https://doi.org/10.1186/s12935-023-03183-3. PMID: 38183112; Top of Form.
36. Martinez-Cannon BA, Colombo I. The evolving role of immune checkpoint inhibitors in cervical and endometrial cancer. Cancer Drug Resist. 2024;7:23. https://doi.org/10.20517/cdr.2023.120. PMID: 39050882.
37. Zafar A, Rashid AA, Moeed A, Tahir MJ, Khan AJ, Shrateh ON, Ahmed A. Safety and efficacy of PD-1/PD-L1 immune checkpoint inhibitors in patients with pre-treated advanced stage malignant mesothelioma: a systematic review and meta-analysis. BMC Cancer. 2024;24(1):1353. https://doi.org/10.1186/s12885-024-13127-3. PMID: 39501196.
38. Shiravand Y, Khodadadi F, Kashani SMA, Hosseini-Fard SR, Hosseini S, Sadeghirad H, Ladwa R, O'Byrne K, Kulasinghe A. Immune checkpoint inhibitors in cancer therapy. Curr Oncol. 2022;29(5):3044–60. https://doi.org/10.3390/curroncol29050247. PMID: 35621637.
39. Conroy S, Jubber I, Noon AP, Rosario DJ, Griffin J, Morgan S, Hubbard R, Kennish S, Mitchell S, Venugopal S, Linton K, Rajasundaram R, Hussain SA, Catto JWF. Real-world outcomes for high-risk non-muscle-invasive bladder cancer: screened patients for the BRAVO trial. BJU Int. 2025;135(2):329–38. https://doi.org/10.1111/bju.16516. Epub 2024 Sep 26. PMID: 39324506.
40. Shen YC, Huang YL, Kang YN, Chiu WK, Hoang KD, Wang HJ, Chen C. Effectiveness and safety of talimogene laherparepvec and granulocyte-macrophage colony-stimulating factor for metastatic melanoma: a systematic review and network meta-analysis of randomized controlled trials. Melanoma Res. 2025;35(1):60–6. https://doi.org/10.1097/CMR.0000000000001010. Epub 2024 Dec 24. PMID: 39787519.
41. Heath EI, Thakur A, Chen W, Hwang C, Paller CJ, Cackowski FC, Boerner JL, Heilbrun L, Smith MP, Schalk DL, Schienschang A, Whitaker SA, Polend A, Smith D, Vaishampayan UN, Dickow B, Lum LG. Race-related differences in sipuleucel-T response among men with metastatic castrate-resistant prostate cancer. Cancer Res Commun. 2024;4(7):1715–25. https://doi.org/10.1158/2767-9764.CRC-24-0112. PMID: 38856749.
42. Wolf J, Kist LF, Pereira SB, Quessada MA, Petek H, Pille A, Maccari JG, Mutlaq MP, Nasi LA. Human papillomavirus infection: epidemiology, biology, host interactions, cancer development, prevention, and therapeutics. Rev Med Virol. 2024;34(3):e2537. https://doi.org/10.1002/rmv.2537. PMID: 38666757.
43. Aggarwal S, Agarwal P, Singh AK. Human papilloma virus vaccines: a comprehensive narrative review. Cancer Treat Res Commun. 2023;37:100780. https://doi.org/10.1016/j.ctarc.2023.100780. Epub 2023 Nov 21. PMID: 38006748.
44. Al-Hawary SIS, Saleh EAM, Mamajanov NA, Gilmanova SN, Alsaab HO, Alghamdi A, Ansari SA, Alawady AHR, Alsaalamy AH, Ibrahim AJ. Breast cancer vaccines; a comprehensive and updated review. Pathol Res Pract. 2023;249:154735. https://doi.org/10.1016/j.prp.2023.154735. Epub 2023 Aug 4. PMID: 37611432.
45. Strika Z, Petković K, Likić R. Effectiveness and safety of mRNA vaccines in the therapy of glioblastoma. J Pers Med. 2024;14(9):993. https://doi.org/10.3390/jpm14090993. PMID: 39338247; PMCID: PMC11433450.
46. Xiong Z, Raphael I, Olin M, Okada H, Li X, Kohanbash G. Glioblastoma vaccines: past, present, and opportunities. EBioMedicine. 2024;100:104963. https://doi.org/10.1016/j.ebiom.2023.104963. Epub 2024 Jan 5. PMID: 38183840.
47. Haanen J, Los C, Phan GQ, Betof WA. Adoptive cell therapy for solid tumors: current status in melanoma and next-generation therapies. Am Soc Clin Oncol Educ Book. 2024;44(3):e431608. https://doi.org/10.1200/EDBK_431608. PMID: 38776509.
48. Wang J, Shen F, Yao Y, Wang LL, Zhu Y, Hu J. Adoptive cell therapy: a novel and potential immunotherapy for glioblastoma. Front Oncol. 2020;10:59. https://doi.org/10.3389/fonc.2020.00059. PMID: 32083009.
49. Parums DV. A review of CAR T cells and adoptive T-cell therapies in lymphoid and solid organ malignancies. Med Sci Monit. 2025;31:e948125. https://doi.org/10.12659/MSM.948125. PMID: 39893510.

50. Hu Q, Xuan J, Wang L, Shen K, Gao Z, Zhou Y, Wei C, Gu J. Application of adoptive cell therapy in malignant melanoma. J Transl Med. 2025;23(1):102. https://doi.org/10.1186/s12967-025-06093-2. PMID: 39844295.
51. Natarelli N, Aleman SJ, Mark IM, Tran JT, Kwak S, Botto E, Aflatooni S, Diaz MJ, Lipner SR. A review of current and pipeline drugs for treatment of melanoma. Pharmaceuticals (Basel). 2024;17(2):214. https://doi.org/10.3390/ph17020214. PMID: 38399429.
52. Reschke R, Enk AH, Hassel JC. Chemokines and cytokines in immunotherapy of melanoma and other tumors: from biomarkers to therapeutic targets. Int J Mol Sci. 2024;25(12):6532. https://doi.org/10.3390/ijms25126532. PMID: 38928238.
53. Wang Y, Suarez ER, Kastrunes G, de Campos NSP, Abbas R, Pivetta RS, Murugan N, Chalbatani GM, D'Andrea V, Marasco WA. Evolution of cell therapy for renal cell carcinoma. Mol Cancer. 2024;23(1):8. https://doi.org/10.1186/s12943-023-01911-x. PMID: 38195534.
54. Berraondo P, Sanmamed MF, Ochoa MC, Etxeberria I, Aznar MA, Pérez-Gracia JL, Rodríguez-Ruiz ME, Ponz-Sarvise M, Castañón E, Melero I. Cytokines in clinical cancer immunotherapy. Br J Cancer. 2019;120(1):6–15. https://doi.org/10.1038/s41416-018-0328-y. Epub 2018 Nov 9. PMID: 30413827.
55. Albarrán V, San Román M, Pozas J, Chamorro J, Rosero DI, Guerrero P, Calvo JC, González C, García de Quevedo C, Pérez de Aguado P, Moreno J, Cortés A, Soria A. Adoptive T cell therapy for solid tumors: current landscape and future challenges. Front Immunol. 2024;15:1352805. https://doi.org/10.3389/fimmu.2024.1352805. PMID: 38550594; PMCID: PMC10972864.
56. de Oliveira GAF, de Oliveira DA, Nisimoto MYSM, Rubinho R, Gomes HC, Marti LC, de Oliveira Filho RS. Advances in tumor-infiltrating lymphocyte (TIL) as a prognostic factor and for treating invasive cutaneous melanoma. Int J Mol Sci. 2024;25(23):12596. https://doi.org/10.3390/ijms252312596.
57. Lin MJ, Svensson-Arvelund J, Lubitz GS, Marabelle A, Melero I, Brown BD, Brody JD. Cancer vaccines: the next immunotherapy frontier. Nat Can. 2022;3(8):911–26. https://doi.org/10.1038/s43018-022-00418-6. Epub 2022 Aug 23.
58. Lorentzen CL, Haanen JB, Met Ö, Svane IM. Clinical advances and ongoing trials on mRNA vaccines for cancer treatment. Lancet Oncol. 2022;23(10):e450–8. https://doi.org/10.1016/S1470-2045(22)00372-2. Erratum in: Lancet Oncol. 2022;23(11):e492. https://doi.org/10.1016/S1470-2045(22)00608-8. PMID: 36174631; PMCID: PMC9512276.
59. Strzelec M, Detka J, Mieszczak P, Sobocińska MK, Majka M. Immunomodulation—a general review of the current state-of-the-art and new therapeutic strategies for targeting the immune system. Front Immunol. 2023;14:1127704. https://doi.org/10.3389/fimmu.2023.1127704. PMID: 36969193; PMCID: PMC10033545.
60. Goswami A, Goyal S, Khurana P, Singh K, Deb B, Kulkarni A. Small molecule innate immune modulators in cancer therapy. Front Immunol. 2024;15:1395655. https://doi.org/10.3389/fimmu.2024.1395655. PMID: 39318624; PMCID: PMC11419979.
61. Hiam-Galvez KJ, Allen BM, Spitzer MH. Systemic immunity in cancer. Nat Rev Cancer. 2021;21(6):345–59. https://doi.org/10.1038/s41568-021-00347-z. Epub 2021 Apr 9. PMID: 33837297; PMCID: PMC8034277.
62. Gotwals P, Cameron S, Cipolletta D, Cremasco V, Crystal A, Hewes B, Mueller B, Quaratino S, Sabatos-Peyton C, Petruzzelli L, Engelman JA, Dranoff G. Prospects for combining targeted and conventional cancer therapy with immunotherapy. Nat Rev Cancer. 2017;17(5):286–301. https://doi.org/10.1038/nrc.2017.17. Epub 2017 Mar 24. PMID: 28338065.
63. Joshi S, Durden DL. Combinatorial approach to improve cancer immunotherapy: rational drug design strategy to simultaneously hit multiple targets to kill tumor cells and to activate the immune system. J Oncol. 2019;2019:5245034. https://doi.org/10.1155/2019/5245034. PMID: 30853982; PMCID: PMC6377965.
64. Genova C, Dellepiane C, Carrega P, Sommariva S, Ferlazzo G, Pronzato P, Gangemi R, Filaci G, Coco S, Croce M. Therapeutic implications of tumor microenvironment in lung cancer: focus on immune checkpoint blockade. Front Immunol. 2022;12:799455. https://doi.org/10.3389/fimmu.2021.799455. PMID: 35069581; PMCID: PMC8777268.

65. Cheng W, Kang K, Zhao A, Wu Y. Dual blockade immunotherapy targeting PD-1/PD-L1 and CTLA-4 in lung cancer. J Hematol Oncol. 2024;17(1):54. https://doi.org/10.1186/s13045-024-01581-2. PMID: 39068460; PMCID: PMC11283714.
66. Finn RS, Qin S, Ikeda M, Galle PR, Ducreux M, Kim TY, Kudo M, Breder V, Merle P, Kaseb AO, Li D, Verret W, Xu DZ, Hernandez S, Liu J, Huang C, Mulla S, Wang Y, Lim HY, Zhu AX, Cheng AL. IMbrave150 investigators. Atezolizumab plus bevacizumab in unresectable hepatocellular carcinoma. N Engl J Med. 2020;382(20):1894–905. https://doi.org/10.1056/NEJMoa1915745. PMID: 32402160.
67. Kulkarni AV, Tevethia H, Kumar K, Premkumar M, Muttaiah MD, Hiraoka A, Hatanaka T, Tada T, Kumada T, Kakizaki S, Vogel A, Finn RS, Rao PN, Pillai A, Reddy DN, Singal AG. Effectiveness and safety of atezolizumab-bevacizumab in patients with unresectable hepatocellular carcinoma: a systematic review and meta-analysis. EClinicalMedicine. 2023;63:102179. https://doi.org/10.1016/j.eclinm.2023.102179. PMID: 37680945; PMCID: PMC10480543.
68. Cushman TR, Gomez D, Kumar R, Likacheva A, Chang JY, Cadena AP, Paris S, Welsh JW. Combining radiation plus immunotherapy to improve systemic immune response. J Thorac Dis. 2018;10(Suppl 3):S468–79. https://doi.org/10.21037/jtd.2018.01.130. PMID: 29593892; PMCID: PMC5861265.
69. Wisdom AJ, Barker CA, Chang JY, Demaria S, Formenti S, Grassberger C, Gregucci F, Hoppe BS, Kirsch DG, Marciscano AE, Mayadev J, Mouw KW, Palta M, Wu CC, Jabbour SK, Schoenfeld JD. The next chapter in immunotherapy and radiation combination therapy: cancer-specific perspectives. Int J Radiat Oncol Biol Phys. 2024;118(5):1404–21. https://doi.org/10.1016/j.ijrobp.2023.12.046. Epub 2024 Jan 5. PMID: 38184173.
70. Sharma P, Hu-Lieskovan S, Wargo JA, Ribas A. Primary, adaptive, and acquired resistance to cancer immunotherapy. Cell. 2017;168(4):707–23. https://doi.org/10.1016/j.cell.2017.01.017. PMID: 28187290; PMCID: PMC5391692.
71. Tufail M, Hu JJ, Liang J, He CY, Wan WD, Huang YQ, Jiang CH, Wu H, Li N. Hallmarks of cancer resistance. iScience. 2024;27(6):109979. https://doi.org/10.1016/j.isci.2024.109979. PMID: 38832007; PMCID: PMC11145355.
72. Salgia R, Kulkarni P. The genetic/non-genetic duality of drug 'resistance' in cancer. Trends Cancer. 2018;4(2):110–8. https://doi.org/10.1016/j.trecan.2018.01.001. Epub 2018 Feb 3. PMID: 29458961; PMCID. PMC5822736.
73. Zhou J, Liu C, Tang Y, Li Z, Cao Y. Phenotypic switching as a non-genetic mechanism of resistance predicts antibody therapy regimens. iScience. 2024;27(4):109450. https://doi.org/10.1016/j.isci.2024.109450. PMID: 38544569; PMCID: PMC10966312.
74. Dunn GP, Old LJ, Schreiber RD. The immunobiology of cancer immunosurveillance and immunoediting. Immunity. 2004;21(2):137–48. https://doi.org/10.1016/j.immuni.2004.07.017. PMID: 15308095.
75. Schreiber RD, Old LJ, Smyth MJ. Cancer immunoediting: integrating immunity's roles in cancer suppression and promotion. Science. 2011;331(6024):1565–70. https://doi.org/10.1126/science.1203486. PMID: 21436444.
76. Borroni EM, Grizzi F. Cancer immunoediting and beyond in 2021. Int J Mol Sci. 2021;22(24):13275. https://doi.org/10.3390/ijms222413275. PMID: 34948072.
77. Gubin MM, Vesely MD. Cancer immunoediting in the era of immuno-oncology. Clin Cancer Res. 2022;28(18):3917–28. https://doi.org/10.1158/1078-0432.CCR-21-1804. PMID: 35594163; PMCID: PMC9481657.
78. Salgia R, Kulkarni P. Integrating clinical and translational research networks-building team medicine. J Clin Med. 2020;9(9):2975. https://doi.org/10.3390/jcm9092975. PMID: 32942638; PMCID: PMC7563426.
79. Kulkarni P, Mohanty A, Bhattacharya S, Singhal S, Guo L, Ramisetty S, Mirzapoiazova T, Mambetsariev B, Mittan S, Malhotra J, Gupta N, Kim P, Babikian R, Rajurkar S, Subbiah S, Tan T, Nguyen D, Merla A, Kollimuttathuillam SV, Phillips T, Baik P, Tan B, Vashi P, Shrestha S, Leach B, Garg R, Rich PL, Stewart FM, Pisick E, Salgia R. Addressing drug resistance in

cancer: a team medicine approach. J Clin Med. 2022;11(19):5701. https://doi.org/10.3390/jcm11195701. PMID: 36233569; PMCID: PMC9572909.
80. Nakamura T. Team medicine and multidisciplinary education. In: Japan nutrition. Singapore: Springer; 2022.
81. Kulkarni P, Salgia R. On the virtues of "team medicine"—a City of Hope perspective. J Clin Med. 2023;12(15):4897. https://doi.org/10.3390/jcm12154897. PMID: 37568299; PMCID: PMC10419954.
82. Crossman BE, Harmon RL, Kostecki KL, McDaniel NK, Iida M, Corday LW, Glitchev CE, Crow MT, Harris MA, Lin CY, Adams JM, Longhurst CA, Nickel KP, Ong IM, Alexandridis RA, Yu M, Yang DT, Hu R, Morris ZS, Hartig GK, Glazer TA, Ramisetty S, Kulkarni P, Salgia R, Kimple RJ, Bruce JY, Harari PM, Wheeler DL. From bench to bedside: a team's approach to multidisciplinary strategies to combat therapeutic resistance in head and neck squamous cell carcinoma. J Clin Med. 2024;13(20):6036. https://doi.org/10.3390/jcm13206036. PMID: 39457986; PMCID: PMC11508784.
83. Bosserman LD, Cianfrocca M, Yuh B, Yeon C, Chen H, Sentovich S, Polverini A, Zachariah F, Deaville D, Lee AB, Sedrak MS, King E, Gray S, Morse D, Glaser S, Bhatt G, Adeimy C, Tan T, Chao J, Nam A, Paz IB, Kruper L, Rao P, Sokolov K, Kulkarni P, Salgia R, Yamzon J, Johnson D. Integrating academic and community cancer care and research through multidisciplinary oncology pathways for value-based care: a review and the City of Hope experience. J Clin Med. 2021;10(2):188. https://doi.org/10.3390/jcm10020188. PMID: 33430334; PMCID: PMC7825796.
84. Koh B, Tan DJH, Ng CH, Fu CE, Lim WH, Zeng RW, Yong JN, Koh JH, Syn N, Meng W, et al. Patterns in cancer incidence among people younger than 50 years in the US, 2010 to 2019. JAMA Netw Open. 2023;6:e2328171. https://doi.org/10.1001/jamanetworkopen.2023.28171.
85. Ledford H. Why are so many young people getting cancer? What the data say. Nature. 2024;627:258–60. https://doi.org/10.1038/d41586-024-00720-6.
86. Jianhui Z, Liying X, Jing S, Mingyang S, Lijuan W, Shuai Y, Yingshuang Z, Zhengwei W, Susanna L, Konstantinos T, et al. Global trends in incidence, death, burden and risk factors of early-onset cancer from 1990 to 2019. BMJ Oncol. 2023;2:e000049. https://doi.org/10.1136/bmjonc-2023-000049.
87. Zhu S, Zhang T, Zheng L, Liu H, Song W, Liu D, Li Z, Pan CX. Combination strategies to maximize the benefits of cancer immunotherapy. J Hematol Oncol. 2021;14(1):156. https://doi.org/10.1186/s13045-021-01164-5. PMID: 34579759; PMCID: PMC8475356.

# Artificial Intelligence and Machine Learning Approaches in Designing Immunotherapy in Cancer

# 2

Lokesh Seth, Colton Ladbury, and Arya Amini

## Abbreviations

| | |
|---|---|
| AI | artificial intelligence |
| ANN | artificial neural networks |
| DL | deep learning |
| IO | immuno-oncology |
| ML | machine learning |

## 2.1 Introduction

Great progress has been made in studying cancer immunology and the development of immunotherapies. The complexity of the immune system and the duplicity of cancer, plus the expense of treatments and variable patient responses, make for a perfect data storm. Artificial intelligence (AI), machine learning (ML), deep learning (DL), and artificial neural networks (ANN) are poised to help unlock cancer's secrets, identify, and validate immuno-oncology (IO) targets, evaluate assets, and apply effective immunotherapies. However, optimally utilizing and effectively mining these large diverse data sets is daunting. The combined efforts of researchers, clinicians, and data scientists are required.

L. Seth · C. Ladbury · A. Amini (✉)
Department of Medical Oncology, City of Hope National Medical Center, Duarte, CA, USA
e-mail: aamini@coh.org



R. Salgia, P. Kulkarni (eds.), *Immunotherapies in Solid Tumors*, Cancer Treatment and Research 129, https://doi.org/10.1007/978-3-031-97242-3_2

## 2.2 The Role of AI in Antibody Design

Therapeutic monoclonal antibodies (mAbs) represent a critical class of drugs used in the treatment of various diseases, including cancers, autoimmune disorders, and infectious diseases. The traditional methods of developing these antibodies are often labor-intensive, time-consuming, and costly. AI, however, offers a revolutionary approach to streamline and enhance the design and development of these therapeutic agents through predictive modeling, innovative design techniques, and integrative data approaches [1].

AI, especially ML and DL, enables the analysis of vast datasets essential for deciphering the complexities of antibody-antigen interactions. By predicting these interactions, AI helps researchers identify antibody candidates with high specificity and strong binding affinity. Training AI models on known antibody-antigen datasets allow for the generation of novel antibody candidates and the prediction of their efficacy, significantly reducing reliance on empirical screening. Predictive modeling through AI facilitates the identification of high-affinity binders and optimizes antibody properties, ultimately enhancing clinical efficacy [1, 2]. For example, Mason et al. utilized DL to predict antigen specificity from antibody sequences, demonstrating significant advancements in therapeutic antibodies optimization. Their model uses known sequences to predict interactions accurately, streamlining the antibody optimization process and significantly reducing the reliance on empirical screenings [2]. In another study by Lim et al., DL was employed to predict antibody binders and generate synthetic antibodies. This approach utilized a dataset comprising multiple antibody structures and demonstrated how AI can forecast antibody interactions with higher precision than traditional methods [1]. This AI-driven methodology not only identified high-affinity binders but also optimized antibody properties to enhance clinical efficacy, allowing for a more refined and targeted approach to therapeutic development [2]. Moreover, Saka et al. explored the use of long short-term memory (LSTM)-based deep generative models for affinity maturation. By leveraging phage display libraries, this model focused on improving affinities and diversities of antibodies, which are critical for functional therapeutic applications [1].

## 2.3 Protein Structure Prediction

The advent of AI-driven tools like AlphaFold2 [3], renowned for its near-experimental accuracy in protein-folding predictions, has been a game-changer. This technology enables precise antibody structure prediction, which is crucial for designing antibodies with optimal specificity and affinity for their targets. Accurate structural predictions streamline the understanding of antibody-antigen interactions at the molecular level [2].

Beyond AlphaFold2, AI-based models such as the Bio-Inspired Antibody Language Model (BALM) have been developed to predict antibody structures directly from sequences. In certain benchmarks, BALM has outperformed traditional methods, facilitating rapid and accurate modeling of antibody structures and aiding in the rational design of therapeutics [4].

## 2.4 Generative Models in Antibody Design

Generative models, including generative adversarial networks (GANs) and variational autoencoders (VAEs), are at the forefront of designing new antibody sequences. These models learn from existing antibody sequences and structures to generate new candidates that mimic desired properties, such as high specificity and low immunogenicity [1]. The design of complementarity-determining regions (CDRs), which are crucial for antigen binding, greatly benefits from these technologies by introducing mutations that may enhance binding efficiency [2]. Shanehsazzadeh et al. (2023) demonstrated the use of deep generative models for the de novo design of antibodies against the human epidermal growth factor receptor 2 (HER2), achieving high binding affinities without additional optimization [5]. Liu et al. (2020) explored DL methods for designing antibody regions, particularly the complementarity-determining regions (CDRs), which are crucial for targeting specific antigens such as HER2 [6]. Jin et al. (2021) employed iterative refinement of graph neural networks for antibody sequence-structure co-design, a method adaptable for designing antibodies against specific targets [7].

## 2.5 Enhancements in Developability

AI technologies play a vital role in addressing developability challenges such as solubility, stability, and manufacturability. Predictive models can assess how structural modifications impact an antibody's aggregation propensity and stability, ensuring lead candidates are suitable for large-scale production [1]. Several computational tools have been developed to enhance the design and manufacturability of antibody therapeutics. CamSol is a method designed for the rational engineering of protein mutants with improved solubility [8]. SOLart is a state-of-the-art model that predicts protein solubility and aggregation based on structural information, outperforming other models in accuracy [9]. AGGRESCAN 3D (A3D) focuses on predicting and optimizing aggregation-prone regions within proteins, aiding in the design of antibodies with reduced aggregation propensity [10]. PfAbNet-viscosity, a 3D convolutional neural network, predicts the viscosity of antibody solutions, a critical factor for high-concentration formulations [11]. Lastly, ABodyBuilder2 enhances the prediction of complex structural regions, such as the HCDR3 loop, directly impacting the manufacturability and stability of antibody therapeutics. These tools collectively contribute to advancing the development of more effective and stable antibody-based treatments [12].

Beyond discovery, AI also optimizes antibody properties to enhance therapeutic potential. ML algorithms can predict the effects of specific mutations on stability, solubility, and immunogenicity. For example, AI-driven platforms have been developed to autonomously balance multiple developability parameters, improving antibody design efficiency and minimizing the need for extensive wet-lab experiments [13].

## 2.6 Multi-omics Integration for Insightful Discovery

Integrating data from genomics, proteomics, and other omic fields provides a comprehensive understanding of antibody functions and interactions. AI excels at synthesizing these data, uncovering patterns and interactions that are not evident through conventional analyses. By leveraging these datasets, AI can facilitate the identification of novel therapeutic targets and refine the design of antibodies [1, 14]. AI-driven multi-omics approaches are increasingly being utilized in lung cancer research to improve treatment predictions and patient outcomes. One example involves a study of non-small cell lung cancer (NSCLC) patients treated with anti-programmed cell death protein-1 (PD-1) and anti-programmed cell death ligand-1 (PD-L1) agents, where a model integrated ribonucleic acid (RNA) sequencing, deoxyribonucleic acid (DNA) sequencing, and immunohistochemistry (IHC) data to predict drug sensitivity [15]. Yang et al. (2021) implemented a multi-omics-based deep learning approach to assess clinical outcomes of anti-PD-1/PD-L1 immunotherapy in patients with advanced NSCLC. By integrating various data sources, including genomics, radiomics, and clinical data, the study demonstrated that this comprehensive approach significantly improved prediction accuracy, outperforming models that relied on a single modality [16]. Similarly, Park et al. (2020) developed AI models that utilized quantitative flow cytometry and RNA sequencing immune profiles derived from fluoro-deoxyglucose-positron emission tomography (FDG-PET) imaging to predict immunotherapy outcomes in lung adenocarcinoma. Their findings highlighted the advantages of integrating imaging data with genomic profiles, providing deeper insights into tumor behavior and therapy response while enhancing patient stratification for treatment [17]. Expanding on this multimodal approach, Mu et al. (2020) employed a DL model that combined genomics, PET radiomics, and clinical data to predict treatment responses in NSCLC. Their study validated the efficacy of multimodal integration, demonstrating improved accuracy in predicting treatment outcomes for patients receiving immune checkpoint inhibitors and targeted therapies [18]. These studies collectively underscore the potential of AI-driven multimodal approaches in advancing personalized medicine for lung cancer treatment.

## 2.7 Challenges and Future Outlook

Despite impressive progress, challenges remain in fully harnessing AI for antibody design. The complexity of accurately modeling biological systems and the reliance on high-quality training datasets are significant hurdles. The AI models require continuous refinement and validation to ensure that they accurately predict real-world biological behaviors. Furthermore, the integration of AI in drug development demands adaptations in regulatory pathways to accommodate AI-generated therapeutics [1, 2].

## 2.8 Conclusions

The integration of AI into mAb design represents a paradigm shift, transforming traditional methodologies and paving the way for innovative therapeutic solutions. With AI capabilities evolving rapidly, the potential for these technologies to redefine drug design and development is immense. Continued advancements in AI must be coupled with suitable regulatory adaptations and comprehensive understanding of biological complexities to fully realize these benefits in therapeutic contexts [1, 2].

## 2.9 AI for Predicting Immunotherapy Response Clinically and Radiographically

Advancements in AI and ML have ushered in a transformative era in oncology, particularly in the field of immunotherapy for cancer treatment. Immunotherapy has shown considerable promise, yet its effectiveness is often hampered by the variability in patient responses. To optimize therapeutic outcomes, AI-based models have emerged as critical tools for predicting immunotherapy responses, both clinically and radiographically. Radiographic techniques, augmented by AI, offer non-invasive means to predict therapeutic response. Nonetheless, interpreting radiographic findings after initiating immunotherapy and other modalities including radiation can be challenging due to pseudoprogression, where an apparent increase in tumor size does not indicate disease progression but rather a treatment-related inflammatory response. AI may aid in differentiating tumor progression from pseudoprogression by integrating various parameters, potentially improving treatment decision-making. Radiomics, a field where AI is used to extract a large number of features from radiographic medical images, provides insights into tumor heterogeneity and microenvironment characteristics that are not discernible by the human eye [19]. These features can include tumor shape irregularity, texture, and intensity variations, which AI models correlate with clinical outcomes, enhancing the stratification of patients who are likely to benefit from immunotherapy [19].

AI-based clinical decision support systems (CDSS) are being developed to assist oncologists in identifying patients who are likely to experience durable responses to immunotherapy, thereby avoiding the unnecessary side effects of ineffective treatments. For instance, a study by Ahn et al. investigated the use of an ML-based CDSS to assess clinical response to PD-1 therapy in patients with NSCLC, demonstrating significant prediction improvements for treatment response [20]. Another study discussed the application of AI in identifying protein signatures to predict immunotherapy responses in NSCLC patients. The derived serum protein classifier successfully stratified patients' resistance or sensitivity to treatment with a satisfactory prediction accuracy [21]. These AI systems continuously improve by learning from vast datasets, which allows for real-time, data-driven recommendations for example AI systems like IBM Watson For Oncology (WFO) have vast amounts of medical data, including patient records and research papers, to assist doctors in diagnosing diseases and suggesting treatment options [22].

Moreover, the integration of AI in pathology through digital image analysis provides additional avenues for response prediction. AI can analyze histopathological slides to assess tumor-infiltrating lymphocytes (TILs), which play a vital role in mediating the effects of immunotherapy. This integration not only enhances the accuracy of predicting responses but also complements traditional diagnostic methods, providing a more holistic view of patient prognosis.

Despite promising results, challenges remain in translating these AI-driven insights into routine clinical practice. Issues such as data heterogeneity, model interpretability, and the need for large, diverse datasets for training and validation are significant hurdles. However, ongoing research and technological advancements continue to refine AI models, enhancing their reliability and applicability [23].

In summary, AI and ML are invaluable in the quest to predict immunotherapy responses, offering the potential to tailor treatments to individual patients and improve clinical outcomes. The synergy of clinical data, radiographic imaging, and AI technologies heralds a new era of precision medicine, poised to transform cancer treatment paradigms [24].

## 2.10 Identifying Additional Biomarkers Associated with an Immune Response

In the realm of cancer immunotherapy, identifying predictive biomarkers is essential for personalizing treatment and improving patient outcomes. While PD-L1 is a well-known biomarker, not all patients with high PD-L1 expression respond to immune checkpoint inhibitors (ICIs), highlighting the need for additional biomarkers. The complex and dynamic nature of tumor-immune interactions necessitates more robust biomarkers to accurately identify patients likely to derive benefit from immunotherapy.

This section explores various biomarkers beyond PD-L1 that are associated with immunotherapy response, including tumor mutational burden (TMB), microsatellite instability (MSI), immune cell infiltration, multi-omics approaches, and others.

## 2.11 Tumor Mutational Burden (TMB)

Tumor mutational burden (TMB) refers to the number of mutations within a tumor's DNA. It has been recognized as a significant biomarker for predicting response to ICIs. Studies indicate that a higher TMB often correlates with better responses to immunotherapy, as more mutations may result in neoantigen formation, thus enhancing immunogenicity [25]. However, while TMB is promising, it is not universally predictive across all cancer types, with efficacy varying significantly [23].

## 2.12 Microsatellite Instability (MSI)

Microsatellite instability, resulting from defective DNA mismatch repair, is another critical biomarker for immune checkpoint blockade success. Tumors characterized by MSI exhibit a high number of mutations, similar to those with high TMB, and show enhanced responses to ICIs [23]. MSI has been extensively validated as a biomarker for predicting favorable outcomes in different types of cancer, including colorectal and endometrial cancers [25].

## 2.13 Immune Cell Infiltration

The presence and composition of tumor-infiltrating lymphocytes (TILs) within the tumor microenvironment are critical indicators of immunotherapy efficacy. Particularly, the density of CD8+ T cells, which are cytotoxic, is associated with positive responses to ICIs [23]. Advanced technologies, such as spatial analysis of tumor samples infused with AI, are being employed to correlate immune cell spatial distribution with therapeutic response [26]. Currently, there is ongoing phase I clinical trial [27] focused on the therapeutic potential of TILs in primary hepatocellular carcinoma (HCC). TILs were harvested from patients, expanded ex vivo, and reintroduced after tumor resection. The study demonstrated that TIL-based therapy was feasible, as TILs were successfully expanded in 88% of patients and infused with minimal toxicity, such as mild flu-like symptoms. Immunologically, the infused TILs exhibited strong antitumor characteristics, including high cytokine production, particularly of IFN-$\gamma$ and TNF-$\alpha$. These findings highlight the role of TILs in immunotherapy for HCC, paving the way for larger trials to explore their efficacy further.

## 2.14 Additional Biomarkers

Several genomic alterations are also explored as potential biomarkers for predicting immunotherapy outcomes. Genetic variations such as mutations in STK11, KEAP1, and TP53 can influence response rates. For example, mutations in KEAP1 and STK11 are often associated with resistance to PD-1 blockade. As part of the TNM-I trial, machine learning models have been developed to classify immune phenotypes in NSCLC. These models showed that tumors with STK11/KEAP1 co-mutations tend to exhibit altered immune microenvironments and are prone to poorer outcomes, highlighting the significance of these genomic alterations in influencing treatment responses [28].

Furthermore, epigenetic markers such as DNA methylation profiles have been identified as potential indicators. These biomarkers can modulate gene expression without altering the DNA sequence, influencing the immune system's ability to recognize cancer cells [29].

## 2.15 Multi-omics Approaches

Multi-omics approaches, combining genomic, transcriptomic, proteomic, metabolomic data and radiomic data, along with AI, facilitate a comprehensive analysis of tumor biology. These strategies help identify new biomarkers and provide a deeper understanding of the tumor microenvironment, further refining predictions of immunotherapy success [24]. These approaches uncover novel biomarkers that may not be evident with single-omic analyses [23]. Machine learning models that integrate multi-omic data can uncover complex interactions and novel biomarkers associated with immunotherapy response [25, 29]. The use of AI tools has also led to the identification of previously unknown biomarkers. For instance, an ML approach helped in discovering RNA-based biosignatures like the immune-related lncRNA signature (IRLS), that have shown potential in predicting ICI efficacy [26]. In another study, ML models integrated radiomic features extracted from computerized tomography (CT) images with TMB data to create a composite biomarker capable of stratifying NSCLC patients into risk categories with differing prognoses—facilitating the clinical selection of appropriate ICIs [24].

## 2.16 Conclusions

AI/ML holds significant potential in enhancing cancer immunotherapy through precise biomarker identification, aiding in personalized treatment strategies and optimizing patient outcomes. Traditionally, biomarkers such as PD-L1 have been employed to guide immunotherapy, yet their limitations necessitate the exploration of additional biomarkers due to variability in patient responses. Identifying and validating biomarkers beyond PD-L1 is crucial for the advancement of immunotherapy in cancer treatment. Continued research into these and additional biomarkers, augmented by multi-omics approaches and AI-driven analyses, will enhance predictive accuracy and lead to more personalized and effective cancer treatments [25, 29]. AI/ML can significantly advance these efforts by integrating complex, multidimensional datasets from various omics paradigms including genomics, proteomics, metabolomics, and radiomics, offering comprehensive insights into tumor biology and immune interactions. AI models enhance the predictive power of biomarkers such as TMB and MSI. By analyzing vast datasets, AI algorithms can detect intricate patterns linking high TMB or MSI status with improved responses to immune checkpoint inhibitors (ICIs), aiding in stratification of patients likely to benefit from such therapies. For instance, machine learning techniques proficiently synthesize genomic data to uncover signatures associated with immune efficacy.

## 2.17 Cancer Immunoediting Platforms to Help Identify T-Cell Targets

The complex interplay between the immune system and cancer cells represents one of the most promising frontiers in contemporary oncology research. Cancer immunoediting, a concept that has transformed our understanding of tumor immunology, provides a framework for understanding how the immune system both controls and shapes developing tumors. Recent technological advances have enabled the development of sophisticated platforms to identify T-cell targets, with Gritstone's EDGE™ (Epitope Discovery in cancer GEnomes) artificial intelligence system representing a cutting-edge approach. These platforms are revolutionizing personalized cancer immunotherapy by enabling precise identification of tumor-specific antigens that can be targeted by T cells.

## 2.18 The Conceptual Framework of Cancer Immunoediting

Cancer immunoediting represents a dynamic process comprising three distinct phases: elimination, equilibrium, and escape [30]. In the elimination phase, innate and adaptive immune mechanisms identify and destroy emerging tumor cells before they manifest clinically. Tumor cells that survive this initial assault enter the equilibrium phase, where the immune system contains but does not completely eradicate the cancer, creating selective pressure that shapes tumor immunogenicity. Eventually, some cancer cells may acquire mechanisms to evade immune recognition or suppress immune responses, entering the escape phase and leading to clinically apparent malignancy [31].

A central tenet of cancer immunoediting is that T-cell recognition of tumor antigens drives the immunological destruction or sculpting of a developing cancer [32]. Through this process, the immune system effectively functions as an extrinsic tumor suppressor while simultaneously sculpting tumor immunogenicity. Although initially demonstrated in mouse models, compelling evidence now indicates that immunoediting occurs in human cancers, with CD8+ T cells playing a particularly important role in tumors exhibiting an adaptive immune resistance phenotype [31].

The fundamental mechanisms underlying cancer immunoediting have been elucidated through innovative research approaches. Matsushita and colleagues used exome sequencing (cDNA capture sequencing) to define the mutational profile of unedited methylcholanthrene-induced sarcomas from immunodeficient $Rag2^{-/-}$ mice [30]. By integrating sequencing data with major histocompatibility complex (MHC) class I epitope prediction algorithms, they identified mutant spectrin-β2 as a potential rejection antigen of the d42m1 sarcoma and validated this prediction using conventional antigen expression cloning and detection [32]. This pivotal work demonstrated that cancer immunoediting occurs via a T-cell-dependent immunoselection process that promotes outgrowth of pre-existing tumor cell clones lacking highly antigenic mutant proteins [32].

The immunoediting process profoundly influences the antigen landscape of tumors. Researchers have found evidence of immunoediting via neoantigen loss in various solid tumor types in human cancer patients [33]. By comparing the rate of predicted neoantigens formed from non-silent mutations to the observed mutational rate of silent mutations in The Cancer Genome Atlas (TCGA) datasets, fewer predicted neoantigens than expected were found in colorectal and kidney clear cell cancers, suggesting that tumor neoantigens were subject to immune selection pressure [33].

Identifying relevant T-cell targets within this complex landscape presents significant challenges. The antigen landscape—as opposed to the mutational landscape—of human cancers represents a critical dimension for understanding tumor immunology and developing effective immunotherapies [30]. Recent advances in genome sequencing have created unprecedented opportunities to assess genetic influences on disease development and identify potential tumor-specific antigens that can serve as targets for immune-mediated elimination [30].

## 2.19 Evolution of Platforms for T-Cell Target Identification

Traditional approaches to identifying tumor antigens relied heavily on laborious experimental methods with limited throughput. The emergence of genomic and proteomic approaches has revolutionized tumor antigen discovery, enabling comprehensive profiling of tumor-specific mutations and their expression. High-throughput DNA and RNA sequencing technologies allow for detailed characterization of the tumor mutanome, while mass spectrometry-based approaches permit direct identification of peptides presented by MHC molecules on tumor cells.

Computational prediction has become increasingly important in epitope identification. Early algorithms primarily focused on MHC binding affinity, but more sophisticated approaches now incorporate multiple aspects of antigen processing and presentation, including proteasomal cleavage, peptide transport, and T-cell receptor recognition probability. Despite these advances, prediction accuracy remains a significant challenge, with high false-positive rates limiting clinical utility.

The demonstration that T-cell recognition of mutant spectrin-β2 serves as a rejection antigen in the d42m1 sarcoma model provided a concrete example of how computational prediction can be validated through conventional antigen expression cloning and detection [32]. This work showed that cancer immunoediting occurs through selection against strong antigens, highlighting the importance of accurate epitope prediction for understanding tumor immunology and developing effective immunotherapies [32].

## 2.20 Next-Generation Platforms for Neoantigen Discovery

Advanced sequencing technologies have significantly enhanced our ability to identify potential T-cell targets. Whole exome sequencing (WES) and RNA sequencing (RNA-seq) allow comprehensive profiling of tumor-specific mutations and their expression levels. These data provide the foundation for neoantigen prediction by identifying mutations that alter protein sequences and are expressed in tumor cells. AI and ML applications have dramatically improved epitope prediction accuracy. These approaches can integrate multiple features beyond MHC binding, including aspects of antigen processing, presentation, and T-cell recognition. By training on large datasets of experimentally validated epitopes, these algorithms can identify complex patterns and relationships that improve prediction accuracy.

Integration of multiple data types has further enhanced prediction performance. Modern platforms combine genomic data (WES, RNA-seq), proteomic data (mass spectrometry), and immunological data (T-cell receptors repertoire sequencing) to provide a more comprehensive view of the tumor-immune interface. This multimodal approach helps prioritize the most promising T-cell targets for further investigation or therapeutic development. The importance of accurate epitope prediction is underscored by the observation that strong immunogenicity of unedited tumors can be ascribed to the expression of highly antigenic mutant proteins [32]. By precisely identifying the most immunogenic epitopes, next-generation platforms can guide the development of more effective cancer immunotherapies that leverage the cancer immunoediting framework.

## 2.21 Gritstone's EDGE™ Platform: A Next-Generation Approach

Gritstone bio has developed the EDGE™ AI system as a proprietary platform for precise identification of epitopes and design of immunogens, which are critical components for creating highly effective vaccines [34, 35]. This cutting-edge technology enables Gritstone to target specific disease-causing elements with unprecedented precision, paving the way for vaccines that are not only effective but also tailored to individual patient needs.

The EDGE™ platform represents a significant advancement in the field of immunotherapy by leveraging AI to improve the accuracy of epitope discovery and design. Traditional epitope prediction methods often focus primarily on MHC binding affinity, but EDGE™ integrates multiple data types and features to enhance prediction performance. By leveraging machine learning algorithms trained on large datasets of experimentally validated epitopes, the system can identify characteristics that distinguish immunogenic epitopes from non-immunogenic ones, improving prediction accuracy compared to earlier approaches. Unlike conventional approaches that may rely on limited datasets or simplified models of antigen presentation, EDGE™ employs deep learning techniques to capture the complex relationships between tumor mutations, antigen processing, MHC presentation, and T-cell recognition. This comprehensive approach enables more precise identification of epitopes likely to elicit potent anti-tumor immune responses.

The integration of EDGE™-identified epitopes with next-generation delivery vectors further enhances the platform's utility. Gritstone has developed innovative vectors, including chimpanzee adenovirus (ChAd) and self-amplifying mRNA (samRNA), engineered to elicit robust and durable immune responses [35]. These advanced delivery systems overcome limitations of traditional vectors, potentially improving the effectiveness of vaccines developed using the EDGE™ platform.

## 2.22 Clinical Applications and Validation of EDGE™

Gritstone's clinical programs demonstrate the practical applications of the EDGE™ platform in cancer immunotherapy. The GRANITE program focuses on individualized neoantigen vaccines for solid tumors, with early-phase trials [36] showing promising results. This approach leverages the EDGE™ platform's ability to identify patient-specific neoantigens for personalized immunotherapy, potentially offering new treatment options for patients with difficult-to-treat malignancies.

The SLATE program [37] represents an alternative approach, using EDGE™ to identify shared neoantigens present in tumors from multiple patients. This off-the-shelf strategy targets recurrent mutations in driver oncogenes, such as KRAS and TP53, offering a more standardized and potentially more accessible form of neoantigen-targeted immunotherapy. The flexibility to support both personalized and shared antigen approaches highlights the versatility of the EDGE™ platform in addressing diverse clinical needs.

Validation of the EDGE™ platform's performance is essential for establishing its clinical utility. While specific performance metrics for EDGE™ are proprietary, the underlying approach of combining advanced sequencing technologies with AI-driven epitope prediction has shown promise in academic research. Studies have demonstrated that AI-based neoantigen prediction can identify clinically relevant T-cell targets and guide the development of effective immunotherapies (Table 2.1).

**Table 2.1** Gritstone bio's immunoediting platforms [37–39]

| Platform | Primary target(s) | Key technology/ approach | Potential applications | Stage of development |
|---|---|---|---|---|
| EDGE | Neoantigens | Advanced prediction algorithms, multi-omic data integration | Personalized cancer vaccines, adoptive cell therapies | Preclinical/ clinical |
| GRANITE | Personalized tumor-specific antigens | Broad antigen discovery, tailored to individual patients | Highly personalized immunotherapies | Preclinical/ clinical |
| SLATE | Shared tumor antigens | Identification of common antigens across patient subsets | "Off-the-shelf" immunotherapies for specific cancer types | Preclinical |

## 2.23 Integration with the cGAS-STING Pathway and Broader Immunotherapy Approaches

The efficacy of platforms like EDGE™ can be further enhanced through integration with complementary immunotherapeutic approaches. The cyclic GMP-AMP synthase (cGAS) and stimulator of interferon genes (STING) pathway represents one such complementary approach, functioning as a linchpin of innate immunity against cancer [40]. Activation of this signaling pathway orchestrates the production of type I interferon (IFN-α/β), fostering the maturation, differentiation, and mobilization of immune effectors in the tumor microenvironment [40].

The cGAS-STING pathway facilitates the release and presentation of tumor antigens, making it an attractive target for cancer immunotherapy [40]. Activation of this pathway has shown favorable tumor regression effects in clinical models by evoking systemic anti-tumor responses, particularly when combined with immune checkpoint inhibitors [40]. These combination approaches have achieved remarkable improvements in survival rates in phase I clinical trials, highlighting the potential for synergistic effects when integrating EDGE™-guided antigen selection with innate immune activation [40].

T cells play essential roles in the immune response against cancer cells, primarily by recognizing tumor-specific antigens presented on MHC-I molecules via their T-cell receptors [40]. Multiple studies have demonstrated the importance of STING pathway activation in increasing cytotoxic T lymphocyte (CTL) engagement and eliciting robust anti-tumor responses [40]. By integrating EDGE™-guided antigen selection with STING pathway activation, it may be possible to enhance both the precision and potency of cancer immunotherapy, potentially overcoming resistance mechanisms that limit current approaches.

## 2.24 Challenges and Future Directions

Despite significant progress, several challenges remain in the development and application of cancer immunoediting platforms for T-cell target identification. Tumor heterogeneity presents a significant obstacle, as different regions of the same tumor may express different antigens, complicating target selection. Immune evasion mechanisms, including loss of antigen presentation machinery and establishment of an immunosuppressive microenvironment, can limit the effectiveness of T-cell-directed therapies even when appropriate targets are identified.

Technical challenges in neoantigen prediction also persist. Current algorithms may not fully capture the complex determinants of immunogenicity, leading to both false-positive and false-negative predictions. The validation of predicted neoantigens remains time-consuming and labor-intensive, limiting the scalability of personalized approaches. Integration of multi-omic data types holds promise for improving prediction accuracy but introduces additional computational complexity.

Future directions for cancer immunoediting platforms like EDGE™ include refinement of prediction algorithms through incorporation of additional data types and features, expansion to additional cancer types and clinical contexts, and integration with complementary therapeutic modalities. The combination of precise antigen identification with strategies to overcome immune suppression in the tumor microenvironment may yield synergistic effects and improve clinical outcomes.

## 2.25 Conclusions

Cancer immunoediting platforms for T-cell target identification, exemplified by Gritstone's EDGE™ system, represent a significant advancement in our ability to harness the immune system for cancer therapy. By identifying the most relevant epitopes, these platforms enable the development of more effective immunotherapies, whether personalized or off-the-shelf. The integration of artificial intelligence with advanced genomic and proteomic technologies has dramatically improved our ability to identify tumor-specific antigens that can serve as effective targets for T-cell-mediated anti-tumor immunity.

The evolution from traditional experimental methods to sophisticated AI-driven platforms reflects our deepening understanding of the complex interplay between cancer and the immune system. As this field continues to advance, we can anticipate further innovations that improve prediction accuracy, expand application to diverse cancer types, and overcome current limitations. With continued research and development, cancer immunoediting platforms like EDGE™ have the potential to significantly enhance our arsenal against cancer and improve outcomes for patients with difficult-to-treat malignancies.

## References


1. Kim DN, McNaughton AD, Kumar N. Leveraging artificial intelligence to expedite antibody design and enhance antibody–antigen interactions. Bioengineering. 2024;11(2):185.
2. Kim J, McFee M, Fang Q, Abdin O, Kim PM. Computational and artificial intelligence-based methods for antibody development. Trends Pharmacol Sci. 2023;44(3):175–89.
3. Jumper J, Evans R, Pritzel A, Green T, Figurnov M, Ronneberger O, et al. Highly accurate protein structure prediction with AlphaFold. Nature. 2021;596(7873):583–9.
4. Jing H, Gao Z, Xu S, Shen T, Peng Z, He S, et al. Accurate prediction of antibody function and structure using bio-inspired antibody language model. Brief Bioinform. 2024;25(4):bbae245.
5. Shanehsazzadeh A, McPartlon M, Kasun G, Steiger AK, Sutton JM, Yassine E, et al. Unlocking de novo antibody design with generative artificial intelligence [Internet]. bioRxiv; 2024 [cited 2025 Mar 15]. p. 2023.01.08.523187. Available from: https://www.biorxiv.org/content/10.1101/2023.01.08.523187v4.
6. Liu G, Zeng H, Mueller J, Carter B, Wang Z, Schilz J, et al. Antibody complementarity determining region design using high-capacity machine learning. Valencia A, editor. Bioinformatics. 2020;36(7):2126–33.
7. Jin W, Wohlwend J, Barzilay R, Jaakkola T. Iterative refinement graph neural network for antibody sequence-structure co-design [Internet]. arXiv; 2022 [cited 2025 Mar 24]. Available from: http://arxiv.org/abs/2110.04624.
8. Sormanni P, Aprile FA, Vendruscolo M. The CamSol method of rational design of protein mutants with enhanced solubility. J Mol Biol. 2015;427(2):478–90.

9. Hou Q, Kwasigroch JM, Rooman M, Pucci F. SOLart: a structure-based method to predict protein solubility and aggregation. Bioinformatics. 2020;36(5):1445–52.
10. Pujols J, Iglesias V, Santos J, Kuriata A, Kmiecik S, Ventura S. A3D 2.0 Update for the prediction and optimization of protein solubility. In: Garcia Fruitós E, Arís Giralt A, editors. Insoluble proteins: methods and protocols [Internet]. New York: Springer US; 2022 [cited 2025 Mar 24]. p. 65–84. Available from: https://doi.org/10.1007/978-1-0716-1859-2_3.
11. Rai BK, Apgar JR, Bennett EM. Low-data interpretable deep learning prediction of antibody viscosity using a biophysically meaningful representation. Sci Rep. 2023;13(1):2917.
12. Abanades B, Wong WK, Boyles F, Georges G, Bujotzek A, Deane CM. ImmuneBuilder: deep-learning models for predicting the structures of immune proteins. Commun Biol. 2023;6(1):1–8.
13. Zheng J, Wang Y, Liang Q, Cui L, Wang L. The application of machine learning on antibody discovery and optimization. Molecules. 2024;29(24):5923.
14. Santuari L, Bachmann Salvy M, Xenarios I, Arpat B. AI-accelerated therapeutic antibody development: practical insights. Front Drug Discov [Internet]. 2024 [cited 2025 Mar 15];4. Available from: https://www.frontiersin.org/journals/drug-discovery/articles/10.3389/fddsv.2024.1447867/full.
15. Molecular characterization of clinical responses to PD-1/PD-L1 inhibitors in non-small cell lung cancer: predictive value of multidimensional immunomarker detection for the efficacy of PD-1 inhibitors in Chinese patients—Song—2019—Thoracic cancer—Wiley Online Library [Internet]. [cited 2025 Mar 24]. Available from: https://onlinelibrary.wiley.com/doi/10.1111/1759-7714.13078.
16. Yang Y, Yang J, Shen L, Chen J, Xia L, Ni B, et al. A multi-omics-based serial deep learning approach to predict clinical outcomes of single-agent anti-PD-1/PD-L1 immunotherapy in advanced stage non-small-cell lung cancer. Am J Transl Res. 2021;13(2):743–56.
17. Park C, Na KJ, Choi H, Ock CY, Ha S, Kim M, et al. Tumor immune profiles noninvasively estimated by FDG PET with deep learning correlate with immunotherapy response in lung adenocarcinoma. Theranostics. 2020;10(23):10838–48.
18. Mu W, Jiang L, Zhang J, Shi Y, Gray JE, Tunali I, et al. Non-invasive decision support for NSCLC treatment using PET/CT radiomics. Nat Commun. 2020;11(1):5228.
19. Trebeschi S, Drago SG, Birkbak NJ, Kurilova I, Călin AM, Delli Pizzi A, et al. Predicting response to cancer immunotherapy using noninvasive radiomic biomarkers. Ann Oncol. 2019;30(6):998–1004.
20. Ahn BC, So JW, Synn CB, Kim TH, Kim JH, Byeon Y, et al. Clinical decision support algorithm based on machine learning to assess the clinical response to anti–programmed death-1 therapy in patients with non–small-cell lung cancer. Eur J Cancer. 2021;153:179–89.
21. A serum protein classifier identifying patients with advanced non–small cell lung cancer who derive clinical benefit from treatment with immune checkpoint inhibitors | Clinical cancer research | American Association for Cancer Research [Internet]. [cited 2025 Mar 24]. Available from: https://aacrjournals.org/clincancerres/article-abstract/26/19/5188/82820/A-Serum-Protein-Classifier-Identifying-Patients?redirectedFrom=fulltext.
22. Wang L, Chen X, Zhang L, Li L, Huang Y, Sun Y, et al. Artificial intelligence in clinical decision support systems for oncology. Int J Med Sci. 2023;20(1):79–86.
23. Roisman LC, Kian W, Anoze A, Fuchs V, Spector M, Steiner R, et al. Radiological artificial intelligence—predicting personalized immunotherapy outcomes in lung cancer. npj Precis Oncol. 2023;7(1):1–7.
24. Yin X, Liao H, Yun H, Lin N, Li S, Xiang Y, et al. Artificial intelligence-based prediction of clinical outcome in immunotherapy and targeted therapy of lung cancer. Semin Cancer Biol. 2022;86:146–59.
25. Rakaee M, Tafavvoghi M, Ricciuti B, Alessi JV, Cortellini A, Citarella F, et al. Deep learning model for predicting immunotherapy response in advanced non−small cell lung cancer. JAMA Oncol. 2025;11(2):109–18.

26. Prelaj A, Miskovic V, Zanitti M, Trovo F, Genova C, Viscardi G, et al. Artificial intelligence for predictive biomarker discovery in immuno-oncology: a systematic review. Ann Oncol. 2024;35(1):29–65.
27. Jiang SS, Tang Y, Zhang YJ, Weng DS, Zhou ZG, Pan K, et al. A phase I clinical trial utilizing autologous tumor-infiltrating lymphocytes in patients with primary hepatocellular carcinoma. Oncotarget. 2015;6(38):41339–49.
28. Rakaee M, Andersen S, Giannikou K, Paulsen EE, Kilvaer TK, Busund LTR, et al. Machine learning-based immune phenotypes correlate with STK11/KEAP1 co-mutations and prognosis in resectable NSCLC: a sub-study of the TNM-I trial. Ann Oncol. 2023;34(7):578–88.
29. Kong J, Ha D, Lee J, Kim I, Park M, Im SH, et al. Network-based machine learning approach to predict immunotherapy response in cancer patients. Nat Commun. 2022;13(1):3703.
30. Vesely MD, Schreiber RD. Cancer immunoediting: antigens, mechanisms and implications to cancer immunotherapy. Ann N Y Acad Sci. 2013;1284(1):1–5.
31. Teng MWL, Galon J, Fridman WH, Smyth MJ. From mice to humans: developments in cancer immunoediting. J Clin Invest. 2015;125(9):3338–46.
32. Matsushita H, Vesely MD, Koboldt DC, Rickert CG, Uppaluri R, Magrini VJ, et al. Cancer exome analysis reveals a T-cell-dependent mechanism of cancer immunoediting. Nature. 2012;482(7385):400–4.
33. Gubin MM, Vesely MD. Cancer immunoediting in the era of immuno-oncology. Clin Cancer Res. 2022;2022:clincanres.1804.2022.
34. BioSpace [Internet]. 2024 [cited 2025 Apr 15]. Gritstone bio presents improvements to EDGE™ platform at AACR 2024. Available from: https://www.biospace.com/gritstone-bio-presents-improvements-to-edge-platform-at-aacr-2024.
35. FirstWord [Internet]. [cited 2025 Apr 15]. Available from: https://firstwordpharma.com/story/5714565.
36. Gritstone bio, Inc. An international phase 1/2 study of GRT-C901/GRT-R902, a neoantigen cancer vaccine, in combination with immune checkpoint blockade for patients with advanced solid tumors [Internet]. clinicaltrials.gov; 2023 [cited 2025 Apr 15]. Report No.: NCT03639714. Available from: https://clinicaltrials.gov/study/NCT03639714.
37. BioSpace [Internet]. 2024 [cited 2025 Apr 15]. Nature medicine publishes interim results from gritstone bio's phase 1/2 study of "off-the-shelf" neoantigen vaccine platform (SLATE). Available from: https://www.biospace.com/nature-medicine-publishes-interim-results-from-gritstone-bio-s-phase-1-2-study-of-off-the-shelf-neoantigen-vaccine-platform-slate.
38. Palmer CD, Rappaport AR, Davis MJ, Hart MG, Scallan CD, Hong SJ, et al. Individualized, heterologous chimpanzee adenovirus and self-amplifying mRNA neoantigen vaccine for advanced metastatic solid tumors: phase 1 trial interim results. Nat Med. 2022;28(8):1619–29.
39. Rappaport AR, Kyi C, Lane M, Hart MG, Johnson ML, Henick BS, et al. A shared neoantigen vaccine combined with immune checkpoint blockade for advanced metastatic solid tumors: phase 1 trial interim results. Nat Med. 2024;30(4):1013–22.
40. Zhang J, Yu S, Peng Q, Wang P, Fang L. Emerging mechanisms and implications of cGAS-STING signaling in cancer immunotherapy strategies. Cancer Biol Med. 2024;21(1):45–64.

# Recent Advancements in Immunotherapy for the Treatment of Metastatic Breast Cancer

3

B. Madhu Krishna, Pankaj Garg, Sravani Ramisetty, Meera Nair, and Sharad S. Singhal

## Abbreviations

| | |
|---|---|
| BC | breast cancer |
| BRCA | breast cancer gene |
| CAR-T | chimeric antigen receptor T-cell |
| CDK | cyclin-dependent kinase |
| DFS | disease-free survival |
| CTLA-4 | cytotoxic T-lymphocyte-associated protein-4 |
| EMT | epithelial-to-mesenchymal transition |
| ICIs | immune checkpoint inhibitors |
| IFNγ | interferon-gamma |
| ORR | objective response rate |
| OS | overall survival |
| PARP | poly (ADP-ribose) polymerase |
| PD-1/PD L1 | programed cell death protein-1/programmed death ligand-1 |
| PFS | progression-free survival |
| TAMs | tumor-associated macrophages |
| TIL | tumor-infiltrating lymphocytes |
| TME | tumor microenvironment |
| Treg | regulatory T-cell |
| TNBC | triple-negative breast cancer |

B. Madhu Krishna · S. Ramisetty · S. S. Singhal (✉)
Department of Medical Oncology, Beckman Research Institute, City of Hope Comprehensive Cancer Center and National Medical Center, Duarte, CA, USA
e-mail: ssinghal@coh.org

P. Garg
Department of Chemistry, GLA University, Mathura, Uttar Pradesh, India

M. Nair
William J. Brennan High School, San Antonio, TX, USA



R. Salgia, P. Kulkarni (eds.), *Immunotherapies in Solid Tumors*, Cancer Treatment and Research 129, https://doi.org/10.1007/978-3-031-97242-3_3

## 3.1 Introduction

Breast cancer (BC) remains one of the primary causes of cancer-related deaths among women in the United States, with an estimated 319,750 new invasive cases diagnosed and approximately 42,680 fatalities expected in 2025 alone [1]. Despite the recent advancements in conventional therapies, BC is significantly associated with high morbidity and mortality [2, 3]. While advancements in early detection and treatment strategies have contributed to a 38% reduction in BC mortality rates, the prognosis for metastatic BC remains poor, with a 5-year survival rate below 25% [4, 5]. The complexity of BC, characterized by its heterogeneous nature, diverse mutational profiles, varied patient responses to neoadjuvant therapies, and increasing chemoresistance, highlights the urgent demand for innovative therapeutic strategies aimed at minimizing relapse and enhancing disease-free survival (DFS) [6].

Given the critical role of the immune system in cancer surveillance and elimination, researchers have explored its potential to target tumor cells [7]. Immunotherapy has emerged as a key approach in the management of multiple cancer types, including melanoma, lung cancer, and, more recently, triple-negative breast cancer (TNBC) [8, 9]. Current research is focused on integrating immunotherapy with conventional treatment modalities for BC, and recent findings indicate its promising potential in improving therapeutic outcomes. Various immunotherapeutic strategies, including immune checkpoint inhibitors (ICIs), monoclonal antibodies, cyclin-dependent kinase (CDK) 4/6 inhibitors, and antibody-drug conjugates (ADCs), have been explored for BC treatment [10]. However, challenges associated with these approaches must be carefully addressed to optimize their clinical efficacy [11].

This review aims to provide a comprehensive analysis of the immune system's role in BC progression, treatment response, and therapeutic resistance. Additionally, it will discuss the current status of immunotherapy in BC, key barriers to its success, and potential strategies to overcome these challenges. Harnessing the immune system to generate an effective antitumor response in BC could pave the way for novel therapeutic protocols with improved efficacy and prolonged survival outcomes.

## 3.2 Immune System in Normal Breast Development

A diverse immune cell population is actively present in the breast stroma during different developmental stages, playing a fundamental role in regulating normal breast maturation and protection. CD4+ T-helper type-1 (Th1) cells engage with mammary CD11c+ antigen-presenting cells, negatively influencing mammary organogenesis via IFN$\gamma$ signaling. This interaction contributes to epithelial remodeling, luminal differentiation, and mammary organogenesis in murine models. Notably, when the MHC-II-dependent CD4+ T-cell response was suppressed, alveolar branching increased, indicating that CD4+ T cells provide an intrinsic regulatory function in normal breast development. However, blocking MHC-I-mediated CD8+ T-cell activation did not impact mammary gland growth in mice [12]. Macrophages and eosinophils are also key regulators of mammary ductal expansion during puberty, secreting specific cytokines and chemokines that modulate this process [13]. The breast undergoes further structural modifications throughout pregnancy, lactation, and post-lactational regression, with alveolar branching and milk production being tightly regulated [14]. During post-lactational involution, macrophage infiltration facilitates apoptosis in milk-producing epithelial cells, contributing to milk clearance and the cessation of lactation [15].

Mammary gland involution is believed to activate both innate and adaptive immune responses. According to gene expression studies conducted by Fornetti et al. neutrophil and macrophage infiltration significantly increases from the initial stages of involution [16]. Pro-inflammatory pathways, particularly those driven by STAT3 and NFκβ activation, promote the migration of macrophages, eosinophils, plasma cells, and B lymphocytes from peri-ductal regions into the ductal lumen during this period [17]. Additionally, macrophages within involuting lobules exhibit elevated levels of Arginase-1, a marker of the M2 macrophage phenotype, commonly associated with tissue remodeling. In human breast tissue, the general leukocyte marker CD45 progressively increases within involuting lobules over the first 12 months postpartum. Immunohistochemistry (IHC) staining has revealed a marked rise in CD4+, CD8+, and CD19+ cells, underscoring the involvement of T- and B-cell-mediated immune responses in breast involution [16]. Given that breast involution requires tightly coordinated immune responses and controlled cell death, any dysregulation in these processes could create a microenvironment conducive to tumorigenesis. An imbalance in inflammatory signaling or immune cell infiltration during involution may contribute to the initiation and progression of BC.

## 3.3 BC Development and Progression

*Oncodrivers in BC:* Oncogenic drivers play a pivotal role in promoting tumor growth and survival, making them promising therapeutic targets for BC treatment. Among the key oncodrivers identified in BC, notable examples include EGFR, HER2, HER3, MET, and mucin-1 (MUC1). The ERBB receptor family, which consists of EGFR, HER2, HER3, and HER4, is known to be significantly upregulated and plays a crucial role in normal breast development, particularly during puberty, pregnancy, and lactation [18]. The activation of EGFR through ligand binding is essential for mammary epithelial growth and ductal differentiation, with its effects being most prominent from puberty to adulthood [19]. Interestingly, HER2 expression has been found to peak during puberty and adulthood, where it is associated with ductal outgrowth and the development of terminal end buds [20]. According to Eccles, HER3 (ERBB3) expression is largely confined to pregnancy, whereas HER4 (ERBB4) remains active throughout pregnancy and lactation, playing a critical role in lobular alveolar development and lactation maintenance [21]. Additionally, MET signaling has been implicated in facilitating luminal cell expansion and ductal branching during breast development [22]. In the context of BC, HER2's constitutive activation has been shown to drive tumor cell proliferation and survival, ultimately contributing to therapeutic resistance, increased invasiveness, and metastatic progression in HER2-positive BC [23]. Notably, HER3 has been identified as a major activator of the PI3K/AKT signaling pathway, with its overexpression linked to trastuzumab resistance, further supporting its role as an oncodriver in BC [24].

A poor 5-year DFS rate and a reduced 10-year overall survival (OS) in TNBC, which lacks surface receptors for targeted therapies, have been correlated with elevated HER3 levels [25, 26]. While EGFR overexpression has been observed across all BC subtypes, it is particularly prevalent in aggressive TNBC and invasive breast carcinomas, where it is strongly linked to larger tumor size and unfavorable clinical outcomes [27, 28]. Studies have shown that TNBCs exhibit high expression of hepatocyte growth factor receptor/receptor tyrosine kinase MET (HGFR/MET), with MET being recognized as an independent prognostic marker for disease recurrence and a predictor of shorter survival [29]. It is speculated that molecular crosstalk between MET and the ERBB receptor family signaling pathways may contribute to resistance against EGFR- and HER2-targeted therapies, suggesting that MET inhibition could hold potential as a therapeutic strategy in oncodriver-targeted treatments [30]. Given the presence of multiple oncodrivers in BC, integrating immunotherapy with oncodriver-targeted approaches may offer a promising avenue for TNBC treatment, which currently lacks effective therapeutic options.

Beyond classical genetic and epigenetic drivers of tumor progression such as oncogene activation, tumor suppressor gene inactivation, abnormal cellular transformation, and aneuploidy, the immune system plays a crucial role in BC development, progression, and metastasis. Research indicates that BC driven by carcinogens is associated with tumor proliferation and immune suppression. For instance, in a dimethylbenz(a)anthracene (DMBA)-induced BC model, thymic atrophy was observed, leading to reduced IL2 expression and impaired T-cell activation [31]. Additionally, dysregulated cytokine signaling may result in abnormal cell proliferation and differentiation. Various immune cells secrete TGFβ, an anti-inflammatory cytokine, whose signaling is mediated via type I and type II TGFβ receptors [32]. Mutations or deletions in these receptors have been linked to increased invasiveness and poorer prognosis in BC. Furthermore, IL10, a cytokine secreted by monocytes and lymphocytes, modulates major histocompatibility complex Class-I (MHC-I) expression on tumor cells, which is essential for natural killer (NK) cell-mediated cytolysis. Reduced IL10 expression in breast carcinomas has been associated with immune evasion and unchecked cellular proliferation, enabling tumors to bypass the anti-tumor immune response [33, 34].

Although the pro-inflammatory cytokine IL6 is essential for modulating immune responses against infections, it can also drive pro-tumorigenic effects by promoting the survival of malignant cells in hostile environments. As a result, elevated IL6 levels are considered a biomarker for advanced-stage cancers [35]. Additionally, IL6 has been implicated in the epithelial-to-mesenchymal transition (EMT) of normal breast cells, fostering cancer stem cell-like traits. Xie et al. demonstrated that IL6 contributes to generating a highly tumorigenic cell pool with the ability to differentiate into diverse tumor cell types [36]. Beyond cytokine-driven inflammation, immune cell infiltration and the tumor microenvironment (TME) composition play a critical role in oncogenic transformation. The presence of CD4+ T-helper cells, CD8+ cytotoxic T lymphocytes, B lymphocytes, M1 macrophages, and NK cells within the tumor milieu is typically associated with improved progression-free survival (PFS) and OS in BC patients [37–39]. These immune infiltrates contribute to the anti-tumor immune response through cytokine-mediated signaling and direct cytotoxic activity. However, regulatory T-cell (Treg) infiltration in the TME suppresses T-cell activation and deactivates effector T cells, leading to immune evasion, increased tumor progression, and poor prognosis [39–41].

The TME is also enriched with M2 macrophages, or tumor-associated macrophages (TAMs), which have been shown to facilitate tumor growth and metastasis. A phenotypic shift from M1 (tumor-suppressive) to M2 (tumor-promoting) macrophages enhances angiogenesis, tumor cell motility, and overall survival of malignant cells, thereby driving metastasis. Additionally, TAMs promote immunosuppression by upregulating TGFβ and IL10, further supporting tumor progression [42–45]. Several studies have explored therapeutic strategies targeting TAM recruitment inhibition or M2-to-M1 repolarization, with varying degrees of success [46, 47]. The role of tumor-infiltrating B cells (TIBs) in BC remains poorly understood. In non-breast tumor tissues, B-cell infiltration has been detected in approximately 70% of cases, with ductal carcinoma *in situ* (DCIS) and non-malignant breast lesions exhibiting B-cell predominance. This suggests a potential role for B cells in early-stage oncogenic transformation and immune surveillance [48]. In certain BC subtypes, a robust B-cell-mediated anti-tumor response has been associated with improved patient outcomes, likely due to antigen recognition and subsequent activation of anti-tumor immunity [49]. While pro-tumorigenic B cell activity has not been observed in BC, this phenomenon has been reported in other malignancies. For instance, Ou et al. reported an increased B-cell infiltration in bladder cancer, leading to the upregulation of IL-8/androgen receptor signaling and overexpression of metastasis-associated matrix metalloproteinases (MMPs) [50].

## 3.4 The Immune System's Paradoxical Role in BC

The immune system exerts both protective and tumor-promoting influences in BC [51]. The concept of cancer immunoediting underscores the evolving interplay between tumor cells and host immunity [52]. In early tumorigenesis, acute inflammation activates innate immune pathways, facilitating tumor cell eradication. This process enhances dendritic cell maturation, leading to the activation of tumor-specific T cells. At this stage, the immune system may either eliminate malignant cells or exert selective pressure, driving tumor evolution toward immune resistance. However, persistent inflammation fosters a complex TME enriched with stromal components (e.g., fibroblasts, endothelial cells) and immunosuppressive factors, including Tregs, myeloid-derived suppressor cells (MDSCs), and B lymphocytes, all of which contribute to immune evasion and tumor progression [53, 54].

As the immune response intensifies in early tumor development, tumor and immune cells upregulate immune checkpoint proteins, while immune-suppressive metabolic pathways become more pronounced. Concurrently, the CD4+ T-cell response shifts from a Th1-dominant (pro-inflammatory, tumor-suppressive) profile to a Th2-skewed (immune-tolerant) state, further dampening anti-tumor immunity [55–58]. This progressive immune suppression within the TME weakens the host's natural defenses, allowing tumor growth to continue unchecked. According to Schreiber et al., tumor cells evade immune destruction through three primary mechanisms [59]. First, they downregulate MHC class I molecules, modify antigen presentation pathways, and reduce tumor antigen expression, thereby avoiding detection by dendritic cells and cytotoxic T lymphocytes. Second, cancer cells develop resistance to cytotoxic immune responses through persistent oncogenic signaling, including STAT3 activation, HER2 and EGFR overexpression, and upregulation of anti-apoptotic proteins like BCL2. Lastly, tumors establish an immunosuppressive TME by secreting inhibitory cytokines (e.g., TGFβ, VEGF), altering metabolic pathways (e.g., indoleamine 2,3-dioxygenase [IDO]), expanding Tregs and MDSCs, and expressing ICIs such as CTLA-4, PD-1, and Tim-3 (Fig. 3.1). These adaptations collectively enable tumor cells to persist despite immune surveillance, facilitating disease progression.

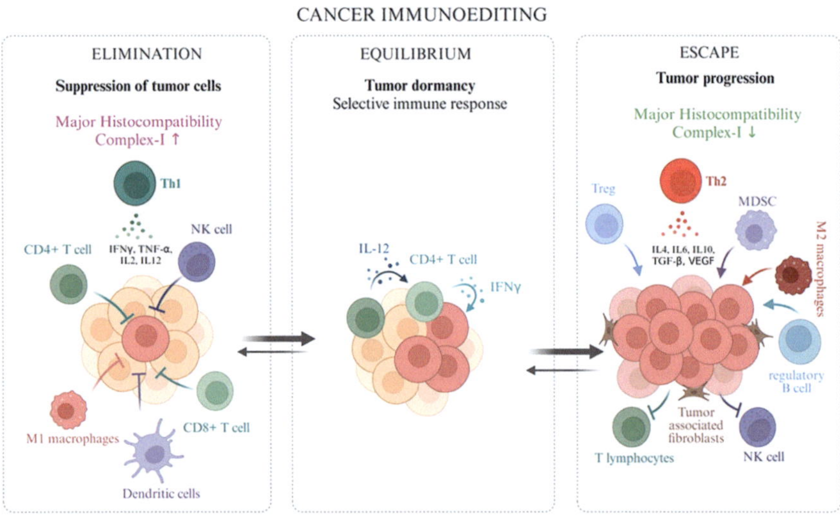


**Fig. 3.1** The immune system exhibits a dualistic role in BC. During tumor elimination, interleukins, IFNγ, and TNFα get secreted at tumor sites, which in turn facilitate maturation of dendritic cells. Matured dendritic cells process tumor-associated antigens efficiently and present them to $CD4^+$ and $CD8^+$ T cells, resulting in the lysis of tumor cells. However, some tumor cells escape this immune response through immunoediting and maintain tumor dormancy until they find a favorable condition. The suppressive TME is comprised of tumor cells, immune cells, tumor-associated fibroblast cells, interleukin 4, 6, 10, and TGFβ. These cells suppress the activation of T lymphocytes and natural killing cells, which leads to the evasion of tumor cells

## 3.5 Immunosurveillance and Immunoediting in BC

The idea that the immune system plays a role in cancer prevention was first proposed by Paul Ehrlich over a century ago, suggesting that immune defenses could limit carcinoma development [60]. This concept was later formalized by Burnet and Thomas in the cancer immunosurveillance hypothesis, which posited that the immune system not only combats malignant transformation but also maintains tissue equilibrium [61–63]. However, due to the absence of suitable animal models, this hypothesis initially faced skepticism. The development of immune-deficient mouse models reignited interest in the field, demonstrating the crucial role of interferon-gamma (IFNγ) in tumor suppression. Experimental studies showed that IFNγ effectively inhibited fibrosarcoma development in mice, regardless of whether tumors were spontaneous, chemically induced, or transplanted [64]. Further investigations using genetically modified mouse models with disrupted IFNγ and/or STAT1 signaling revealed that mice lacking these pathways exhibited a nearly threefold increase in chemically induced tumor formation compared to their wild-type counterparts. These findings underscored the essential role of IFNγ and lymphocyte-mediated mechanisms in controlling tumorigenesis [65]. Subsequent research with these models provided the basis for immunologic sculpting, a concept describing how the immune system influences tumor antigenicity, antigen processing, and IFNγ signaling. Building on this, Schreiber et al. refined the cancer immunoediting framework, emphasizing the immune system's dual function in both eliminating tumor cells and shaping their evolutionary trajectory over time [59].

## 3.6 Immune Biomarkers for Prognosis and Therapy in BC

BC is a highly heterogeneous malignancy categorized into three primary subtypes based on receptor status: (a) hormone receptor-positive (HR-positive), which includes luminal subtypes expressing estrogen receptor (ER) and/or progesterone receptor (PR); (b) human epidermal growth factor receptor 2 (HER2)-positive; and (c) TNBC, which lacks ER, PR, and HER2 expression [66]. These subtypes differ in biological behavior and therapeutic responses because of variations in receptor signaling. Among these subtypes, tumor-infiltrating lymphocytes (TILs) are more frequently observed in HER2-positive BC and TNBC at diagnosis compared to luminal BC. Elevated levels of TILs are indicative of better prognoses in early-stage diseases, irrespective of the treatment approach: A significant presence of TILs within the tumor correlates with enhanced 5-year OS (74.3% for the high TIL cohort compared to 52.0% for the low TIL cohort), increased rates of pathological complete response (pCR; 40–50% in the high TIL group post-chemotherapy), and improved DFS, particularly in TNBC [67, 68]. The presence of TILs within the tumor stroma has demonstrated significant prognostic relevance, correlating with clinical outcomes [64]. Recent studies indicate a direct correlation between stromal tumor-infiltrating lymphocytes (sTILs) and patient outcomes in early-stage TNBC, where individuals with 50% or more sTILs and T1c tumors experienced a 10-year survival rate of 95% without chemotherapy, which improved to 98% with sTILs of 75% or higher. These results further reinforce the role of sTILs as a potential biomarker for de-escalation treatment strategies [69, 70]. Additionally, HER2-positive BC and TNBC exhibit higher levels of programmed death ligand-1 (PD-L1) expression in the TME compared to luminal BC [71, 72]. A higher density of TILs at diagnosis has been linked to favorable responses to both neoadjuvant and adjuvant therapies, contributing to improved PFS and OS. Furthermore, an increased CD8+ cytotoxic T-cell to regulatory T-cell (Treg) ratio has been associated with a higher likelihood of achieving a complete pathological response (cPR) following neoadjuvant chemotherapy [73]. Given the expression of PD-L1 in certain BC subtypes, immune checkpoint blockade targeting the programmed cell death-1 (PD-1)/PD-L1 axis has emerged as a promising therapeutic approach. Clinical trials have demonstrated the effectiveness of checkpoint inhibitors in various PD-L1-positive solid tumors, suggesting that this strategy may provide substantial therapeutic benefits for select BC subtypes as well [74].

## 3.7 Tumor Antigens and Their Significance in BC Vaccine Development

The immune system recognizes tumor antigens through MHC molecules, with MHC class I presenting to CD8+ T cells and MHC class II engaging CD4+ T cells. This process initiates cross-priming, leading to T-cell activation and subsequent tumor elimination. BC vaccines aim to elicit tumor-specific T-cell responses that selectively target and destroy malignant cells. These vaccines typically focus on tissue-specific antigens that are either unique to breast tissue or overexpressed in tumors relative to normal cells (Fig. 3.2). A significant challenge in BC vaccine development arises from the fact that shared tumor antigens are often recognized as self-antigens. To prevent autoimmunity, high-avidity T cells targeting these antigens are deleted during thymic selection, leaving only low-avidity T cells to mount tumor-directed immune responses. Various vaccine strategies have been explored in clinical trials, including peptide- and protein-based vaccines targeting HER2 and Mucin-1, dendritic cell (DC)-based vaccines specific for HER2, cell-based poly-antigen vaccines secreting granulocyte-macrophage colony-stimulating factor (GM-CSF), and viral vector vaccines delivering carcinoembryonic antigen (CEA), Mucin-1, and T-cell activation molecules. Although these vaccines have been shown to be safe and capable of eliciting immune responses, their therapeutic efficacy has remained limited, often generating only weak T-cell activation.

A promising strategy to address these limitations is targeting neoantigens tumor-specific mutated proteins that the immune system perceives as foreign. Unlike shared tumor antigens, neoantigens can activate high-avidity T cells, making them attractive therapeutic targets [75]. This approach is supported by observations that tumors with

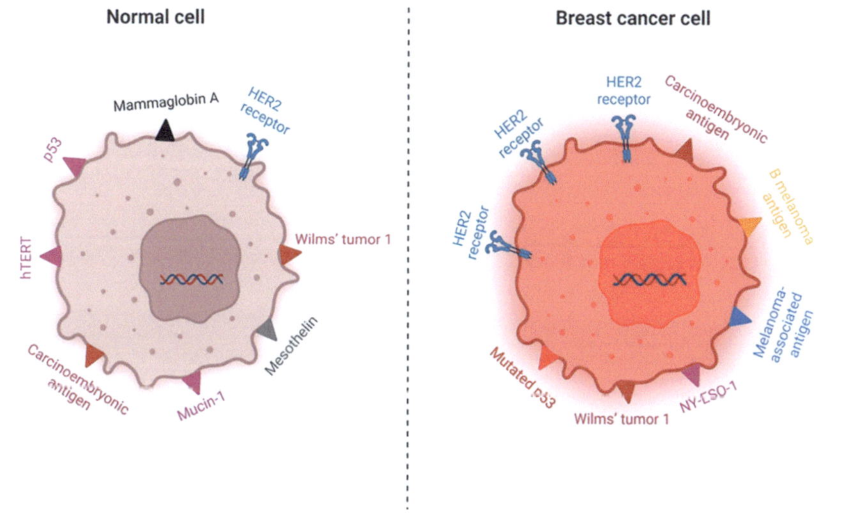


**Fig. 3.2** Tumor-specific antigens facilitate minimal immune tolerance. Antigens commonly expressed by both normal and breast tumor cells establish immune tolerance. Although mutations/polymorphisms and elevated levels of these antigens lead to a better recognition of tumor cells in comparison with normal cells, the discovery of neoantigens unique to tumor cells becomes essential. These neoantigens could possibly induce more of an immune response due to lack of predetermined intolerance towards them

a high mutational burden tend to respond better to immune checkpoint blockade therapies [76]. Ongoing research efforts are focused on developing personalized BC vaccines by sequencing individual tumors to identify unique mutations. However, the extent to which mutational burden directly influences clinical response in BC remains uncertain [77]. Both generalized and patient-specific vaccines have encountered obstacles due to immune checkpoint pathways and other suppressive mechanisms that limit vaccine-induced T-cell activity [51]. To improve vaccine efficacy, several clinical trials have investigated combining BC vaccines with chemotherapy. High-dose chemotherapy has been utilized to reduce tumor burden, enhance antigen release, and counteract immune suppression within the TME. In contrast, low-dose chemotherapy has been employed to selectively diminish Treg-mediated immune suppression (Table 3.1) [78–80]. Additionally, peptide- and cell-based vaccines targeting HER2 have been tested in combination with trastuzumab, either alone to promote immune priming, CD8+ T-cell activation, and immune memory, or alongside trastuzumab and low-dose cyclophosphamide, which helps suppress Treg activity [81–83]. These approaches have led to improved vaccine-induced immune responses. A particularly promising research direction involves integrating BC vaccines with ICIs targeting CTLA-4 or PD-1/PD-L1. This combination aims to counteract immune-suppressive signals that deactivate vaccine-induced T cells within the TME, thereby enhancing the overall efficacy of cancer vaccines.

**Table 3.1** Clinical trials of anti-PD-1/PD-L1 in metastatic BC

| S. no | Study | Phase | Population | No of patients | Safety profile | ORR % | PFS (months) | OS (months) | References |
|---|---|---|---|---|---|---|---|---|---|
| 1 | Pembrolizumab Keynote-12 | Phase 1b | Metastatic TNBC, PD-L1+ | 27 | 3–5 Grade adverse events: 5.6%; 5 Grade 3 Adverse events: anemia, aseptic meningitis, lymphopenia, headache, pyrexia; death (DIC):1 | 18.5 | 1.9 | 11.2 | [99] |
| 2 | Pembrolizumab Keynote-086 Cohort A | Phase 2 | Metastatic TNBC,PD-L1+/– | 170 | Grade 3–4 adverse events: 12%; immune-related adverse events of any grade: 19%, of which Grade 3–4 is of 1.2%: (hypothyroidism/ hyperthyroidism, pneumonitis) | 4.7 (4.8/4.7: PD-L1+/ PD-L1−) | 2.1 | NA | [101] |
| 3 | Pembrolizumab Keynote-086 Cohort B | Phase 2 | Metastatic TNBC, PD-L1+ | 84 | Grade 3–4 adverse events: 10%; Deaths due to treatment-related adverse events: 0 | 23.1 | 2 | 8.9 | [100] |
| 4 | Pembrolizumab Keynote-028 | Phase 1b | HER+ metastatic BC, PD-L1+ | 25 | Grade 3–4 adverse events: 16%, immune-related adverse events included hepatitis, pneumonitis, hyperthyroidism/hypothyroidism | 12 | 1.8 | 8.6 | [105] |
| 5 | Pembrolizumab Keynote-355 | Phase 3 | Metastatic TNBC, PD-L1+ | 847 | Grade 3–4 adverse events: 0% immune-related adverse events: 5.3% | 53% (PD-L1+) | 7.6 | 17.6 | [111] |
| 6 | IMpassion132 | Phase 3 | Advanced, Early-Relapsing TNBC <12 months | 354 | Grade 3–4 adverse events: 67%, Treatment-related grade 3/4 adverse events: 62% | 40% | 4 | <12 | [98] |
| 7 | Avelumab JAVELIN | Phase 1b | Metastatic BC, PD-L1+/– | 168 | Grade 3–5 adverse events: 14.3%, immune-related adverse events: autoimmune hepatitis:1.8%; treatment-related deaths: 2 | 4.8 (33/2.4/5.2/2.8/0: PD-L1+/PD-L1−/ TNBC/ HER+/ ERBB2−/ERBB2+) | 5.9 | 8.1 | [92] |

| | | | | | | | | | |
|---|---|---|---|---|---|---|---|---|---|
| 8 | Atezolizumab | Phase 1a | Metastatic TNBC,PD-L1+/– | 115 | Grade 3/4 treatment-related adverse events: 11%, Grade 5 treatment-related adverse events: 2% (1 pulmonary hypertension, 1 unspecified) | 10 (12/0: PD-L1+ / PD-L1−) | 1.4 | 8.9 | [97] |
| 9 | Pembrolizumab + Eribulin | Phase 1b/2 | Metastatic TNBC,PD-L1+/– | 107 | No dose-limiting toxic effect, Grade 3–4 adverse events: 66.7%; most common, neutropenia and fatigue; most common immune-related adverse events hypothyroidism/hyperthyroidism, rash, hyperglycemia, and pneumonitis | 26.4 | 4.2 | 17.7 | [110] |
| 10 | Pembrolizumab + Abemaciclib | Phase 2 | HR+, ERBB2– metastatic BC | 28 | Serious adverse events: 28.6%, Grade 5 adverse events: 3.6%; Grade 4 adverse events: 0; Grade 3 adverse events: diarrhea:10.7%, neutropenia: 28.6%, aspartate aminotransferase increase: 14.3%, alanine aminotransferase: 10.7% | 28.6 | NA | NA | [123] |
| 11 | Durvalumab + Olaparib | Phase 2 | Mutated BRCA1/2, metastatic HER2 BC | 25 | Grade 3–4 adverse events: anemia: 8%, neutropenia: 8%, hemolysis: 4%, dyspnea: 4%, pancreatitis: 4%, fatigue: 4%, lymphopenia: 4%, and leukopenia: 4% | 52 | NA | NA | [129] |
| 12 | Tremelimumab + Exemestane | Phase 1 | HR+ metastatic BC | 26 | 5 dose-limiting toxic effects | 0 | NA | NA | [87] |
| 13 | Atezolizumab + nab paclitaxel | Phase 1b | Metastatic TNBC,PD-L1+/– | 33 | Grade 3–4 treatment-related adverse events: 73%, most common: neutropenia, anemia, thrombocytopenia, diarrhea, pneumonia. | 39 | 5.5 | 14.7 | [109] |

## 3.8 Advancements in Immunotherapy for BC

The development of ICIs targeting CTLA-4, PD-1, and PD-L1 has revolutionized cancer treatment, offering durable responses and, in some cases, improving OS across various malignancies [84, 85]. Despite the widespread approval of ICIs for multiple cancer types, their role in BC remains relatively restricted. Clinical trials assessing CTLA-4 inhibitors, such as tremelimumab and ipilimumab, have shown encouraging immunomodulatory effects in BC. Additionally, early-stage studies indicate that PD-1/PD-L1 blockade may hold therapeutic potential for specific BC subtypes, including estrogen receptor-positive (ER+) HER2-negative BC and metastatic TNBC, where a subset of patients has exhibited prolonged responses.

### 3.8.1 Targeting CTLA-4 in BC

CTLA-4 functions as a critical immune checkpoint receptor that is upregulated following T-cell activation. By competing with CD28 for binding to CD80/CD86, CTLA-4 serves as a negative regulator that suppresses excessive immune activation, thereby preventing autoimmunity [86]. However, in cancer, this mechanism can inhibit effective anti-tumor immune responses. To counteract this immunosuppressive effect, monoclonal antibodies (mAbs) targeting CTLA-4 have been developed for clinical applications.

#### 3.8.1.1 Tremelimumab in BC Therapy

Tremelimumab, an anti-CTLA-4 monoclonal antibody, is under clinical evaluation for its efficacy in multiple cancer types, including BC. A Phase I study investigating tremelimumab in combination with exemestane in patients with ER-positive, HER2-negative BC enrolled 26 participants [87]. The trial identified dose-limiting toxicities (DLTs) in five individuals, with adverse effects including elevated liver transaminases (one case) and diarrhea (four cases). Based on these findings, the maximum tolerated dose (MTD) was established at 6 mg/kg administered every 90 days. Immunophenotyping of treated patients revealed an increase in ICOS+ FoxP3+ CD4+ T cells, suggesting an immune-modulating effect. Additionally, 42% of participants achieved stable disease (SD) for a minimum duration of 12 weeks, indicating a partial but measurable immunotherapeutic benefit.

#### 3.8.1.2 Ipilimumab: A CTLA-4-Targeting Immunotherapy in BC

Ipilimumab, an anti-CTLA-4 monoclonal antibody, is FDA-approved for melanoma and is currently being evaluated in combination with PD-1/PD-L1 inhibitors for various malignancies, including BC [85]. In a clinical study investigating its potential in BC, 12 patients with early-stage disease received a single neoadjuvant dose of ipilimumab, either as monotherapy or in combination with cryoablation prior to mastectomy. An additional six patients underwent cryoablation alone as a control group [88]. Immune profiling of tumor samples revealed that ipilimumab, when combined with cryoablation, led to a significant increase in the CD8+

T-cell-to-FoxP3+Treg ratio within the TME. Moreover, systemic immune responses were enhanced, as evidenced by the expansion of circulating ICOS+ Ki67+ CD4+ and ICOS+ Ki67+ CD8+ T cells, along with increased secretion of Th1 cytokines, suggesting a shift toward a pro-inflammatory, anti-tumor immune response. Hematoxylin and eosin (H&E) staining of tumor-infiltrating lymphocytes (TILs) demonstrated a positive correlation between TIL density and the clonal expansion of tumor-reactive T cells, as confirmed by T-cell receptor (TCR) DNA sequencing [89]. Building on these findings, a clinical trial is currently underway to investigate a combination strategy integrating cryoablation, CTLA-4 blockade with ipilimumab (1 mg/kg), and PD-1 inhibition with nivolumab (3 mg/kg) (NCT02833233).

### 3.8.2 Targeting the PD-1/PD-L1 Axis in BC

The PD-1 receptor, upon interaction with its ligands PD-L1 or PD-L2, transmits inhibitory signals that downregulate T-cell activation, thereby attenuating anti-tumor immunity [86]. To counteract this immune evasion mechanism, multiple humanized monoclonal antibodies (mAbs) have been developed to inhibit the PD-1/PD-L1 axis, including PD-L1-targeting agents (avelumab, atezolizumab) and PD-1 inhibitors (pembrolizumab). Clinical trials evaluating these ICIs in metastatic BC, particularly in TNBC, have shown encouraging therapeutic potential [90]. However, as observed in other malignancies, PD-1/PD-L1 blockade in BC is associated with immune-related adverse effects, which require careful monitoring and management.

#### 3.8.2.1 Avelumab in BC Immunotherapy

The JAVELIN clinical trial (Phase Ia/Ib) evaluated the safety and efficacy of avelumab, an anti-PD-L1 monoclonal antibody, across multiple cancer types, including BC [91]. In the Phase Ib expansion cohort, 168 BC patients were enrolled regardless of their PD-L1 status or molecular subtype [92]. Among these participants, 42.9% had estrogen receptor-positive (ER+)/progesterone receptor-positive (PR+)/HER2-negative BC, 34.5% were diagnosed with TNBC, 15.5% had HER2-positive BC, and 7.1% were classified as undetermined. Notably, more than half of the patients had undergone at least three prior lines of systemic therapy for metastatic disease.

The overall response rate (ORR) in the full cohort was 4.8%, comprising one complete response (CR), seven partial responses (PRs), and 39 cases of stable disease (SD), leading to a disease control rate (DCR) of 28%. While responses were observed across all BC subtypes, they were most pronounced in TNBC. Among the 58 TNBC patients, the ORR was 8.6%, with five PRs, 13 SDs, no CRs, and a DCR of 31%. PD-L1 expression analysis was conducted in 136 patients, revealing that only 12 had ≥10% PD-L1+ immune cells within the TME, while 124 exhibited PD-L1 expression below this threshold. The PR rate varied significantly between these subgroups, with 33.3% in the PD-L1-high group versus 2.4% in the PD-L1-low group. A more focused analysis of TNBC patients showed that among 48 evaluable cases, 39 were PD-L1-negative, and nine were PD-L1-positive, with ORRs of 2.6% and 44.4%, respectively. Building on these findings, a Phase III clinical trial

(NCT02926196) is currently investigating avelumab as an adjuvant therapy over 1 year for patients with high-risk, early-stage TNBC, with OS and DFS as primary and secondary endpoints. Additionally, avelumab is being tested in combination with an anti-41BB (CD137) agonist antibody in a Phase Ib/II study for advanced malignancies, including TNBC (NCT02554812). Anti-41BB agents enhance T-cell co-stimulatory signaling, potentially augmenting anti-tumor immune responses [93].

#### 3.8.2.2 Atezolizumab in TNBC

Atezolizumab, a PD-L1 inhibitor, was assessed as a monotherapy in a Phase Ia trial involving 115 patients with TNBC [94, 95]. PD-L1 expression was evaluated using the SP142 antibody, with tumors classified as PD-L1-positive if at least 5% of tumor-infiltrating immune cells expressed PD-L1[96]. Initially, enrollment was restricted to PD-L1+ patients, but the criteria were later broadened to include all TNBC patients. The study found that 62% of participants were PD-L1+, 32% were PD-L1-negative, and 4% had an undetermined PD-L1 status. Most patients had undergone extensive prior treatment, with a median of seven previous lines of therapy. However, 17% of participants received atezolizumab as their first-line therapy for metastatic TNBC. The ORR was 10% among 112 evaluable patients, with a higher ORR of 13% in PD-L1+ cases compared to 5% in PD-L1-negative patients. Notably, patients who received atezolizumab as a first-line therapy experienced an ORR of 26%, significantly higher than the 4–8% ORR observed in those receiving second- or third-line treatments. The disease control rate (DCR) was 23% overall, with 27% in PD-L1+ cases and 16% in PD-L1-negative cases. The median OS was 9.3 months, with a median follow-up period of 15.2 months. Patients who achieved complete response (CR) or partial response (PR) had a remarkable 100% survival rate beyond 2–3 years, while the overall 1-year survival rate was 41%. Interestingly, approximately 11% of patients classified as having progressive disease per RECIST criteria exhibited atypical responses, such as pseudo-progression, yet experienced prolonged survival. A subsequent analysis of the Phase I trial reaffirmed the ORR of 10% across all evaluable patients, regardless of PD-L1 status [97].

The potential advantage of atezolizumab in early-relapsing TNBC, a high-risk group characterized by an early relapse (<12 months) after the last chemotherapy or surgery for early-stage disease, was assessed in the Phase III IMpassion132 trial. This study which included 354 patients who had not received prior immunotherapy were randomly assigned to receive chemotherapy of the physician's choice along with either atezolizumab or a placebo. Although patients with any PD-L1 status were included initially, the study was further restricted to patients with PD-L1 > 1%. Approximately 67% of patients had a disease-free interval (DFI) of less than 6 months. No significant difference in median DFI or OS was observed [98]. These findings, along with the exploratory analysis of relapses occurring within 12 months in KEYNOTE-355, indicate that some patients with rapidly relapsing TNBC may possess an inherent resistance to immunotherapy. Nevertheless, the current standard of care for first-line treatment in early-stage TNBC now incorporates immunotherapy, meaning that few patients will enter the early-relapsed category without having received prior immunotherapy.

#### 3.8.2.3 Pembrolizumab in TNBC

Pembrolizumab, a PD-1 inhibitor, has been extensively studied across various cancer types, including TNBC. The KEYNOTE-012 Phase Ib trial specifically evaluated pembrolizumab monotherapy in advanced PD-L1+ TNBC [99]. PD-L1 expression was determined using the 22C3 antibody, with positivity defined as ≥1% PD-L1 staining in tumor cells or PD-L1+ immune cells. Among 111 prescreened patients, 58.7% (65 individuals) had PD-L1+ tumors, and 32 were enrolled. In 27 efficacy-evaluable patients, pembrolizumab achieved an ORR of 18.6%, including one complete response (CR), four partial responses (PRs), and seven cases of stable disease (SD), leading to a disease control rate (DCR) of 25.8%. The median OS was 10.2 months, with a 1-year survival rate of 41.1%. Notably, the median duration of response (DOR) was not yet reached. The Phase II KEYNOTE-086 trial further assessed pembrolizumab in metastatic TNBC, both as a first line therapy for PD-L1+ cases (cohort B) and as salvage therapy for previously treated patients, regardless of PD-L1 status (cohort A) [100, 101]. In cohort A (170 patients), 62% (105 individuals) had PD-L1+ tumors, and over 40% had received at least three prior lines of therapy. Interestingly, PD-L1 expression levels did not significantly correlate with clinical benefit, as ORRs ranged from 4.6% to 4.7%, with a median PFS of 1.9–2.0 months and an OS of 8.3–10.0 months. However, patients who achieved CR or PR had a 100% OS at 9 months, compared to 89.6% for those with SD and 39% for those with progressive disease (PD). Notably, cohort B patients, who received pembrolizumab as a first-line therapy, had a higher ORR of 23.1%, supporting the idea that first-line PD-1 blockade improves response rates in metastatic TNBC [96].

Despite these findings, a randomized clinical trial (NCT02555657) comparing pembrolizumab to chemotherapy in TNBC patients did not demonstrate a significant OS advantage [102]. Research is ongoing to evaluate pembrolizumab in both neoadjuvant and adjuvant settings. Preliminary results from the I-SPY trial indicate that adding pembrolizumab to neoadjuvant paclitaxel substantially improves predicted pathologic complete response (pCR) rates: 48% vs. 17% in HER2-negative TNBC, 61% vs. 21% in ER+/PR+/HER2-negative cases, and 35% vs. 14% in other HER2-negative subtypes [103]. These data suggest that pembrolizumab could enhance treatment outcomes in HER2-negative BC. Additionally, the KEYNOTE-173 trial is investigating pembrolizumab in combination with chemotherapy for neoadjuvant TNBC therapy, with preliminary results indicating better responses in PD-L1+ cases [104]. Pembrolizumab has also been explored in ER+/HER2- BC. The KEYNOTE-028 trial, which examined pembrolizumab monotherapy in a small cohort of advanced ER+/HER2- patients, reported an ORR of 12% and a clinical benefit rate (CBR) of 21% [105]. Among 248 prescreened patients, 19.5% (48 individuals) were PD-L1+, and 25 received pembrolizumab, all of whom had undergone at least one prior line of therapy, with 45% having received five previous treatments. This study observed four SDs, three PRs, and no CRs.

Recent studies demonstrated that pembrolizumab combined with standard neoadjuvant chemotherapy exhibited enhanced DFS in individuals with high-risk early-stage TNBC. Although most patients with residual disease have benefited from post-neoadjuvant pembrolizumab administration, 5-year data from the KEYNOTE-522 trial reveals that the effect of post-neoadjuvant pembrolizumab therapy is less robust compared to its effectiveness during the neoadjuvant therapy. The most substantial advantage from pembrolizumab was seen in the RCB-2 category, with a notable disparity in 3-year event-free survival (EFS) between RCB-1 (~84%) and RCB-3 (~30%) [106]. However, since all participants in the KEYNOTE 522 trial received adjuvant immunotherapy, it remains unclear whether certain patients could skip this aspect of treatment, which is an area currently under investigation to further tailor the treatment for individuals with early breast cancer [106, 107].

## 3.9 Coalescing Chemotherapy with Immunotherapy

The interaction between chemotherapy and the immune system is complex, shaped by factors such as drug type, dosage, and treatment duration. Unlike immunotherapy, which directly stimulates or modulates immune responses, chemotherapy can have dual effects—it may suppress immune function or, conversely, enhance anti-tumor immunity by increasing antigen release, modulating dendritic cell activity, and disrupting immunosuppressive signals within the TME (Fig. 3.3) [108]. Given these potential immunomodulatory effects, ongoing clinical trials are exploring chemotherapy and PD-1/PD-L1 inhibitor combinations to improve immune priming and sustain anti-tumor responses. Early findings suggest that chemotherapeutic agents like eribulin and nab-paclitaxel may work synergistically with ICIs. One Phase Ib trial evaluated the combination of atezolizumab (840 mg every 2 weeks) with nab-paclitaxel (125 mg/m$^2$ on days 1, 8, and 15 of a 28-day cycle) in patients with metastatic TNBC, regardless of PD-L1 status [109]. Among 32 patients assessed, the combination achieved an ORR of 37% at a median follow-up of 5 months, including one complete response (CR), eleven partial responses (PRs), and two non-classical responses. Although more than half of the patients experienced grade 3 or 4 hematologic toxicities, these adverse effects were considered manageable. Notably, responses were observed in both PD-L1-positive and PD-L1-negative patients, with those receiving the combination as a first-line treatment showing a higher response rate than previously treated patients.

A large-scale, randomized, double-blind, placebo-controlled Phase III trial (NCT02425891) is currently investigating atezolizumab in combination with nab-paclitaxel as a first-line treatment for metastatic TNBC. Additionally, another ongoing study is evaluating pembrolizumab (200 mg intravenously every 3 weeks) with eribulin (1.4 mg/m$^2$ on days 1 and 8 of a 21-day cycle) in 95 patients with metastatic TNBC who already received at least two prior chemotherapy regimens [110]. An interim analysis of 39 patients showed that the combination was well tolerated, with common side effects including fatigue, alopecia, nausea, neutropenia, and peripheral neuropathy. Among the 17 patients receiving first-line treatment, the ORR was 41.1%, with a clinical benefit rate (CBR) of 41%. In those treated in the second or third line, the ORR was 27.4%, with 12 PRs and one CR. Interestingly, response rates were not significantly impacted by PD-L1 status—PD-L1-positive patients had

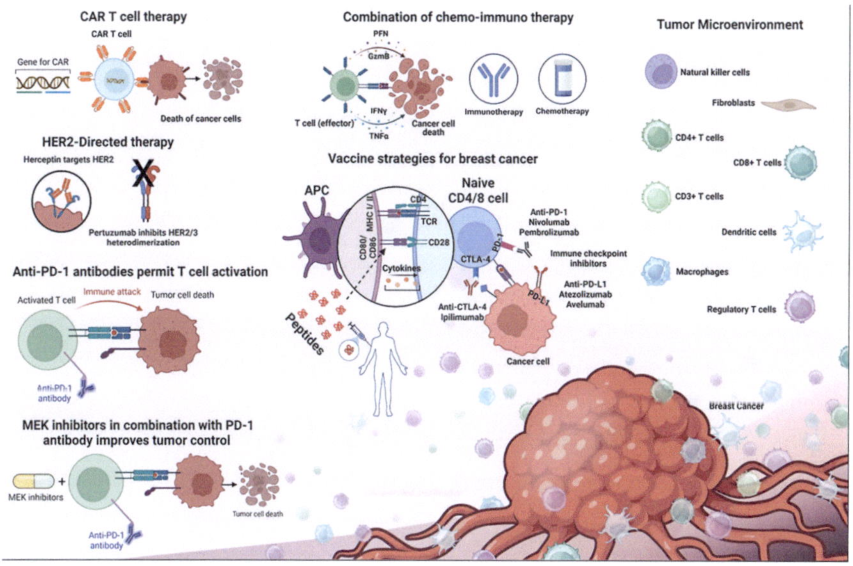


**Fig. 3.3** Immunotherapy-combinatorial strategies for targeting BC malignancy. Emerging therapeutic strategies are designed to counteract immunosuppressive mechanisms within the TME, thereby enhancing anti-tumor immune activity and improving treatment efficacy in BC. These approaches encompass immunomodulatory therapies, including ICIs, cytokine-based treatments, CAR T-cell therapy, and HER2-directed therapy. Additionally, combination treatments, such as immunotherapy-based regimens, vaccines, and chemo-immunotherapy, aim to overcome immune resistance. These advancements pave the way for more precise and personalized therapeutic approaches in BC management

an ORR and CBR of 29.3% and 35.4%, while PD-L1-negative patients had slightly higher rates at 33.2% and 44.5%, respectively. Beyond TNBC, researchers are now investigating similar immunotherapy-chemotherapy combinations in metastatic estrogen receptor-positive (ER+)/HER2-negative (HER2−) BC. The ongoing KEYNOTE-355 Phase III trial (NCT02819518) is assessing pembrolizumab with chemotherapy as a first-line treatment for advanced TNBC, comparing its efficacy against chemotherapy alone [111]. These studies are expected to further refine the role of immunotherapy-chemotherapy integration, paving the way for more effective and personalized treatment strategies in BC. A wide range of combination strategies are being explored to enhance immunotherapy efficacy in BC, including checkpoint blockade, PARP inhibition, IDO inhibition, and radiation therapy (Table 3.2).

### 3.9.1 Advances in HER2-Directed Therapy

Trastuzumab, a humanized monoclonal antibody that selectively binds to HER2 homodimers, remains the cornerstone of treatment for HER2-overexpressing BC in both early and advanced stages [112]. When combined with standard chemotherapy,

**Table 3.2** Immunotherapy strategies in BC—mechanisms, advances, and clinical insights

| Therapeutic strategy | Mechanism of action | Key findings in BC | Ongoing clinical trials/ applications |
|---|---|---|---|
| Checkpoint Inhibition (PD-1/ PD-L1, CTLA-4 inhibitors) | Blocks inhibitory immune checkpoints to restore T-cell activity | PD-L1 inhibitors show clinical benefit in metastatic TNBC; synergy with chemotherapy and PARP inhibitors | Multiple trials exploring combination with chemotherapy, radiation, and targeted therapies |
| PARP Inhibition + Immunotherapy | PARP inhibitors induce DNA damage, leading to immune activation and PD-L1 upregulation | Enhances response to PD-L1 blockade; significant tumor suppression in BRCA-mutated BC models | Trials combining PARP inhibitors with ICIs and VEGF-targeting agents |
| IDO Inhibition + Checkpoint Blockade | Suppresses tryptophan metabolism to reverse immune evasion | IDO inhibitors enhance checkpoint blockade efficacy in BC | Pembrolizumab + IDO inhibitor trials ongoing |
| Adenosine Pathway Inhibition | Blocks adenosine-mediated immune suppression (via CD39/ CD73 inhibitors, A2a receptor blockade) | CPI-444 shows activity in TNBC, especially in PD-L1-resistant cases | Investigational trials combining A2aR antagonists with ICIs |
| Radiotherapy + Immunotherapy | Radiation-induced antigen release boosts immune priming and T-cell infiltration | Abscopal effect observed in BC; enhances efficacy of ICIs | Hypofractionated radiation + ICI trials ongoing |
| Cancer Vaccination + ICIs | Enhances tumor antigen presentation and T-cell priming while overcoming checkpoint suppression | Neoantigen-based vaccines show promise; DC-based vaccines in testing | TRICOM, peptide, viral vector, and STING-based vaccine trials |
| Personalized Immunotherapy | Tailors immunotherapy to a patient's specific tumor antigen profile | Neoantigen prediction strategies in BC progressing | Advances in AI-driven biomarker discovery and single-cell sequencing |
| Microbiome & Metabolism in Immunotherapy | Gut microbiome and metabolic factors modulate immune responses to ICIs | Evidence of microbiome-driven immune response variation | Ongoing studies on metabolic reprogramming and microbiota interventions |

trastuzumab significantly reduces recurrence risk by nearly 50% in early-stage disease and improves survival in metastatic cases. Another HER2-specific monoclonal antibody, pertuzumab, enhances treatment efficacy by blocking HER2/HER3 heterodimerization, a key driver of tumor progression. Clinical studies have shown that adding pertuzumab to trastuzumab and taxotere in first-line metastatic HER2-positive BC prolongs OS [113]. Incorporating cisplatin into this regimen has also yielded some of the highest reported pathological complete response (pCR) rates [114]. For patients whose disease progresses despite trastuzumab and taxane therapy, ado-trastuzumab emtansine (T-DM1) provides an essential treatment option. This antibody-drug conjugate (ADC) links trastuzumab to the cytotoxic agent emtansine, offering superior PFS and OS compared to the lapatinib-capecitabine combination [115]. Beyond its direct anti-tumor effects, trastuzumab has immune-modulatory properties, including the ability to induce antibody-dependent cellular cytotoxicity (ADCC) and enhance HER2-specific T-cell responses [116, 117]. Interestingly, the emtansine component in T-DM1 may further contribute to immune activation by modulating dendritic cell function. Preclinical studies in HER2-transgenic mouse models suggest that T-DM1 treatment enhances effector T-cell activity, sustains memory T-cell responses, and promotes Fc-mediated dendritic cell priming [118].

Emerging evidence indicates that combining T-DM1 with ICIs could enhance treatment efficacy. In HER2-positive tumor models, dual blockade with anti-CTLA-4 and anti-PD-1 antibodies alongside T-DM1 has achieved survival rates exceeding 90%. Additionally, studies suggest that pairing PD-1 inhibitors with a trastuzumab-like antibody improves tumor clearance [119]. Several clinical trials are actively exploring PD-1/PD-L1 inhibitors in combination with HER2-targeted therapies for locally advanced and metastatic HER2-positive BC. One such trial, a Phase II randomized, double-blind, placebo-controlled study (NCT02924883) is evaluating whether adding atezolizumab to T-DM1 can further improve outcomes in patients with metastatic HER2-positive BC who have previously received trastuzumab and taxane-based therapy. As these trials advance, they are expected to refine the role of immune checkpoint blockade in HER2-targeted treatment, potentially reshaping the therapeutic landscape for HER2-positive BC.

### 3.9.2 MEK Inhibitors: Targeting the Ras Pathway for Immune Modulation

The Ras signaling pathway, frequently dysregulated in various cancers, has been a key target in therapeutic development. MEK inhibitors, which act by blocking mitogen-activated protein kinase (MAPK) kinase (MEK), have demonstrated potential in counteracting oncogenic Ras mutations. While these inhibitors may impair naïve T-cell priming in tumor-bearing models, they have also been found to enhance the function of effector CD8+ T cells by mitigating activation-induced cell death. This preservation of T-cell activity within the TME suggests a complex but potentially beneficial role for MEK inhibition in cancer immunotherapy [120]. Notably, combining MEK inhibitors with PD-L1 blockade has yielded synergistic and durable anticancer effects, further reinforcing their promise as an immunotherapeutic strategy. In the context of TNBC, emerging research has provided deeper insights into this approach. Studies analyzing residual disease following neoadjuvant chemotherapy have shown a strong correlation between TILs and favorable clinical outcomes. However, Ras/MAPK pathway dysregulation has been linked to diminished TIL presence, suggesting that targeting this signaling cascade may help restore immune infiltration and improve therapeutic responses [121]. Preclinical studies have demonstrated that MEK inhibition upregulates MHC class I and II molecules, along with PD-L1 expression, on TNBC cells. Moreover, combining MEK inhibitors with PD-1 pathway antagonists has been shown to enhance tumor-specific immune responses and improve tumor control in BC models. Several clinical trials are currently underway to evaluate the efficacy of MEK inhibitors in combination with PD-1 blockade, with the potential to redefine treatment strategies for BC. These investigations could ultimately lead to more effective immunotherapeutic approaches, particularly in tumors with Ras pathway alterations.

### 3.9.3 CDK4/6 Inhibitors: Bridging Targeted and Immune-Based Therapies

Cyclin-dependent kinase 4/6 (CDK4/6) inhibitors have become a cornerstone in the management of estrogen receptor-positive (ER+) metastatic BC. When used in combination with fulvestrant (Faslodex) or an aromatase inhibitor, these agents have shown significant efficacy in both first- and second-line treatment settings [122]. Beyond their established role in endocrine therapy, emerging evidence suggests that CDK4/6 inhibitors may also influence the tumor immune landscape by promoting the recruitment of TILs, highlighting a potential immunomodulatory function [123]. ER+/HER2− breast tumors are typically categorized as immunologically "cold," characterized by low TIL infiltration and limited responsiveness to PD-1/PD-L1 blockade as monotherapy [105]. However, the capacity of CDK4/6 inhibitors to enhance TIL infiltration raises the possibility of transforming these tumors into an inflamed phenotype, thereby improving their sensitivity to ICIs. Given this potential, ongoing research is focused on integrating PD-1/PD-L1 blockade with CDK4/6 inhibitors and endocrine therapy in preclinical models to evaluate their combined therapeutic efficacy. If successful, this approach could establish a new paradigm in ER+ BC treatment by effectively bridging targeted therapy with immunotherapy.

### 3.9.4 Synergizing Immunotherapy with Epigenetic Modulation

The role of epigenetic therapy in enhancing the response of BC to immunotherapy has gained considerable attention. Epigenetic modifications can reprogram the TME, restoring T-helper type 1 (Th1) cytokine and chemokine production while activating a type I interferon response, which is an essential mechanism for robust anti-tumor immunity [124]. In preclinical models, the combination of entinostat, a histone deacetylase (HDAC) inhibitor, with CTLA-4 and PD-1 checkpoint inhibitors demonstrated remarkable efficacy, eradicating both primary and metastatic breast tumors. This therapeutic effect was largely attributed to a reduction in granulocytic MDSCs, a key immunosuppressive component within the TME [125]. Clinically, a Phase II trial evaluating entinostat with exemestane in advanced ER+ BC patients reported an 8.3-month improvement in median OS compared to exemestane alone. Additionally, analysis of blood samples from 34 patients showed a decline in MDSC levels, increased CD40 expression, and enhanced MHC class II presentation on CD14+ monocytes within 2 weeks of treatment, though T-cell phenotypes remained unchanged [126]. In light of these promising findings, multiple clinical trials are currently investigating whether dual checkpoint blockade (CTLA-4 and PD-1/PD-L1 inhibitors) combined with epigenetic therapies can overcome resistance to immunotherapy. If successful, epigenetic modulation could provide a novel strategy for expanding immunotherapeutic options for BC patients.

### 3.9.5 Integrating Immunotherapy with PARP Inhibition

Recent studies indicate that PARP inhibitors not only impair DNA repair in cancer cells but also influence the tumor immune microenvironment. Research in BC cell lines and animal models suggests that PARP inhibition increases PD-L1 expression, potentially enhancing tumor susceptibility to immune checkpoint blockade [127]. Notably, PD-L1 inhibitors amplify T-cell-mediated cytotoxicity against cancer cells pretreated with PARP inhibitors. An inverse correlation has been identified between PD-L1 expression and polymeric adenosine diphosphate ribose (poly(ADP-ribose) or PAR) levels in human BC samples. In murine BC models, combining PD-L1 blockade with PARP inhibition led to significantly greater tumor suppression than either therapy alone. A similar synergistic effect has been reported in BRCA-deficient ovarian cancer, where CTLA-4 checkpoint inhibition enhanced the efficacy of PARP inhibitors [128]. Expanding on this concept, clinical studies have demonstrated promising outcomes when PD-L1 inhibitors are combined with PARP inhibitors or VEGF-targeting agents in breast and ovarian cancer patients [129]. These findings support ongoing research into the therapeutic potential of PARP inhibitors in combination with ICIs and antiangiogenic agents, particularly in BRCA-mutated cancers.

### 3.9.6 Combining Immune Checkpoint Blockade with IDO Inhibitors

Indoleamine 2,3-dioxygenase (IDO) is a key mediator of immune evasion, depleting tryptophan in the TME and increasing kynurenine levels, which suppress T-cell activity and promote immune tolerance [130]. Similar to PD-L1, IDO expression is upregulated in response to IFNγ secretion by T cells, suggesting potential redundancy between these pathways in breast tumors with TILs. Given its immunosuppressive role, strategies combining IDO inhibition with immune checkpoint blockade are under active investigation. The oral IDO inhibitor indoximod, in combination with taxotere, has been evaluated in solid tumors, including BC, with preliminary findings indicating clinical efficacy and manageable safety, as demonstrated by partial responses and mild tumor regressions [131]. Several clinical trials are currently assessing dual blockade of the PD-1 and IDO pathways across multiple cancers, including BC. A particularly promising approach involves combining pembrolizumab (PD-1 inhibitor) with indoximod, which has already yielded encouraging clinical responses in melanoma [132]. These findings underscore the potential of IDO inhibitors as complementary agents to immune checkpoint therapy, warranting further exploration in BC and other malignancies.

### 3.9.7 Adenosine Signaling Inhibition and PD-1/PD-L1 Blockade

Adenosine is a potent immunosuppressive metabolite within the TME [133]. Tumor cells release ATP, which undergoes sequential degradation by ectonucleotidases CD39 and CD73—CD39 converts ATP to AMP, while CD73 hydrolyzes AMP into adenosine. This accumulation of adenosine suppresses anti-tumor immune responses by activating A2a receptors (A2aR) on immune cells. To counteract adenosine-mediated immunosuppression, several therapeutic strategies are being explored, including monoclonal antibodies targeting CD39 and CD73, as well as small-molecule inhibitors of adenosine receptor signaling. CPI-444, an A2aR antagonist, is currently being evaluated in a multicohort clinical trial involving patients with advanced, treatment-resistant malignancies, including TNBC. CPI-444 is being tested both as a monotherapy and in combination with the PD-L1 inhibitor atezolizumab [134]. Early clinical data suggest that this combination exhibits anti-tumor activity, even in patients resistant to PD-1/PD-L1 blockade, with a favorable safety profile. Ongoing trials continue to investigate adenosine-targeting therapies across various tumor types.

### 3.9.8 Integrating Immune Checkpoint Blockade with Radiation Therapy

The abscopal effect refers to a phenomenon where localized radiation therapy induces systemic tumor regression, likely through immune-mediated mechanisms. Emerging evidence indicates that radiation enhances anti-tumor immunity via multiple pathways [85, 135]. It facilitates T-cell priming by releasing tumor antigens, thereby allowing dendritic cells to process and cross-present them more effectively. Additionally, radiation upregulates MHC molecules, stress-induced ligands, and death receptors on cancer cells, increasing their immunogenicity. It also stimulates the secretion of chemokines and vascular adhesion molecules, improving T-cell infiltration into tumors. Despite these promising effects, the optimal radiation dose and scheduling for maximizing immune responses remain unclear. In lung cancer and melanoma, hypo-fractionated radiation combined with the CTLA-4 inhibitor ipilimumab has shown encouraging abscopal effects [85]. Several ongoing clinical trials are currently investigating the integration of radiation therapy with PD-1/PD-L1 inhibitors to enhance therapeutic efficacy and improve clinical outcomes in multiple cancer types.

### 3.9.9 Vaccination Strategies Utilizing Immune Checkpoint Blockade

Cancer vaccines have shown the ability to activate immune responses but have demonstrated limited clinical efficacy, especially in advanced disease when used alone or alongside conventional chemotherapy. A key challenge is immune checkpoint signaling, particularly through the PD-1 pathway, which suppresses anti-tumor immunity. Administering a vaccine without addressing these immune checkpoints is akin to pressing the immune system's accelerator while the brakes remain engaged. However, the success of ICIs has renewed interest in combining vaccines with these agents to enhance T-cell priming and activation while overcoming immune suppression. This approach holds the most promise when dendritic cell-based vaccines, genetically engineered poly-antigen vaccines such as TRICOM, or whole-cell tumor vaccines are combined with PD-1 inhibitors or other agents targeting immune suppression pathways. However, a major limitation of these vaccine strategies is their reliance on known tumor antigens, which are often recognized as self-antigens, reducing immune response efficacy. This limitation has driven interest in personalized neoantigen-based vaccines, as responses to immune checkpoint blockade are strongly linked to immune recognition of neoantigens, particularly in tumors with high mutational burdens [75].

Several platforms for neoantigen-based vaccines in BC are currently under investigation, including peptide-based vaccines, genetically modified bacterial or viral vectors, and nucleic acid-based vaccines [51]. Additionally, cryoablation, a technique previously discussed, has been explored as a method to trigger tumor-specific immunity and has already been tested in BC patients in combination with CTLA-4 inhibition [88, 89]. Another promising approach is intratumoral delivery of innate immune agonists, such as those targeting the STING (stimulator of interferon genes) pathway. The STING agonist ADU-S100 has been shown to induce IFNβ production, dendritic cell maturation, and chemokine-driven T-cell recruitment at the tumor site [136]. Moreover, preclinical studies in a tolerized mouse model of BC indicate that combining ADU-S100 with PD-L1 inhibition and OX40 receptor stimulation can overcome antigen-specific tolerance and drive tumor regression [136]. Clinical trials evaluating ADU-S100 as a monotherapy are currently underway (NCT02675439), with future studies exploring its potential in combination immunotherapies.

## 3.10 Conclusions and Future Prospects

Immunotherapy, particularly ICIs, has emerged as a transformative strategy in BC treatment, offering a means to harness the immune system against the disease. In metastatic TNBC, therapies targeting the PD-1/PD-L1 axis have demonstrated durable clinical benefits in select patients. Ongoing research aims to validate these findings and extend immunotherapy applications to luminal and HER2-positive BC, where immune responses may be modulated differently. Additionally, clinical trials are actively assessing the adjuvant and neoadjuvant use of immunotherapy, potentially expanding its impact across various BC subtypes. Looking ahead, combination immunotherapies hold significant promise in converting immunologically "cold" tumors into immune-responsive ones, thereby enhancing treatment efficacy. The field of personalized immunotherapy is advancing rapidly, with ongoing efforts to develop tumor-specific neoantigen vaccines and immune-modulating agents tailored to an individual's tumor profile. Furthermore, researchers are exploring how external factors—including the microbiome, metabolic and hormonal influences, and concurrent pharmacological treatments—shape immune responses and influence therapeutic outcomes. A key challenge remains the identification of predictive biomarkers to improve treatment selection and overcome resistance [137]. Advances in single-cell sequencing, artificial intelligence (AI)-driven biomarker discovery, and spatial transcriptomics are expected to refine patient stratification and therapeutic targeting. By integrating cancer vaccination strategies with cutting-edge immunotherapy advancements, the field continues to move closer to the ultimate goal of immune-based BC prevention and treatment.

## 3.11 Clinical Significance

- The immune system plays a dualistic role in the initiation, development, progression, and elimination of BC.
- Immune checkpoint inhibition has shown promising results in treating metastatic TNBC patients.
- The PD-1/PD-L1 pathway has been demonstrated as a promising therapeutic target for the treatment of TNBCs.
- Integration of immunotherapy with adjuvant and neoadjuvant therapeutic strategies will reduce tumor burden significantly and improve survival.
- Personalized immunotherapy including vaccines, immune-modulating agents, and tumor-specific neoantigens will be the future prospect in BC treatment.

**Acknowledgments** We truly appreciate Dr. Ravi Salgia's support of our study and his role as Professor and Chair of the Department of Medical Oncology at City of Hope National Medical Center, Duarte, CA. The figures were made using https://biorender.com.

**Conflicts of Interest** The authors have no conflicts of interest to disclose.

**Declaration of Competing Interest** The authors have no conflicts of interest to disclose.

**Consent for Publication** Not applicable.

**Ethics Approval** Not applicable.

**Availability of Data and Material** No new data was created or analyzed in this study. Data sharing is not applicable to this article.

**Authors Contributions**

BMK; SSS: had the idea for the article and performed the literature search, and writing—original draft preparation.

SR; PG; MN: review and editing.

All authors read and approved the final manuscript.

**Funding** The National Cancer Institute of the National Institutes of Health (P30CA33572) and the United States Department of Defense (W81XWH-16-1-0641, W81XWH-22-1-0331, HT9425-25-1-0500) provided funding for this project. Also appreciated is financial support from City of Hope's Beckman Research Institute.

## References

1. Siegel RL, Kratzer TB, Giaquinto AN, Sung H, Jemal A. Cancer statistics. CA Cancer J Clin. 2025;75(2025):10–45.
2. A.C. Society. Breast cancer statistics; 2024.
3. Xu S, Murtagh S, Han Y, Wan F, Toriola AT. Breast cancer incidence among US women aged 20 to 49 years by race, stage, and hormone receptor status. JAMA Netw Open. 2024;7:e2353331.
4. McCormack V, McKenzie F, Foerster M, Zietsman A, Galukande M, Adisa C, Anele A, Parham G, Pinder LF, Cubasch H, Joffe M, Beaney T, Quaresma M, Togawa K, Abedi-Ardekani B, Anderson BO, Schuz J, Dos-Santos-Silva I. Breast cancer survival and survival gap apportionment in sub-Saharan Africa (ABC-DO): a prospective cohort study. Lancet Glob Health. 2020;8:e1203–12.
5. Birnbaum JK, Duggan C, Anderson BO, Etzioni R. Early detection and treatment strategies for breast cancer in low-income and upper middle-income countries: a modelling study. Lancet Glob Health. 2018;6:e885–93.
6. Guo L, Kong D, Liu J, Zhan L, Luo L, Zheng W, Zheng Q, Chen C, Sun S. Breast cancer heterogeneity and its implication in personalized precision therapy. Exp Hematol Oncol. 2023;12:3.
7. Kumar AR, Devan AR, Nair B, Vinod BS, Nath LR. Harnessing the immune system against cancer: current immunotherapy approaches and therapeutic targets. Mol Biol Rep. 2021;48:8075–95.
8. Sordo-Bahamonde C, Lorenzo-Herrero S, Gonzalez-Rodriguez AP, Martinez-Perez A, Rodrigo JP, Garcia-Pedrero JM, Gonzalez S. Chemo-immunotherapy: a new trend in cancer treatment. Cancers (Basel). 2023;15:2912.
9. Abdou Y, Goudarzi A, Yu JX, Upadhaya S, Vincent B, Carey LA. Immunotherapy in triple negative breast cancer: beyond checkpoint inhibitors. NPJ Breast Cancer. 2022;8:121.
10. U.S.F.D. Administration. Oncology (cancer)/hematologic malignancies approval notifications. U.S.F.D. Administration; 2024.
11. Debien V, De Caluwe A, Wang X, Piccart-Gebhart M, Tuohy VK, Romano E, Buisseret L. Immunotherapy in breast cancer: an overview of current strategies and perspectives. NPJ Breast Cancer. 2023;9:7.
12. Plaks V, Boldajipour B, Linnemann JR, Nguyen NH, Kersten K, Wolf Y, Casbon AJ, Kong N, van den Bijgaart RJ, Sheppard D, Melton AC, Krummel MF, Werb Z. Adaptive immune regulation of mammary postnatal organogenesis. Dev Cell. 2015;34:493–504.
13. Gouon-Evans V, Lin EY, Pollard JW. Requirement of macrophages and eosinophils and their cytokines/chemokines for mammary gland development. Breast Cancer Res. 2002;4:155–64.
14. Watson CJ, Khaled WT. Mammary development in the embryo and adult: a journey of morphogenesis and commitment. Development. 2008;135:995–1003.

15. McDaniel SM, Rumer KK, Biroc SL, Metz RP, Singh M, Porter W, Schedin P. Remodeling of the mammary microenvironment after lactation promotes breast tumor cell metastasis. Am J Pathol. 2006;168:608–20.
16. Fornetti J, Martinson HA, Betts CB, Lyons TR, Jindal S, Guo Q, Coussens LM, Borges VF, Schedin P. Mammary gland involution as an immunotherapeutic target for postpartum breast cancer. J Mammary Gland Biol Neoplasia. 2014;19:213–28.
17. Watson CJ, Kreuzaler PA. Remodeling mechanisms of the mammary gland during involution. Int J Dev Biol. 2011;55:757–62.
18. Stern DF. ErbBs in mammary development. Exp Cell Res. 2003;284:89–98.
19. Morato A, Martignani E, Miretti S, Baratta M, Accornero P. External and internal EGFR-activating signals drive mammary epithelial cells proliferation and viability. Mol Cell Endocrinol. 2021;520:111081.
20. Jackson-Fisher AJ, Bellinger G, Ramabhadran R, Morris JK, Lee KF, Stern DF. ErbB2 is required for ductal morphogenesis of the mammary gland. Proc Natl Acad Sci USA. 2004;101:17138–43.
21. Eccles SA. The epidermal growth factor receptor/Erb-B/HER family in normal and malignant breast biology. Int J Dev Biol. 2011;55:685–96.
22. Ho-Yen CM, Jones JL, Kermorgant S. The clinical and functional significance of c-Met in breast cancer: a review. Breast Cancer Res. 2015;17:52.
23. Nocera NF, Lee MC, De La Cruz LM, Rosemblit C, Czerniecki BJ. Restoring lost anti-HER-2 Th1 immunity in breast cancer: a crucial role for Th1 cytokines in therapy and prevention. Front Pharmacol. 2016;7:356.
24. Zhang N, Chang Y, Rios A, An Z. HER3/ErbB3, an emerging cancer therapeutic target. Acta Biochim Biophys Sin Shanghai. 2016;48:39–48.
25. Giltnane JM, Moeder CB, Camp RL, Rimm DL. Quantitative multiplexed analysis of ErbB family coexpression for primary breast cancer prognosis in a large retrospective cohort. Cancer. 2009;115:2400–9.
26. Bae SY, La Choi Y, Kim S, Kim M, Kim J, Jung SP, Choi MY, Lee SK, Kil WH, Lee JE, Nam SJ. HER3 status by immunohistochemistry is correlated with poor prognosis in hormone receptor-negative breast cancer patients. Breast Cancer Res Treat. 2013;139:741–50.
27. Ueno T, Emi M, Sato H, Ito N, Muta M, Kuroi K, Toi M. Genome-wide copy number analysis in primary breast cancer. Expert Opin Ther Targets. 2012;16(Suppl 1):S31–5.
28. Rimawi MF, Shetty PB, Weiss HL, Schiff R, Osborne CK, Chamness GC, Elledge RM. Epidermal growth factor receptor expression in breast cancer association with biologic phenotype and clinical outcomes. Cancer. 2010;116:1234–42.
29. Zagouri F, Bago-Horvath Z, Rossler F, Brandstetter A, Bartsch R, Papadimitriou CA, Dimitrakakis C, Tsigginou A, Papaspyrou I, Giannos A, Dimopoulos MA, Filipits M. High MET expression is an adverse prognostic factor in patients with triple-negative breast cancer. Br J Cancer. 2013;108:1100–5.
30. Minuti G, Landi L. MET deregulation in breast cancer. Ann Transl Med. 2015;3:181.
31. Gallo F, Morale MC, Sambataro D, Farinella Z, Scapagnini U, Marchetti B. The immune system response during development and progression of carcinogen-induced rat mammary tumors: prevention of tumor growth and restoration of immune system responsiveness by thymopentin. Breast Cancer Res Treat. 1993;27:221–37.
32. Levy L, Hill CS. Alterations in components of the TGF-beta superfamily signaling pathways in human cancer. Cytokine Growth Factor Rev. 2006;17:41–58.
33. Kundu N, Fulton AM. Interleukin-10 inhibits tumor metastasis, downregulates MHC class I, and enhances NK lysis. Cell Immunol. 1997;180:55–61.
34. Zheng LM, Ojcius DM, Garaud F, Roth C, Maxwell E, Li Z, Rong H, Chen J, Wang XY, Catino JJ, King I. Interleukin-10 inhibits tumor metastasis through an NK cell-dependent mechanism. J Exp Med. 1996;184:579–84.
35. Hodge DR, Hurt EM, Farrar WL. The role of IL-6 and STAT3 in inflammation and cancer. Eur J Cancer. 2005;41:2502–12.

36. Xie G, Yao Q, Liu Y, Du S, Liu A, Guo Z, Sun A, Ruan J, Chen L, Ye C, Yuan Y. IL-6-induced epithelial-mesenchymal transition promotes the generation of breast cancer stem-like cells analogous to mammosphere cultures. Int J Oncol. 2012;40:1171–9.
37. Bhan AK, DesMarais CL. Immunohistologic characterization of major histocompatibility antigens and inflammatory cellular infiltrate in human breast cancer. J Natl Cancer Inst. 1983;71:507–16.
38. Gil Del Alcazar CR, Huh SJ, Ekram MB, Trinh A, Liu LL, Beca F, Zi X, Kwak M, Bergholtz H, Su Y, Ding L, Russnes HG, Richardson AL, Babski K, Min Hui Kim E, McDonnell CH 3rd, Wagner J, Rowberry R, Freeman GJ, Dillon D, Sorlie T, Coussens LM, Garber JE, Fan R, Bobolis K, Allred DC, Jeong J, Park SY, Michor F, Polyak K. Immune escape in breast cancer during in situ to invasive carcinoma transition. Cancer Discov. 2017;7:1098–115.
39. Nakasone ES, Hurvitz SA, McCann KE. Harnessing the immune system in the battle against breast cancer. Drugs Context. 2018;7:212520.
40. Xu L, Xu W, Qiu S, Xiong S. Enrichment of CCR6+Foxp3+ regulatory T cells in the tumor mass correlates with impaired CD8+ T cell function and poor prognosis of breast cancer. Clin Immunol. 2010;135:466–75.
41. Watanabe MA, Oda JM, Amarante MK, Cesar Voltarelli J. Regulatory T cells and breast cancer: implications for immunopathogenesis. Cancer Metastasis Rev. 2010;29:569–79.
42. Zhang QW, Liu L, Gong CY, Shi HS, Zeng YH, Wang XZ, Zhao YW, Wei YQ. Prognostic significance of tumor-associated macrophages in solid tumor: a meta-analysis of the literature. PLoS One. 2012;7:e50946.
43. Quatromoni JG, Eruslanov E. Tumor-associated macrophages: function, phenotype, and link to prognosis in human lung cancer. Am J Transl Res. 2012;4:376–89.
44. Qiu SQ, Waaijer SJH, Zwager MC, de Vries EGE, van der Vegt B, Schroder CP. Tumor-associated macrophages in breast cancer: innocent bystander or important player? Cancer Treat Rev. 2018;70:178–89.
45. Noy R, Pollard JW. Tumor-associated macrophages: from mechanisms to therapy. Immunity. 2014;41:49–61.
46. DeNardo DG, Brennan DJ, Rexhepaj E, Ruffell B, Shiao SL, Madden SF, Gallagher WM, Wadhwani N, Keil SD, Junaid SA, Rugo HS, Hwang ES, Jirstrom K, West BL, Coussens LM. Leukocyte complexity predicts breast cancer survival and functionally regulates response to chemotherapy. Cancer Discov. 2011;1:54–67.
47. Xu M, Liu M, Du X, Li S, Li H, Li X, Li Y, Wang Y, Qin Z, Fu YX, Wang S. Intratumoral delivery of IL-21 overcomes anti-Her2/Neu resistance through shifting tumor-associated macrophages from M2 to M1 phenotype. J Immunol. 2015;194:4997–5006.
48. Shimokawara I, Imamura M, Yamanaka N, Ishii Y, Kikuchi K. Identification of lymphocyte subpopulations in human breast cancer tissue and its significance: an immunoperoxidase study with anti-human T- and B-cell sera. Cancer. 1982;49:1456–64.
49. Hansen MH, Nielsen H, Ditzel HJ. The tumor-infiltrating B cell response in medullary breast cancer is oligoclonal and directed against the autoantigen actin exposed on the surface of apoptotic cancer cells. Proc Natl Acad Sci USA. 2001;98:12659–64.
50. Ou Z, Wang Y, Liu L, Li L, Yeh S, Qi L, Chang C. Tumor microenvironment B cells increase bladder cancer metastasis via modulation of the IL-8/androgen receptor (AR)/MMPs signals. Oncotarget. 2015;6:26065–78.
51. Emens LA. Breast cancer immunobiology driving immunotherapy: vaccines and immune checkpoint blockade. Expert Rev Anticancer Ther. 2012;12:1597–611.
52. Smyth MJ, Dunn GP, Schreiber RD. Cancer immunosurveillance and immunoediting: the roles of immunity in suppressing tumor development and shaping tumor immunogenicity. Adv Immunol. 2006;90:1–50.
53. Coussens LM, Pollard JW. Leukocytes in mammary development and cancer. Cold Spring Harb Perspect Biol. 2011;3:a003285.
54. DeNardo DG, Coussens LM. Inflammation and breast cancer. Balancing immune response: crosstalk between adaptive and innate immune cells during breast cancer progression. Breast Cancer Res. 2007;9:212.

55. DeNardo DG, Barreto JB, Andreu P, Vasquez L, Tawfik D, Kolhatkar N, Coussens LM. CD4(+) T cells regulate pulmonary metastasis of mammary carcinomas by enhancing protumor properties of macrophages. Cancer Cell. 2009;16:91–102.
56. Ribas A. Adaptive immune resistance: how cancer protects from immune attack. Cancer Discov. 2015;5:915–9.
57. Ho PC, Kaech SM. Reenergizing T cell anti-tumor immunity by harnessing immunometabolic checkpoints and machineries. Curr Opin Immunol. 2017;46:38–44.
58. Allard B, Beavis PA, Darcy PK, Stagg J. Immunosuppressive activities of adenosine in cancer. Curr Opin Pharmacol. 2016;29:7–16.
59. Schreiber RD, Old LJ, Smyth MJ. Cancer immunoediting: integrating immunity's roles in cancer suppression and promotion. Science. 2011;331:1565–70.
60. Ehrlich P. Ueber den jetzigen Stand der Karzinomforschung. Ned Tijdschr Geneeskd. 1908;5:273–90.
61. Burnet M. Cancer—a biological approach, III. Viruses associated with neoplastic conditions. IV. Practical applications. Br Med J. 1957;1:841–7.
62. Burnet FM. The concept of immunological surveillance. Prog Exp Tumor Res. 1970;13:1–27.
63. Thomas L. Delayed hypersensitivity in health and disease. In: Cellular and humoral aspects of the hypersensitive states. New York: Hoeber-Harper; 1959. p. 529–32.
64. Dighe AS, Richards E, Old LJ, Schreiber RD. Enhanced in vivo growth and resistance to rejection of tumor cells expressing dominant negative IFN gamma receptors. Immunity. 1994;1:447–56.
65. Dunn GP, Bruce AT, Ikeda H, Old LJ, Schreiber RD. Cancer immunoediting: from immunosurveillance to tumor escape. Nat Immunol. 2002;3:991–8.
66. Gradishar WJ, Anderson BO, Balassanian R, Blair SL, Burstein HJ, Cyr A, Elias AD, Farrar WB, Forero A, Giordano SH, Goetz MP, Goldstein LJ, Isakoff SJ, Lyons J, Marcom PK, Mayer IA, McCormick B, Moran MS, O'Regan RM, Patel SA, Pierce LJ, Reed EC, Salerno KE, Schwartzberg LS, Sitapati A, Smith KL, Smith ML, Soliman H, Somlo G, Telli M, Ward JH, Shead DA, Kumar R. NCCN guidelines insights: breast cancer, version 1.2017. J Natl Compr Cancer Netw. 2017;15:433–51.
67. El Bairi K, Haynes HR, Blackley E, Fineberg S, Shear J, Turner S, de Freitas JR, Sur D, Amendola LC, Gharib M, Kallala A, Arun I, Azmoudeh-Ardalan F, Fujimoto L, Sua LF, Liu SW, Lien HC, Kirtani P, Balancin M, El Attar H, Guleria P, Yang W, Shash E, Chen IC, Bautista V, Do Prado Moura JF, Rapoport BL, Castaneda C, Spengler E, Acosta-Haab G, Frahm I, Sanchez J, Castillo M, Bouchmaa N, Zin RRM, Shui R, Onyuma T, Yang W, Husain Z, Willard-Gallo K, Coosemans A, Perez EA, Provenzano E, Ericsson PG, Richardet E, Mehrotra R, Sarancone S, Ehinger A, Rimm DL, Bartlett JMS, Viale G, Denkert C, Hida AI, Sotiriou C, Loibl S, Hewitt SM, Badve S, Symmans WF, Kim RS, Pruneri G, Goel S, Francis PA, Inurrigarro G, Yamaguchi R, Garcia-Rivello H, Horlings H, Afqir S, Salgado R, Adams S, Kok M, Dieci MV, Michiels S, Demaria S, Loi S, G. International Immuno-Oncology Biomarker Working. The tale of TILs in breast cancer: a report from The International Immuno-Oncology Biomarker Working Group. NPJ Breast Cancer. 2021;7:150.
68. Denkert C, von Minckwitz G, Darb-Esfahani S, Lederer B, Heppner BI, Weber KE, Budczies J, Huober J, Klauschen F, Furlanetto J, Schmitt WD, Blohmer JU, Karn T, Pfitzner BM, Kummel S, Engels K, Schneeweiss A, Hartmann A, Noske A, Fasching PA, Jackisch C, van Mackelenbergh M, Sinn P, Schem C, Hanusch C, Untch M, Loibl S. Tumour-infiltrating lymphocytes and prognosis in different subtypes of breast cancer: a pooled analysis of 3771 patients treated with neoadjuvant therapy. Lancet Oncol. 2018;19:40–50.
69. Foldi J, Silber A, Reisenbichler E, Singh K, Fischbach N, Persico J, Adelson K, Katoch A, Horowitz N, Lannin D, Chagpar A, Park T, Marczyk M, Frederick C, Burrello T, Ibrahim E, Qing T, Bai Y, Blenman K, Rimm DL, Pusztai L. Neoadjuvant durvalumab plus weekly nab-paclitaxel and dose-dense doxorubicin/cyclophosphamide in triple-negative breast cancer. NPJ Breast Cancer. 2021;7:9.
70. Geurts VCM, Balduzzi S, Steenbruggen TG, Linn SC, Siesling S, Badve SS, DeMichele A, Ignatiadis M, Leon-Ferre RA, Goetz MP, Wolff AC, Klar N, Michiels S, Loi S, Adams

S, Horlings HM, Sonke GS, Salgado R, Kok M. Tumor-infiltrating lymphocytes in patients with stage I triple-negative breast cancer untreated with chemotherapy. JAMA Oncol. 2024;10:1077–86.

71. Cimino-Mathews A, Thompson E, Taube JM, Ye X, Lu Y, Meeker A, Xu H, Sharma R, Lecksell K, Cornish TC, Cuka N, Argani P, Emens LA. PD-L1 (B7-H1) expression and the immune tumor microenvironment in primary and metastatic breast carcinomas. Hum Pathol. 2016;47:52–63.
72. Li X, Li M, Lian Z, Zhu H, Kong L, Wang P, Yu J. Prognostic role of programmed death ligand-1 expression in breast cancer: a systematic review and meta-analysis. Target Oncol. 2016;11:753–61.
73. Ladoire S, Arnould L, Apetoh L, Coudert B, Martin F, Chauffert B, Fumoleau P, Ghiringhelli F. Pathologic complete response to neoadjuvant chemotherapy of breast carcinoma is associated with the disappearance of tumor-infiltrating foxp3+ regulatory T cells. Clin Cancer Res. 2008;14:2413–20.
74. Tumeh PC, Harview CL, Yearley JH, Shintaku IP, Taylor EJ, Robert L, Chmielowski B, Spasic M, Henry G, Ciobanu V, West AN, Carmona M, Kivork C, Seja E, Cherry G, Gutierrez AJ, Grogan TR, Mateus C, Tomasic G, Glaspy JA, Emerson RO, Robins H, Pierce RH, Elashoff DA, Robert C, Ribas A. PD-1 blockade induces responses by inhibiting adaptive immune resistance. Nature. 2014;515:568–71.
75. Yarchoan M, Johnson BA 3rd, Lutz ER, Laheru DA, Jaffee EM. Targeting neoantigens to augment antitumour immunity. Nat Rev Cancer. 2017;17:209–22.
76. Snyder A, Makarov V, Merghoub T, Yuan J, Zaretsky JM, Desrichard A, Walsh LA, Postow MA, Wong P, Ho TS, Hollmann TJ, Bruggeman C, Kannan K, Li Y, Elipenahli C, Liu C, Harbison CT, Wang L, Ribas A, Wolchok JD, Chan TA. Genetic basis for clinical response to CTLA-4 blockade in melanoma. N Engl J Med. 2014;371:2189–99.
77. Luen S, Virassamy B, Savas P, Salgado R, Loi S. The genomic landscape of breast cancer and its interaction with host immunity. Breast. 2016;29:241–50.
78. Miles D, Roche H, Martin M, Perren TJ, Cameron DA, Glaspy J, Dodwell D, Parker J, Mayordomo J, Tres A, Murray JL, Ibrahim NK. Theratope Study, Phase III multicenter clinical trial of the sialyl-TN (STn)-keyhole limpet hemocyanin (KLH) vaccine for metastatic breast cancer. Oncologist. 2011;16:1092–100.
79. Emens LA, Asquith JM, Leatherman JM, Kobrin BJ, Petrik S, Laiko M, Levi J, Daphtary MM, Biedrzycki B, Wolff AC, Stearns V, Disis ML, Ye X, Piantadosi S, Fetting JH, Davidson NE, Jaffee EM. Timed sequential treatment with cyclophosphamide, doxorubicin, and an allogeneic granulocyte-macrophage colony-stimulating factor-secreting breast tumor vaccine: a chemotherapy dose-ranging factorial study of safety and immune activation. J Clin Oncol. 2009;27:5911–8.
80. Heery CR, Ibrahim NK, Arlen PM, Mohebtash M, Murray JL, Koenig K, Madan RA, McMahon S, Marte JL, Steinberg SM, Donahue RN, Grenga I, Jochems C, Farsaci B, Folio LR, Schlom J, Gulley JL. Docetaxel alone or in combination with a therapeutic cancer vaccine (PANVAC) in patients with metastatic breast cancer: a randomized clinical trial. JAMA Oncol. 2015;1:1087–95.
81. Disis ML, Wallace DR, Gooley TA, Dang Y, Slota M, Lu H, Coveler AL, Childs JS, Higgins DM, Fintak PA, dela Rosa C, Tietje K, Link J, Waisman J, Salazar LG. Concurrent trastuzumab and HER2/neu-specific vaccination in patients with metastatic breast cancer. J Clin Oncol. 2009;27:4685–92.
82. Clifton GT, Litton JK, Arrington K, Ponniah S, Ibrahim NK, Gall V, Alatrash G, Peoples GE, Mittendorf EA. Results of a phase Ib trial of combination immunotherapy with a CD8+ T cell eliciting vaccine and trastuzumab in breast cancer patients. Ann Surg Oncol. 2017;24:2161–7.
83. Chen G, Gupta R, Petrik S, Laiko M, Leatherman JM, Asquith JM, Daphtary MM, Garrett-Mayer E, Davidson NE, Hirt K, Berg M, Uram JN, Dauses T, Fetting J, Duus EM, Atay-Rosenthal S, Ye X, Wolff AC, Stearns V, Jaffee EM, Emens LA. A feasibility study of cyclophosphamide, trastuzumab, and an allogeneic GM-CSF-secreting breast tumor vaccine for HER2+ metastatic breast cancer. Cancer Immunol Res. 2014;2:949–61.

84. Lipson EJ, Forde PM, Hammers HJ, Emens LA, Taube JM, Topalian SL. Antagonists of PD-1 and PD-L1 in cancer treatment. Semin Oncol. 2015;42:587–600.
85. Emens L, Powderly J, Fong L, Brody J, Forde P, Hellmann M, Hughes B, Kummar S, Loi S, Luke J, Mahadevan D, Markman B, McCaffery I, Miller R, Laport G. Abstract CT119: CPI-444, an oral adenosine A2a receptor (A2aR) antagonist, demonstrates clinical activity in patients with advanced solid tumors. Cancer Res. 2017;77:CT119.
86. Pardoll DM. The blockade of immune checkpoints in cancer immunotherapy. Nat Rev Cancer. 2012;12:252–64.
87. Vonderheide RH, LoRusso PM, Khalil M, Gartner EM, Khaira D, Soulieres D, Dorazio P, Trosko JA, Ruter J, Mariani GL, Usari T, Domchek SM. Tremelimumab in combination with exemestane in patients with advanced breast cancer and treatment-associated modulation of inducible costimulator expression on patient T cells. Clin Cancer Res. 2010;16:3485–94.
88. McArthur HL, Diab A, Page DB, Yuan J, Solomon SB, Sacchini V, Comstock C, Durack JC, Maybody M, Sung J, Ginsberg A, Wong P, Barlas A, Dong Z, Zhao C, Blum B, Patil S, Neville D, Comen EA, Morris EA, Kotin A, Brogi E, Wen YH, Morrow M, Lacouture ME, Sharma P, Allison JP, Hudis CA, Wolchok JD, Norton L. A pilot study of preoperative single-dose ipilimumab and/or cryoablation in women with early-stage breast cancer with comprehensive immune profiling. Clin Cancer Res. 2016;22:5729–37.
89. Page DB, Yuan J, Redmond D, Wen YH, Durack JC, Emerson R, Solomon S, Dong Z, Wong P, Comstock C, Diab A, Sung J, Maybody M, Morris E, Brogi E, Morrow M, Sacchini V, Elemento O, Robins H, Patil S, Allison JP, Wolchok JD, Hudis C, Norton L, McArthur HL. Deep sequencing of T-cell receptor DNA as a biomarker of clonally expanded TILs in breast cancer after immunotherapy. Cancer Immunol Res. 2016;4:835–44.
90. Emens LA, Kok M, Ojalvo LS. Targeting the programmed cell death-1 pathway in breast and ovarian cancer. Curr Opin Obstet Gynecol. 2016;28:142–7.
91. Heery CR, O'Sullivan-Coyne G, Madan RA, Cordes L, Rajan A, Rauckhorst M, Lamping E, Oyelakin I, Marte JL, Lepone LM, Donahue RN, Grenga I, Cuillerot JM, Neuteboom B, Heydebreck AV, Chin K, Schlom J, Gulley JL. Avelumab for metastatic or locally advanced previously treated solid tumours (JAVELIN Solid Tumor): a phase 1a, multicohort, dose-escalation trial. Lancet Oncol. 2017;18:587–98.
92. Dirix LY, Takacs I, Jerusalem G, Nikolinakos P, Arkenau HT, Forero-Torres A, Boccia R, Lippman ME, Somer R, Smakal M, Emens LA, Hrinczenko B, Edenfield W, Gurtler J, von Heydebreck A, Grote HJ, Chin K, Hamilton EP. Avelumab, an anti-PD-L1 antibody, in patients with locally advanced or metastatic breast cancer: a phase 1b JAVELIN Solid Tumor study. Breast Cancer Res Treat. 2018;167:671–86.
93. Sanchez-Paulete AR, Labiano S, Rodriguez-Ruiz ME, Azpilikueta A, Etxeberria I, Bolanos E, Lang V, Rodriguez M, Aznar MA, Jure-Kunkel M, Melero I. Deciphering CD137 (4-1BB) signaling in T-cell costimulation for translation into successful cancer immunotherapy. Eur J Immunol. 2016;46:513–22.
94. Emens LA, Braiteh FS, Cassier P, Delord J-P, Eder JP, Fasso M, Xiao Y, Wang Y, Molinero L, Chen DS, Krop I. Abstract 2859: inhibition of PD-L1 by MPDL3280A leads to clinical activity in patients with metastatic triple-negative breast cancer (TNBC). Cancer Res. 2015;75:2859.
95. Schmid P, Cruz C, Braiteh FS, Eder JP, Tolaney S, Kuter I, Nanda R, Chung C, Cassier P, Delord J-P, Gordon M, Li Y, Liu B, O'Hear C, Fasso M, Molinero L, Emens LA. Abstract 2986: atezolizumab in metastatic TNBC (mTNBC): long-term clinical outcomes and biomarker analyses. Cancer Res. 2017;77:2986.
96. Herbst RS, Soria JC, Kowanetz M, Fine GD, Hamid O, Gordon MS, Sosman JA, McDermott DF, Powderly JD, Gettinger SN, Kohrt HE, Horn L, Lawrence DP, Rost S, Leabman M, Xiao Y, Mokatrin A, Koeppen H, Hegde PS, Mellman I, Chen DS, Hodi FS. Predictive correlates of response to the anti-PD-L1 antibody MPDL3280A in cancer patients. Nature. 2014;515:563–7.
97. Emens LA, Cruz C, Eder JP, Braiteh F, Chung C, Tolaney SM, Kuter I, Nanda R, Cassier PA, Delord JP, Gordon MS, ElGabry E, Chang CW, Sarkar I, Grossman W, O'Hear C, Fasso M,

Molinero L, Schmid P. Long-term clinical outcomes and biomarker analyses of atezolizumab therapy for patients with metastatic triple-negative breast cancer: a phase 1 study. JAMA Oncol. 2019;5:74–82.
98. Dent R, Andre F, Goncalves A, Martin M, Schmid P, Schutz F, Kummel S, Swain SM, Bilici A, Loirat D, Villalobos Valencia R, Im SA, Park YH, De Laurentis M, Colleoni M, Guarneri V, Bianchini G, Li H, Kirchmayer Machackova Z, Mouta J, Deurloo R, Gan X, Fan M, Mani A, Swat A, Cortes J. IMpassion132 double-blind randomised phase III trial of chemotherapy with or without atezolizumab for early relapsing unresectable locally advanced or metastatic triple-negative breast cancer. Ann Oncol. 2024;35:630–42.
99. Nanda R, Chow LQ, Dees EC, Berger R, Gupta S, Geva R, Pusztai L, Pathiraja K, Aktan G, Cheng JD, Karantza V, Buisseret L. Pembrolizumab in patients with advanced triple-negative breast cancer: phase Ib KEYNOTE-012 study. J Clin Oncol. 2016;34:2460–7.
100. Adams S, Loi S, Toppmeyer D, Cescon DW, De Laurentiis M, Nanda R, Winer EP, Mukai H, Tamura K, Armstrong A, Liu MC, Iwata H, Ryvo L, Wimberger P, Rugo HS, Tan AR, Jia L, Ding Y, Karantza V, Schmid P. Pembrolizumab monotherapy for previously untreated, PD-L1-positive, metastatic triple-negative breast cancer: cohort B of the phase II KEYNOTE-086 study. Ann Oncol. 2019;30:405–11.
101. Adams S, Schmid P, Rugo HS, Winer EP, Loirat D, Awada A, Cescon DW, Iwata H, Campone M, Nanda R, Hui R, Curigliano G, Toppmeyer D, O'Shaughnessy J, Loi S, Paluch-Shimon S, Tan AR, Card D, Zhao J, Karantza V, Cortes J. Pembrolizumab monotherapy for previously treated metastatic triple-negative breast cancer: cohort A of the phase II KEYNOTE-086 study. Ann Oncol. 2019;30:397–404.
102. Winer EP, Lipatov O, Im SA, Goncalves A, Munoz-Couselo E, Lee KS, Schmid P, Tamura K, Testa L, Witzel I, Ohtani S, Turner N, Zambelli S, Harbeck N, Andre F, Dent R, Zhou X, Karantza V, Mejia J, Cortes J, K. Investigators. Pembrolizumab versus investigator-choice chemotherapy for metastatic triple-negative breast cancer (KEYNOTE-119): a randomised, open-label, phase 3 trial. Lancet Oncol. 2021;22:499–511.
103. Nanda R, Liu MC, Yau C, Shatsky R, Pusztai L, Wallace A, Chien AJ, Forero-Torres A, Ellis E, Han H, Clark A, Albain K, Boughey JC, Jaskowiak NT, Elias A, Isaacs C, Kemmer K, Helsten T, Majure M, Stringer-Reasor E, Parker C, Lee MC, Haddad T, Cohen RN, Asare S, Wilson A, Hirst GL, Singhrao R, Steeg K, Asare A, Matthews JB, Berry S, Sanil A, Schwab R, Symmans WF, van't Veer L, Yee D, DeMichele A, Hylton NM, Melisko M, Perlmutter J, Rugo HS, Berry DA, Esserman LJ. Effect of pembrolizumab plus neoadjuvant chemotherapy on pathologic complete response in women with early-stage breast cancer: an analysis of the ongoing phase 2 adaptively randomized I-SPY2 trial. JAMA Oncol. 2020;6:676–84.
104. Schmid P, Salgado R, Park YH, Munoz-Couselo E, Kim SB, Sohn J, Im SA, Foukakis T, Kuemmel S, Dent R, Yin L, Wang A, Tryfonidis K, Karantza V, Cortes J, Loi S. Pembrolizumab plus chemotherapy as neoadjuvant treatment of high-risk, early-stage triple-negative breast cancer: results from the phase 1b open-label, multicohort KEYNOTE-173 study. Ann Oncol. 2020;31:569–81.
105. Rugo H, Delord J-P, Im S-A, Ott P, Piha-Paul S, Bedard P, Sachdev J, Le Tourneau C, van Brummelen E, Varga A, Saraf S, Pietrangelo D, Karantza V, Tan A. Abstract S5-07: preliminary efficacy and safety of pembrolizumab (MK-3475) in patients with PD-L1–positive, estrogen receptor-positive (ER+)/HER2-negative advanced breast cancer enrolled in KEYNOTE-028. Cancer Res. 2016;76:S5-07–S05-07.
106. Pusztai L, Denkert C, O'Shaughnessy J, Cortes J, Dent R, McArthur H, Kummel S, Bergh J, Park YH, Hui R, Harbeck N, Takahashi M, Untch M, Fasching PA, Cardoso F, Zhu Y, Pan W, Tryfonidis K, Schmid P. Event-free survival by residual cancer burden with pembrolizumab in early-stage TNBC: exploratory analysis from KEYNOTE-522. Ann Oncol. 2024;35:429–36.
107. Schlam I, Dower J, Lynce F. Addressing residual disease in HER2-positive and triple-negative breast cancer: what is next? Curr Oncol Rep. 2024;26:336–45.
108. Emens LA, Middleton G. The interplay of immunotherapy and chemotherapy: harnessing potential synergies. Cancer Immunol Res. 2015;3:436–43.

109. Adams S, Diamond JR, Hamilton EP, Pohlmann PR, Tolaney SM, Molinero L, He X, Waterkamp D, Funke RP, Powderly JD. Phase Ib trial of atezolizumab in combination with nab-paclitaxel in patients with metastatic triple-negative breast cancer (mTNBC). J Clin Oncol. 2016;34:1009.
110. Tolaney S, Kalinsky K, Kaklamani V, Savulsky C, Olivo M, Aktan G, Kaufman P, Xing D, Almonte A, Misir S, Karantza V, Diab S. Abstract PD6-13: phase 1b/2 study to evaluate eribulin mesylate in combination with pembrolizumab in patients with metastatic triple-negative breast cancer. Cancer Res. 2018;78:PD6-13–PD16-13.
111. Cortes J, Rugo HS, Cescon DW, Im SA, Yusof MM, Gallardo C, Lipatov O, Barrios CH, Perez-Garcia J, Iwata H, Masuda N, Torregroza Otero M, Gokmen E, Loi S, Guo Z, Zhou X, Karantza V, Pan W, Schmid P, K. Investigators. Pembrolizumab plus chemotherapy in advanced triple-negative breast cancer. N Engl J Med. 2022;387:217–26.
112. Loibl S, Gianni L. HER2-positive breast cancer. Lancet. 2017;389:2415–29.
113. Swain SM, Baselga J, Kim SB, Ro J, Semiglazov V, Campone M, Ciruelos E, Ferrero JM, Schneeweiss A, Heeson S, Clark E, Ross G, Benyunes MC, Cortes J, C.S. Group. Pertuzumab, trastuzumab, and docetaxel in HER2-positive metastatic breast cancer. N Engl J Med. 2015;372:724–34.
114. Schneeweiss A, Chia S, Hickish T, Harvey V, Eniu A, Hegg R, Tausch C, Seo JH, Tsai YF, Ratnayake J, McNally V, Ross G, Cortes J. Pertuzumab plus trastuzumab in combination with standard neoadjuvant anthracycline-containing and anthracycline-free chemotherapy regimens in patients with HER2-positive early breast cancer: a randomized phase II cardiac safety study (TRYPHAENA). Ann Oncol. 2013;24:2278–84.
115. Verma S, Miles D, Gianni L, Krop IE, Welslau M, Baselga J, Pegram M, Oh DY, Dieras V, Guardino E, Fang L, Lu MW, Olsen S, Blackwell K, E.S. Group. Trastuzumab emtansine for HER2-positive advanced breast cancer. N Engl J Med. 2012;367:1783–91.
116. Arnould L, Gelly M, Penault-Llorca F, Benoit L, Bonnetain F, Migeon C, Cabaret V, Fermeaux V, Bertheau P, Garnier J, Jeannin JF, Coudert B. Trastuzumab-based treatment of HER2-positive breast cancer: an antibody-dependent cellular cytotoxicity mechanism? Br J Cancer. 2006;94:259–67.
117. Muraro E, Comaro E, Talamini R, Turchet E, Miolo G, Scalone S, Militello L, Lombardi D, Spazzapan S, Perin T, Massarut S, Crivellari D, Dolcetti R, Martorelli D. Improved natural killer cell activity and retained anti-tumor CD8(+) T cell responses contribute to the induction of a pathological complete response in HER2-positive breast cancer patients undergoing neoadjuvant chemotherapy. J Transl Med. 2015;13:204.
118. Muller P, Martin K, Theurich S, Schreiner J, Savic S, Terszowski G, Lardinois D, Heinzelmann-Schwarz VA, Schlaak M, Kvasnicka HM, Spagnoli G, Dirnhofer S, Speiser DE, von Bergwelt-Baildon M, Zippelius A. Microtubule-depolymerizing agents used in antibody-drug conjugates induce antitumor immunity by stimulation of dendritic cells. Cancer Immunol Res. 2014;2:741–55.
119. Muller P, Kreuzaler M, Khan T, Thommen DS, Martin K, Glatz K, Savic S, Harbeck N, Nitz U, Gluz O, von Bergwelt-Baildon M, Kreipe H, Reddy S, Christgen M, Zippelius A. Trastuzumab emtansine (T-DM1) renders HER2+ breast cancer highly susceptible to CTLA-4/PD-1 blockade. Sci Transl Med. 2015;7:315ra188.
120. Ebert PJR, Cheung J, Yang Y, McNamara E, Hong R, Moskalenko M, Gould SE, Maecker H, Irving BA, Kim JM, Belvin M, Mellman I. MAP kinase inhibition promotes T Cell and antitumor activity in combination with PD-L1 checkpoint blockade. Immunity. 2016;44:609–21.
121. Loi S, Dushyanthen S, Beavis PA, Salgado R, Denkert C, Savas P, Combs S, Rimm DL, Giltnane JM, Estrada MV, Sanchez V, Sanders ME, Cook RS, Pilkinton MA, Mallal SA, Wang K, Miller VA, Stephens PJ, Yelensky R, Doimi FD, Gomez H, Ryzhov SV, Darcy PK, Arteaga CL, Balko JM. RAS/MAPK activation is associated with reduced tumor-infiltrating lymphocytes in triple-negative breast cancer: therapeutic cooperation between MEK and PD-1/PD-L1 immune checkpoint inhibitors. Clin Cancer Res. 2016;22:1499–509.
122. Finn RS, Aleshin A, Slamon DJ. Targeting the cyclin-dependent kinases (CDK) 4/6 in estrogen receptor-positive breast cancers. Breast Cancer Res. 2016;18:17.

123. Hurvitz S, Martin M, Fernández Abad M, Chan D, Rostorfer R, Petru E, Barriga S, Costigan T, Caldwell C, Nguyen T, Press M, Slamon D. Abstract S4-06: biological effects of abemaciclib in a phase 2 neoadjuvant study for postmenopausal patients with HR+, HER2- breast cancer. Cancer Res. 2017;77:S4-06.
124. Chiappinelli KB, Strissel PL, Desrichard A, Li H, Henke C, Akman B, Hein A, Rote NS, Cope LM, Snyder A, Makarov V, Budhu S, Slamon DJ, Wolchok JD, Pardoll DM, Beckmann MW, Zahnow CA, Merghoub T, Chan TA, Baylin SB, Strick R. Inhibiting DNA methylation causes an interferon response in cancer via dsRNA including endogenous retroviruses. Cell. 2015;162:974–86.
125. Kim K, Skora AD, Li Z, Liu Q, Tam AJ, Blosser RL, Diaz LA Jr, Papadopoulos N, Kinzler KW, Vogelstein B, Zhou S. Eradication of metastatic mouse cancers resistant to immune checkpoint blockade by suppression of myeloid-derived cells. Proc Natl Acad Sci USA. 2014;111:11774–9.
126. Tomita Y, Lee MJ, Lee S, Tomita S, Chumsri S, Cruickshank S, Ordentlich P, Trepel JB. The interplay of epigenetic therapy and immunity in locally recurrent or metastatic estrogen receptor-positive breast cancer: correlative analysis of ENCORE 301, a randomized, placebo-controlled phase II trial of exemestane with or without entinostat. Onco Targets Ther. 2016;5:e1219008.
127. Jiao S, Xia W, Yamaguchi H, Wei Y, Chen MK, Hsu JM, Hsu JL, Yu WH, Du Y, Lee HH, Li CW, Chou CK, Lim SO, Chang SS, Litton J, Arun B, Hortobagyi GN, Hung MC. PARP inhibitor upregulates PD-L1 expression and enhances cancer-associated immunosuppression. Clin Cancer Res. 2017;23:3711–20.
128. Higuchi T, Flies DB, Marjon NA, Mantia-Smaldone G, Ronner L, Gimotty PA, Adams SF. CTLA-4 blockade synergizes therapeutically with PARP inhibition in BRCA1-deficient ovarian cancer. Cancer Immunol Res. 2015;3:1257–68.
129. Lee JM, Cimino-Mathews A, Peer CJ, Zimmer A, Lipkowitz S, Annunziata CM, Cao L, Harrell MI, Swisher EM, Houston N, Botesteanu DA, Taube JM, Thompson E, Ogurtsova A, Xu H, Nguyen J, Ho TW, Figg WD, Kohn EC. Safety and clinical activity of the programmed death-ligand 1 inhibitor durvalumab in combination with poly (ADP-Ribose) polymerase inhibitor olaparib or vascular endothelial growth factor receptor 1-3 inhibitor cediranib in women's cancers: a dose-escalation, phase I study. J Clin Oncol. 2017;35:2193–202.
130. Brochez L, Chevolet I, Kruse V. The rationale of indoleamine 2,3 dioxygenase inhibition for cancer therapy. Eur J Cancer. 2017;76:167–82.
131. Soliman HH, Jackson E, Neuger T, Dees EC, Harvey RD, Han H, Ismail-Khan R, Minton S, Vahanian NN, Link C, Sullivan DM, Antonia S. A first in man phase I trial of the oral immunomodulator, indoximod, combined with docetaxel in patients with metastatic solid tumors. Oncotarget. 2014;5:8136–46.
132. Zakharia Y, McWilliams R, Shaheen M, Grossman K, Drabick J, Milhem M, Rixie O, Khleif S, Lott R, Kennedy E, Munn D, Vahanian N, Link C. Abstract CT117: interim analysis of the phase 2 clinical trial of the IDO pathway inhibitor indoximod in combination with pembrolizumab for patients with advanced melanoma. Cancer Res. 2017;77:CT117.
133. Antonioli L, Blandizzi C, Pacher P, Hasko G. Immunity, inflammation and cancer: a leading role for adenosine. Nat Rev Cancer. 2013;13:842–57.
134. Emens LA, Ascierto PA, Darcy PK, Demaria S, Eggermont AMM, Redmond WL, Seliger B, Marincola FM. Cancer immunotherapy: opportunities and challenges in the rapidly evolving clinical landscape. Eur J Cancer. 2017;81:116–29.
135. Demaria S, Golden EB, Formenti SC. Role of local radiation therapy in cancer immunotherapy. JAMA Oncol. 2015;1:1325–32.
136. Foote JB, Kok M, Leatherman JM, Armstrong TD, Marcinkowski BC, Ojalvo LS, Kanne DB, Jaffee EM, Dubensky TW Jr, Emens LA. A STING agonist given with OX40 receptor and PD-L1 modulators primes immunity and reduces tumor growth in tolerized mice. Cancer Immunol Res. 2017;5:468–79.
137. Kroemer G, Senovilla L, Galluzzi L, Andre F, Zitvogel L. Natural and therapy-induced immunosurveillance in breast cancer. Nat Med. 2015;21:1128–38.

# Breast Cancer Immunotherapy: A Team Science Approach

# 4

Max Duesberg, Alexis LeVee, Hannah Chang, Karen Tsai, Bridget Crossman, Marissa Tadi, Sharon Xu, Deric Wheeler, and Irene Kang

## 4.1 Introduction

### 4.1.1 Rationale for Immune Checkpoint Inhibitors (ICIs) in Breast Cancer

Immune checkpoint inhibitors (ICIs) have revolutionized the treatment landscape for various malignancies by enhancing the host immune response against tumors [1]. Immune checkpoints are regulatory pathways that mediate the immune evasion

M. Duesberg
Department of Internal Medicine, Santa Clara Valley Medical Center, San Jose, CA, USA

A. LeVee · H. Chang
Department of Medical Oncology and Therapeutics Research, City of Hope Comprehensive Cancer Center, Duarte, CA, USA

K. Tsai
Department of Endocrinology, City of Hope Comprehensive Cancer Center, Duarte, CA, USA

B. Crossman
Department of Human Oncology, School of Medicine and Public Health, University of Wisconsin, Madison, WI, USA

M. Tadi · I. Kang (✉)
Department of Medical Oncology and Therapeutics Research, City of Hope Comprehensive Cancer Center, Irvine, CA, USA
e-mail: ikang@coh.org

S. Xu
Department of Pharmacy, City of Hope Comprehensive Cancer Center, Irvine, CA, USA

D. Wheeler
Department of Human Oncology, School of Medicine and Public Health, University of Wisconsin, Madison, WI, USA

Carbone Cancer Center, University of Wisconsin, Madison, WI, USA



R. Salgia, P. Kulkarni (eds.), *Immunotherapies in Solid Tumors*, Cancer Treatment and Research 129, https://doi.org/10.1007/978-3-031-97242-3_4

of tumor cells. One crucial pathway is the programmed death-1 (PD-1) pathway. The PD-1 inhibitory receptor regulates effector T-cell responses and is also expressed in the tumor microenvironment and antigen-presenting cells. Blockade of the PD-1 or PD-L1 molecules with ICIs have demonstrated powerful antitumor responses with the distinct hallmark of durable responses in a subset of patients [2, 3].

In breast cancer, combination therapy with ICIs and chemotherapy has demonstrated clinical benefit and is now incorporated into standard of care in triple-negative breast cancer (TNBC), due to the immunogenic nature of this subtype [4, 5]. TNBC is characterized by the absence of estrogen receptor (ER) and progesterone receptor (PR) expression and lack of human epidermal growth factor receptor-2 (HER2) immunohistochemistry (IHC) and fluorescence in situ hybridization (FISH) [6]. TNBC is generally associated with more aggressive disease and poorer prognosis compared to other breast cancer subtypes [7]. The rationale for using ICIs in TNBC stems from its higher levels of tumor-infiltrating lymphocytes (TILs) and PD-L1 expression compared to other breast cancer subtypes, which suggest a more immunogenic tumor microenvironment [8–10]. The tumor immune microenvironment (TIME) is a key factor in anti-tumor immunity and response to ICI therapy, referred to on a relative scale from "cold," or immune-excluded, to "hot," or highly immune infiltrated. While breast cancers are typically considered cold, the TNBC TIME, while highly heterogeneous, is thought to be hotter relative to hormone receptor-positive breast cancers [8]. ICIs have been studied in other subtypes of breast cancer including hormone receptor-positive (HR+) breast cancer, traditionally characterized by ER and/or PR expression $\geq$1%, as well as HER2-positive breast cancers. These subtypes have historically demonstrated less robust response to ICIs however clinical use in these subtypes continues to develop.

### 4.1.2 Chapter Overview

This chapter will focus on the application of ICIs in TNBC given its more immunogenic profile and current FDA-approval of ICIs in this subtype. TNBC accounts for approximately 15–20% of all breast cancer cases but is responsible for a disproportionate number of breast cancer-related deaths due to its aggressive nature and limited treatment options. The chapter will explore the current evidence supporting the use of ICIs in TNBC, including pivotal clinical trials such as KEYNOTE-522 and KEYNOTE-355, which have demonstrated improvements in clinical outcomes with the addition of pembrolizumab to chemotherapy in early-stage and metastatic TNBC, respectively [4, 5]. Additionally, the chapter will discuss management of toxicities, developing data for the use of ICIs in other breast cancer subtypes, biomarkers for response, and future directions for novel immunotherapy strategies in breast cancer.

## 4.2 Immune Checkpoint Inhibitors in Metastatic TNBC (mTNBC)

### 4.2.1 Rationale for Immunotherapy in Triple-Negative Breast Cancer (TNBC)

Higher Tumor Mutational Burden (TMB): TNBC is characterized by a higher tumor mutational burden compared to other breast cancer subtypes. This increased mutational load results in the generation of more neoantigens, which can be recognized by the immune system, making TNBC more immunogenic and responsive to immunotherapy [10–13].

Increased Programmed Death-Ligand 1 (PD-L1) Expression: TNBC often exhibits higher levels of PD-L1 expression on tumor cells and immune cells within the tumor microenvironment. PD-L1 expression is a critical factor for the efficacy of immune checkpoint inhibitors (ICIs) such as pembrolizumab and atezolizumab, which block the PD-1/PD-L1 pathway, thereby enhancing the anti-tumor immune response [2, 3, 14].

Role of Tumor-Infiltrating Lymphocytes (TILs): TNBC is associated with a higher presence of tumor-infiltrating lymphocytes (TILs). The presence of TILs is indicative of an ongoing immune response against the tumor and has been correlated with better prognosis and response to immunotherapy. TILs can enhance the effectiveness of ICIs by providing a pre-existing immune contexture that can be further activated by these therapies [15–17].

In summary, the rationale for immunotherapy in TNBC is supported by its higher TMB, increased PD-L1 expression, and the presence of TILs, all of which contribute to the immunogenicity of this breast cancer subtype and its responsiveness to immune checkpoint blockade.

### 4.2.2 Landmark Clinical Trials in mTNBC

#### 4.2.2.1 KEYNOTE-012 (Pembrolizumab, Phase Ib)

The KEYNOTE-012 trial investigated pembrolizumab in heavily pre-treated advanced PD-L1 positive (PD-L1+) TNBC and demonstrated an initial signal of activity and a potentially acceptable safety profile of pembrolizumab in this setting [18].

#### 4.2.2.2 KEYNOTE-086 (Pembrolizumab Monotherapy, Phase II)

The KEYNOTE-086 trial evaluated pembrolizumab monotherapy in mTNBC in the first and later-line settings. The trial reported favorable response rates in both treatment settings with a manageable safety profile, demonstrating the potential of pembrolizumab as a treatment strategy in PD-L1+ mTNBC [19].

#### 4.2.2.3 KEYNOTE-355 (Pembrolizumab + Chemotherapy, Phase III)

The KEYNOTE-355 trial was the pivotal phase III study of the addition of pembrolizumab vs placebo to chemotherapy in patients with previously untreated inoperable or mTNBC. The study demonstrated significantly improved PFS (9.7 months vs 5.6 months; hazard ratio (HR), 0.66; 95% confidence interval [CI], 0.50–0.88) and OS (23.0 months vs. 15.1 months; HR, 0.73; 95% CI, 0.55–0.95; $p = 0.0185$) in patients with a PD-L1 combined positive score (CPS) of ≥10 compared to chemotherapy alone. Subsequent analyses demonstrated benefit regardless of chemotherapy partner and no detriment to patient-reported quality of life. This study led to the US Food and Drug Administration (FDA) approval of pembrolizumab in combination with chemotherapy in the first-line setting for mTNBC [5, 20, 21].

#### 4.2.2.4 IMpassion130 (Atezolizumab + Taxane, Phase III) and IMpassion131

The IMpassion130 trial evaluated patients with metastatic TNBC in the first-line setting in which patients were randomized to nab-paclitaxel with atezolizumab or placebo. The trial demonstrated statistically significant improvements in PFS for the ITT and PD-L1+ (Ventana SP142 assay) subgroups (ITT: 7.2 v 5.5 months, hazard ratio [HR], 0.80; 95% CI, 0.69–0.92; $P = .002$; PD-L1+: 7.5 months v 5.0 months, HR, 0.62; 95% CI, 0.49–0.78; $P < .001$). However OS improvement was not demonstrated in the ITT population and, due to a hierarchical statistical approach, could not be formally tested in the PD-L1+ subgroup although it was numerically improved in a post hoc analysis [22, 23].

The IMpassion131 trial was a confirmatory and similarly designed trial randomizing patients in the first setting to paclitaxel with atezolizumab or placebo. Surprisingly, this trial did not demonstrate significant benefits in PFS or OS, contrasting with the positive results of IMpassion130. PD-L1+ group (OS 22.1 v 28.3 months; HR, 1.12; 95% CI, 0.76–1.65) and ITT (OS 19.2 v 22.8 months; HR, 1.11; 95% CI, 0.87–1.42). After an initial FDA approval for atezoliumab with nab-paclitaxel for PD-L1+ mTNBC, this indication was withdrawn due to the lack of confirmatory positive results [24].

#### 4.2.2.5 Newer Trials and Combinations

Recent and ongoing trials are exploring dual checkpoint blockade (e.g., PD-1+ CTLA-4 inhibitors) and combinations with other agents such as antibody-drug conjugates and PARP inhibitors [25, 26]. For example, the phase IB/II MORPHEUS-panBC study reported early data suggesting improved response with atezolizumab plus sacituzumab govitecan compared with atezolizumab plus nab-paclitaxel in the first-line setting [27]. Currently, two phase III studies are looking at the combination of ADC+ ICI in the first-line setting for PD-L1+ TNBC. TROPION-Breast05 (NCT06103864) is a study of datopotamab deruxtecan +/− durvalumab vs chemotherapy + pembrolizumab in patients with PD-L1+ mTNBC [28]. ASCENT04 (NCT05382286) is a phase III study of sacituzumab govitecan with pembrolizumab vs treatment of physician's choice plus pembrolizumab [29]. These strategies aim to enhance the antitumor immune response and overcome resistance mechanisms. Using a team-science-based approach will be key in elucidating mechanisms of resistance as well as designing rational combinations for future therapy.

## 4.3 Immune Checkpoint Inhibitors in Early-Stage TNBC

The KEYNOTE-522 trial demonstrated that the addition of pembrolizumab to chemotherapy in stage II or III TNBC significantly increased pCR rates compared to chemotherapy alone (64.8% vs. 51.2%, respectively). These findings led to the FDA approval of pembrolizumab for early-stage TNBC. Updated results from the trial also demonstrate significant improvements in event-free survival (EFS) and overall survival (OS). With a median duration of follow-up of 75.1 months (range 65.9–84.0), the trial reported an estimated 5-year EFS of 81.2% compared to 72.2% for chemotherapy alone (HR, 0.65; $p < 0.001$). The estimated 5-year OS in the pembrolizumab-chemotherapy group was 86.6% versus 81.7% for the chemotherapy alone group [4, 30].

### 4.3.1 Other Trials of ICI in Early-Stage TNBC

The IMpassion031 trial evaluated the combination of atezolizumab with chemotherapy in the neoadjuvant setting. This phase III study showed an improvement in pCR rates with atezolizumab, although the EFS data were less robust compared to KEYNOTE-522. The trial reported a pCR rate of 57.6% in the atezolizumab group versus 41.1% in the placebo group [31].

The NeoTRIPaPDL1 trial investigated atezolizumab in combination with carboplatin and nab-paclitaxel in patients with high-risk early TNBC. Unlike the previous trials, this study did not show a significant improvement in pCR rates with the addition of atezolizumab. However, survival follow-up is ongoing to assess long-term outcomes [32].

GeparDouze also investigated neoadjuvant atezolizumab with neoadjuvant chemotherapy followed by adjuvant atezolizumab. Although there was an increased pCR from 57% to 63% with the addition of atezolizumab, there was no statistically significant improvement in EFS (the primary endpoint of the study) [33].

#### 4.3.1.1 De-escalation

The NeoPACT trial was a phase II study investigating an anthracycline-free regimen, pembrolizumab with carboplatin plus docetaxel for 6 cycles in early stage TNBC. NeoPACT reported an encouraging pCR rate of 58% with an estimated

3-year EFS of 86% [34]. These encouraging results suggest some patients may be appropriate for a chemotherapy de-escalated strategy. The ongoing SWOG S2212 SCARLET trial (NCT05929768) is evaluating a similar shorter, anthracycline-free regimen (paclitaxel or docetaxel plus carboplatin) combined with pembrolizumab compared to the standard chemotherapy (paclitaxel, carboplatin with pembrolizumab followed by doxorubicin, cyclophosphamide with pembrolizumab).

#### 4.3.1.2 Novel Combinations and Trials for Residual Disease

Additional trials are incorporating immunotherapy in various combinations and strategies to enhance the efficacy and minimize toxicity in early-stage TNBC. These include the use of dual immune checkpoint inhibitors targeting PD-1 and CTLA-4 [35], as well as in combination with ADCs [36], radiation [37], vaccines, or novel agents [38, 39]. For instance, combining pembrolizumab with PARP inhibitors and radiation has shown promise in preclinical studies and early-phase trials.

In the setting of residual disease post neoadjuvant chemotherapy + ICI, prognosis is poor and clinical trials looking to improve outcomes in this space are ongoing. Several phase III trials are looking at ICI combinations with ADCs (Table 4.1).

#### 4.3.1.3 Role of Immune Checkpoint Inhibitors (ICIs) in the Adjuvant Setting

In the adjuvant setting, the utility of ICI is unclear. The Impassion030/ALEXANDRA study examined the addition of atezolizumab to adjuvant anthracycline-based chemotherapy and no benefit in IDFS was demonstrated [40].

Interestingly, the A-BRAVE trial examined adjuvant avelumab in high-risk TNBC patients after completion of locoregional and systemic therapy (neoadjuvant or adjuvant therapy). The primary objective was DFS which demonstrated a numeric but not statistically significant improvement in both the ITT as well as the subgroup that was treated neoadjuvantly. However, the secondary endpoint of OS demonstrated an 8.5% improvement in 3-year OS 84.8% in the avelumab arm compared to 76.3% in the control group with a HR of 0.66 and p-value of 0.035. Suggesting that checkpoint inhibition may have a survival benefit even in the absence of improved disease-free survival [41].

For patients receiving neoadjuvant chemotherapy + immunotherapy, the standard is to continue adjuvant pembrolizumab for an additional 9 cycles based on the

**Table 4.1** Ongoing phase III adjuvant trials with ICI + ADC for residual disease post neoadjuvant therapy

| Trial name/ID | Regimen | Primary endpoint |
|---|---|---|
| ASCENT-05/OptimICE-RD NCT05633654 | SG + Pembro vs Pembro +/− capecitabine | iDFS |
| NCT06393374 | Sacituzumab Tirumotecan + Pembro vs TPC | iDFS |
| TROPION-Breast03 NCT05629585 | Datopotamab +/− durvalumab vs ICT | iDFS Dato-Dxd+Durva vs ICT |

*SG* Sacituzumab govitecan, *Pembro* pembrolizumab, *TPC* treatment of physician's choice, *ICT* investigator's choice of therapy design of the Keynote-522 study. However, the utility of ICI in the adjuvant setting is unclear. The ongoing phase III OPT-PEMBRO (NCT06606730) Alliance trial will answer whether cessation of pembrolizumab in the setting of pCR is appropriate for patients treated with neoadjuvant chemotherapy + ICI. The SWOG S1418/NRG-006 (NCT02954874) will address whether adjuvant pembrolizumab improves outcomes for patients who received neoadjuvant chemotherapy (without ICI) and have residual disease.

In summary, the integration of ICI (e.g., pembrolizumab) into the treatment of early-stage TNBC has significantly improved clinical outcomes. Ongoing research aims to optimize these regimens and explore new combinations to further improve patient outcomes.

## 4.4 Biomarkers of Immune Responsiveness in Triple-Negative Breast Cancer (TNBC)

### 4.4.1 Programmed Death-Ligand 1 (PD-L1) Expression

PD-L1 expression is the only FDA-approved biomarker for predicting response to ICIs in mTNBC. The National Comprehensive Cancer Network (NCCN)/American Society of Clinical Oncology (ASCO) recommends testing for PD-L1 expression using 22C3 antibody to determine eligibility for the addition of pembrolizumab to chemotherapy in the metastatic setting, with a cut-off threshold for positivity of CPS 10 or more [42].

### 4.4.2 Tumor Mutational Burden (TMB) and Microsatellite Instability (MSI)

High TMB ($\geq$10 mutations/Mb) is associated with improved response to pembrolizumab in various cancers, including mTNBC [11–13, 42]. MSI-high status, although rare in TNBC, is another biomarker for pembrolizumab efficacy. NCCN/ASCO guidelines recommend testing for TMB and MSI as tumor-agnostic biomarkers to guide ICI therapy for all advanced solid tumors [42].

### 4.4.3 Tumor-Infiltrating Lymphocytes (TILs) and Immune Gene Signatures

High levels of TILs are associated with better outcomes and response to ICIs in TNBC. TILs can be assessed on hematoxylin and eosin-stained slides and have shown reliable inter-reader reproducibility [43]. Immune gene signatures, which reflect the immune microenvironment, are emerging as potential predictive biomarkers [44, 45].

### 4.4.4 Emerging Biomarkers

Emerging biomarkers predictive of ICI response include the gut microbiome. The gut microbiome has been shown to influence both the efficacy of ICI and play a role in the development of irAE. The gut microbiome interacts closely with the immune system through a number of mechanisms, including maintaining intestinal barrier integrity, impacting the development and activation of immune cells, and producing cytokines and microbial metabolites that have a direct impact on immunogenicity. In several cancer types, studies demonstrate that specific gut profiles are associated with improved responses to ICI, with specific bacteria and bacterial compositions associated with improved responses to anti-PD-1/PD-L1 therapy [46–49]. In breast cancer, studies are ongoing exploring the potential of the gut microbiome as a biomarker of ICI response [50–53].

Spatial transcriptomics and other strategies to better understand the tumor immune microenvironment and identify important molecular pathways within TNBC may help identify other predictive biomarkers [54, 55]. The development of these biomarkers is crucial for optimizing treatment strategies and improving outcomes in mTNBC patients.

### 4.4.5 Predictors of Response in the Neoadjuvant Setting

There are currently no FDA-approved biomarkers to predict ICI response in early-stage TNBC. Biomarkers including PD-L1 expression, tumor-infiltrating lymphocytes (TILs), and tumor mutational burden (TMB) have all been explored. PD-L1 expression has been associated with improved response rates to ICIs; however, KEYNOTE-522 demonstrated that patients benefit from the addition of pembrolizumab regardless of PD-L1 positivity [4, 39]. High levels of TILs and elevated TMB have also been correlated with better responses to ICIs as well as improved prognosis overall [34, 43]. Other immune signatures are underway such as the ImPRINT assay developed from the I-SPY2 trial [56].

## 4.5 Future Directions and Unmet Needs

### 4.5.1 Expanding Immunotherapy to Other Breast Cancer Subtypes

#### 4.5.1.1 Human Epidermal Growth Factor Receptor 2 Positive (HER2+) Breast Cancer

While ICIs have shown to be effective in triple-negative breast cancer (TNBC), their role in HER2+ breast cancer is still under investigation. Current research is exploring the combination of ICIs with HER2-targeted therapies such as trastuzumab and pertuzumab. Early-phase clinical trials have shown promising results, suggesting that combining ICIs with HER2-targeted therapies may enhance anti-tumor immune responses and improve clinical outcomes. The NeoHIP study (NCT03747120) recently presented data on improved pCR rates with the addition of pembrolizumab to neoadjuvant paclitaxel, trastuzumab, and pertuzumab (THP). The rate of pCR was 48.3% in the THP arm and 67.2% in the pembrolizumab-THP arm ($P = .030$) [57]. Additionally, antibody-drug conjugates (ADCs) like trastuzumab deruxtecan are being studied in combination with ICIs to further potentiate the immune response [38]. An ongoing phase Ib study is evaluating the combination of trastuzumab deruxtecan with nivolumab in HER2-expressing metastatic breast or urothelial cancers [58].

#### 4.5.1.2 Hormone Receptor-Positive/Human Epidermal Growth Factor Receptor 2-Negative (HR+/HER2-) Breast Cancer

HR+/HER2- breast cancer is considered to be less immunogenic than TNBC; however, certain subsets of luminal breast cancer may still benefit from ICI. Recently, the Checkmate 7FL and KEYNOTE-756 studies each demonstrated increased pCR rates with the addition of nivolumab or pembrolizumab respectively to neoadjuvant chemotherapy for high-risk early-stage HR+HER2- breast cancer. These studies together demonstrated increasing likelihood of pCR with higher PD-L1 expression. The Checkmate 7FL trial also reported rates of pCR to be higher with stromal TILs >1% compared to sTIL 1% [59, 60]. Similarly, the ISPY2 trial demonstrated an increase in pCR rates when ICIs were added to chemotherapy in high-risk HR+/HER2- breast cancer as defined by Mammaprint [61, 62]. MammaPrint is a multigene assay to determine the recurrence risk in HR+ breast cancers and inform the decisions about use of adjuvant or neoadjuvant chemotherapy [63, 64]. Among MammaPrint High tumors, the ultra-high (MP2) subset is characterized by higher proliferative activity, lower ER-related gene expression, and the poorest prognosis. This MP2 subset has also demonstrated high levels of TILs and immune gene expression profiles similar to what is observed in TNBC [65]. The ongoing study SWOG S2206 (NCT06058377) is using this MP2 designation to select patients with HR+HER2- early-stage breast cancer who may benefit from neoadjuvant ICI. Strategies to enhance the immunotherapeutic activity in this subtype include combining ICIs with endocrine therapy, PARP inhibitors, HDAC inhibitors, CDK4/6 inhibitors, and radiotherapy [46]. These combinations aim to modulate the tumor microenvironment and overcome the immunosuppressive barriers characteristic of HR+/HER2- breast cancer.

### 4.5.2 Emerging Strategies

Novel approaches such as cancer vaccines, bispecific antibodies, and adoptive cell therapies (e.g., CAR-T cells) are being actively investigated across various breast cancer subtypes. These strategies aim to enhance the specificity and efficacy of the immune response against breast cancer cells. Additionally, the identification of predictive biomarkers for response to immunotherapy remains a critical area of research, with the goal of personalizing treatment and improving outcomes for patients with HER2+ and HR+/HER2- breast cancer [66].

In summary, expanding the use of immunotherapy to HER2+ and HR+/HER2- breast cancer subtypes and improving outcomes in TNBC involves exploring combination therapies, novel immunotherapeutic strategies, and the identification of predictive biomarkers to optimize patient selection and treatment efficacy.

#### 4.5.2.1 Bispecific Antibodies

Bispecific antibodies are engineered to simultaneously bind to two different antigens, typically one on the cancer cell and one on the immune cell, thereby bringing the immune cell into close proximity to the cancer cell to enhance its destruction. This approach is being actively researched in breast cancer, with promising preclinical and early clinical trial results—particularly in the HER2-targeted setting [67].

#### 4.5.2.2 T-Cell Engagers

T-cell engagers, such as bispecific T-cell engagers (BiTEs), are a subset of bispecific antibodies that specifically recruit T cells to the tumor site. These molecules have shown potential in preclinical models and are currently being evaluated in clinical trials for their efficacy in breast cancer [38, 68].

#### 4.5.2.3 Cellular Therapies

Cellular therapies in breast cancer involve utilizing or modifying living cells from a patient or donor to combat the cancer cells. Various approaches are under investigation, including chimeric antigen receptor (CAR-T) cells, tumor-infiltrating lymphocytes (TILs), and dendritic cell (DC) vaccines. While these therapies have been approved in other cancer types, they are all still under investigation in breast cancer.

#### 4.5.2.4 Chimeric Antigen Receptor T-Cell (CAR-T) Therapy

CAR-T therapy involves genetically modifying a patient's T cells to express receptors specific to tumor antigens. This approach has shown significant promise in hematologic malignancies and is now being explored in solid tumors, including breast cancer. Early-phase clinical trials are ongoing to determine the safety and efficacy of CAR-T cells targeting various breast cancer antigens [69, 70].

Several challenges have limited the success of CAR-T cell therapy in breast cancer, including limited T-cell trafficking and infiltration into tumors, reduced functional persistence due to T-cell exhaustion, and the tumor heterogeneity characteristic of breast cancer [71, 72].

#### 4.5.2.5 Tumor Infiltrating Lymphocytes (TILs) Therapy

Tumor-infiltrating lymphocytes (TILs) represent another cellular therapy approach in which a patient's immune cells are isolated, expanded ex vivo in a laboratory, and re-infused after lymphodepleting therapy. Current studies are currently exploring the combination of TIL therapy with chemotherapy or immunotherapy to enhance immune responses in advanced breast cancer [73].

#### 4.5.2.6 Dendritic Cell (DC) Immunotherapy

Dendritic cell (DC) immunotherapy in the form of vaccines is an emerging cellular therapy under investigation for breast cancer. Many of these early-phase trials involve peptide- and mRNA-based DC vaccines, which load dendritic cells with specific peptides or mRNA-encoding tumor-associated antigens, such as HER2. These modified dendritic cells are then reintroduced into the patient to elicit a tumor-specific immune response by optimizing antigen recognition [74].

#### 4.5.2.7 Cancer Vaccines

Cancer vaccines aim to stimulate the patient's immune system to recognize and attack cancer cells. Various types of vaccines, including peptide-based, dendritic cell-based, and mRNA vaccines, are under investigation for breast cancer. These vaccines are designed to induce a robust and specific immune response against tumor-associated antigens [38, 75, 76].

## 4.6 Toxicity and Management of Immune Checkpoint Inhibitors

The side effect profile of ICIs are unique from those observed with chemotherapy and in rare cases can be life-threatening. In the KEYNOTE-522 study, a population of patients treated with curative-intent, 35% of patients experienced any grade and 13% experienced high-grade (grade $\geq 3$) irAEs and 2 patients died due to irAE [4]. A study in the metastatic setting, the KEYNOTE-355 study reported immune-related adverse eventsirAEs in 26.5% of patients treated with pembrolizumab-chemotherapy with 5.6% developing grade 3 or 4 events [5]. Some of the most common toxicities include hyper and hypothyroidism, rash, colitis, pneumonitis, and hypophysitis [77]. While endocrine toxicities are often readily manageable and typically do not require cessation of immunotherapy, most endocrine toxicities are permanent. Although rarer irAEs such as colitis and pneumonitis may require hospitalization and steroid treatment, some can necessitate permanent discontinuation of ICI therapy and may even be fatal. This underscores the importance of appropriate patient selection and identification of risk factors all the more pressing as indications for ICIs and immunotherapy expand and more combination therapies with ICIs are developed. Real-world evidence is emerging in this population confirming the relatively high rates of any grade irAEs as well as the rare but severe toxicities [78]. Increased awareness of irAEs is important to facilitate early detection and appropriate treatment management. As cancer treatment becomes increasingly multidisciplinary, a team-based approach to monitoring irAEs—including physicians, advanced practice providers, pharmacists, and nurses—can lead to better patient outcomes.

## 4.7 Conclusion

The addition of ICIs into the treatment landscape of TNBC has improved outcomes in TNBC. TNBC is characterized by a higher TMB, increased PD-L1 expression, and the presence of TILS compared to the other subtypes, which has resulted in the effectiveness of ICIs in both the metastatic and early-stage settings.

In metastatic TNBC, KEYNOTE-355 demonstrated improved PFS and PS in PD-L1–positive patients receiving pembrolizumab in combination with chemotherapy. In early-stage TNBC, KEYNOTE-522 demonstrated that the addition of pembrolizumab to chemotherapy results in improved pCR, EFS, and OS, setting a new standard of care for high-risk patients.

Despite these advances, challenges remain, including optimizing biomarkers for patient selection, managing immune-related toxicities, and overcoming primary and acquired resistance. Ongoing trials are exploring novel ICI combinations and the expansion of immunotherapy to other breast cancer subtypes.

Ultimately, the continued refinement of immunotherapy strategies and biomarker development holds the promise of delivering more durable responses and improved outcomes for patients with TNBC and beyond.

## References

1. Ribas A, Wolchok JD. Cancer immunotherapy using checkpoint blockade. Science. 2018;359(6382):1350–5.
2. Wang X, Yang X, Zhang C, et al. Tumor cell-intrinsic PD-1 receptor is a tumor suppressor and mediates resistance to PD-1 blockade therapy. Proc Natl Acad Sci. 2020;117(12):6640–50. https://doi.org/10.1073/pnas.1921445117.
3. LaFleur MW, Muroyama Y, Drake CG, Sharpe AH. Inhibitors of the PD-1 pathway in tumor therapy. J Immunol. 2018;200(2):375–83. https://doi.org/10.4049/jimmunol.1701044.
4. Schmid P, Cortes J, Pusztai L, et al. Pembrolizumab for early triple-negative breast cancer. N Engl J Med. 2020;382(9):810–21. https://doi.org/10.1056/NEJMoa1910549.
5. Cortes J, Rugo HS, Cescon DW, et al. Pembrolizumab plus chemotherapy in advanced triple-negative breast cancer. N Engl J Med. 2022;387(3):217–26.
6. Ahn SG, Kim SJ, Kim C, Jeong J. Molecular classification of triple-negative breast cancer. J Breast Cancer. 2016;19(3):223.
7. Gucalp A, Traina TA. Triple-negative breast cancer: adjuvant therapeutic options. Chemother Res Pract. 2011;2011(1):696208.
8. Loizides S, Constantinidou A. Triple negative breast cancer: immunogenicity, tumor microenvironment, and immunotherapy. Front Genet. 2023;13:1095839.
9. Luo C, Wang P, He S, Zhu J, Shi Y, Wang J. Progress and prospect of immunotherapy for triple-negative breast cancer. Front Oncol. 2022;12:919072.
10. Agostinetto E, Losurdo A, Nader-Marta G, et al. Progress and pitfalls in the use of immunotherapy for patients with triple negative breast cancer. Expert Opin Investig Drugs. 2022;31(6):567–91.
11. Barroso-Sousa R, Jain E, Cohen O, et al. Prevalence and mutational determinants of high tumor mutation burden in breast cancer. Ann Oncol. 2020;31(3):387–94.
12. O'Meara TA, Tolaney SM. Tumor mutational burden as a predictor of immunotherapy response in breast cancer. Oncotarget. 2021;12(5):394.

13. Sinn HP, Huober J, Becker C, Blohmer J-U, Marmé F, Schmitt WD, Wu S, van Mackelenbergh M, Müller V, Schem C, Stickeler E, Fasching PA, Jackisch C, Untch M, Schneeweiss A, Loibl S. Tumor mutational burden and immune infiltration as independent predictors of response to neoadjuvant immune checkpoint inhibition in early TNBC in GeparNuevo. Ann Oncol. 2020;31(9):1216–22. https://doi.org/10.1016/j.annonc.2020.05.015.
14. Serrano García L, Jávega B, Llombart Cussac A, et al. Patterns of immune evasion in triple-negative breast cancer and new potential therapeutic targets: a review. Front Immunol. 2024;15:1513421.
15. Blackley EF, Loi S. Targeting immune pathways in breast cancer: review of the prognostic utility of TILs in early stage triple negative breast cancer (TNBC). Breast. 2019;48:S44–8.
16. Loi S, Adams S, Schmid P, et al. Relationship between tumor infiltrating lymphocyte (TIL) levels and response to pembrolizumab (pembro) in metastatic triple-negative breast cancer (mTNBC): results from KEYNOTE-086. Ann Oncol. 2017;28:v608.
17. Gao G, Wang Z, Qu X, Zhang Z. Prognostic value of tumor-infiltrating lymphocytes in patients with triple-negative breast cancer: a systematic review and meta-analysis. BMC Cancer. 2020;20:1–15.
18. Nanda R, Chow LQ, Dees EC, et al. Pembrolizumab in patients with advanced triple-negative breast cancer: phase Ib KEYNOTE-012 study. J Clin Oncol. 2016;34(21):2460–7.
19. Adams S, Schmid P, Rugo H, et al. Pembrolizumab monotherapy for previously treated metastatic triple-negative breast cancer: cohort A of the phase II KEYNOTE-086 study. Ann Oncol. 2019;30(3):397–404.
20. Cescon DW, Schmid P, Rugo HS, et al. Health-related quality of life with pembrolizumab plus chemotherapy vs placebo plus chemotherapy for advanced triple-negative breast cancer: KEYNOTE-355. JNCI J Natl Cancer Inst. 2023;116(5):717–27. https://doi.org/10.1093/jnci/djad240.
21. Rugo HS, Schmid P, Cescon DW, et al. Abstract GS3-01: additional efficacy endpoints from the phase 3 KEYNOTE-355 study of pembrolizumab plus chemotherapy vs placebo plus chemotherapy as first-line therapy for locally recurrent inoperable or metastatic triple-negative breast cancer. Cancer Res. 2021;81(4_Suppl):GS3-01.
22. Schmid P, Adams S, Rugo HS, et al. Atezolizumab and nab-paclitaxel in advanced triple-negative breast cancer. N Engl J Med. 2018;379(22):2108–21.
23. Schmid P, Rugo HS, Adams S, et al. Atezolizumab plus nab-paclitaxel as first line treatment for unresectable, locally advanced or metastatic triple-negative breast cancer (IMpassion130): updated efficacy results from a randomised, double-blind, placebo-controlled, phase 3 trial. Lancet Oncol. 2020;21(1):44–59. https://doi.org/10.1016/S1470-2045(19)30689-8.
24. Miles D, Gligorov J, André F, et al. Primary results from IMpassion131, a double-blind, placebo-controlled, randomised phase III trial of first-line paclitaxel with or without atezolizumab for unresectable locally advanced/metastatic triple-negative breast cancer. Ann Oncol. 2021;32(8):994–1004. https://doi.org/10.1016/j.annonc.2021.05.801.
25. Domchek SM, Postel-Vinay S, Im S-A, et al. Olaparib and durvalumab in patients with germline BRCA-mutated metastatic breast cancer (MEDIOLA): an open-label, multicentre, phase 1/2, basket study. Lancet Oncol. 2020;21(9):1155–64. https://doi.org/10.1016/S1470-2045(20)30324-7.
26. Garrido-Castro AC, Kim SE, Desrosiers J, et al. SACI-IO HR+: a randomized phase II trial of sacituzumab govitecan with or without pembrolizumab in patients with metastatic hormone receptor-positive/HER2-negative breast cancer. J Clin Oncol. 2024;42(17_suppl):LBA1004. https://doi.org/10.1200/JCO.2024.42.17_suppl.LBA1004.
27. Schmid P, Loi S, De la Cruz Merino L, et al. 181O Interim analysis (IA) of the atezolizumab (atezo) + sacituzumab govitecan (SG) arm in patients (pts) with triple-negative breast cancer (TNBC) in MORPHEUS-pan BC: a phase Ib/II study of multiple treatment (tx) combinations in pts with locally advanced/metastatic BC (LA/mBC). ESMO Open. 2024;9 https://doi.org/10.1016/j.esmoop.2024.103203.
28. Schmid P, Oliveira M, O'Shaughnessy J, et al. ESMO Open. 2024;9 https://doi.org/10.1016/j.esmoop.2024.103282.

29. Tolaney SM, de Azambuja E, Emens LA, et al. 276TiP ASCENT-04/KEYNOTE-D19: phase III study of sacituzumab govitecan (SG) plus pembrolizumab (pembro) vs treatment of physician's choice (TPC) plus pembro in first-line (1L) programmed death-ligand 1-positive (PD-L1+) metastatic triple-negative breast cancer (mTNBC). Ann Oncol. 2022;33:S664–5. https://doi.org/10.1016/j.annonc.2022.07.1860.
30. Schmid P, Cortes J, Dent R, et al. Overall survival with pembrolizumab in early-stage triple-negative breast cancer. N Engl J Med. 2024;391(21):1981–91.
31. Barrios C, Harbeck N, Zhang HA, et al. LBA1 Final analysis of the placebo-controlled randomised phase III IMpassion031 trial evaluating neoadjuvant atezolizumab (atezo) plus chemotherapy (CT) followed by open-label adjuvant atezo in patients (pts) with early-stage triple-negative breast cancer (eTNBC). ESMO Open. 2023;8(1) https://doi.org/10.1016/j.esmoop.2023.101571.
32. Gianni L, Huang CS, Egle D, et al. Pathologic complete response (pCR) to neoadjuvant treatment with or without atezolizumab in triple-negative, early high-risk and locally advanced breast cancer: NeoTRIP Michelangelo randomized study☆. Ann Oncol. 2022;33(5):534–43. https://doi.org/10.1016/j.annonc.2022.02.004.
33. Geyer C, Valentina N. NSABP B-59/GBG-96-GeparDouze: a randomized double-blind phase III clinical trial of neoadjuvant chemotherapy with atezolizumab or placebo followed by adjuvant atezolizumab or placebo in patients with stage II and III triple-negative breast cancer. J Clin Oncol. 2024; https://doi.org/10.1200/JCO.2018.36.15_suppl.TPS603.
34. Sharma P, Stecklein SR, Yoder R, et al. Clinical and biomarker findings of neoadjuvant pembrolizumab and carboplatin plus docetaxel in triple-negative breast cancer: NeoPACT phase 2 clinical trial. JAMA Oncol. 2024;10(2):227–35. https://doi.org/10.1001/jamaoncol.2023.5033.
35. Nederlof I, Isaeva OI, de Graaf M, et al. Neoadjuvant nivolumab or nivolumab plus ipilimumab in early-stage triple-negative breast cancer: a phase 2 adaptive trial. Nat Med. 2024;30(11):3223–35. https://doi.org/10.1038/s41591-024-03249-3.
36. McArthur HL, Tolaney SM, Dent R, et al. TROPION-Breast04: a randomized phase III study of neoadjuvant datopotamab deruxtecan (Dato-DXd) plus durvalumab followed by adjuvant durvalumab versus standard of care in patients with treatment-naïve early-stage triple negative or HR-low/HER2- breast cancer. Ther Adv Med Oncol. 2025;17:17588359251316176. https://doi.org/10.1177/17588359251316176.
37. Ho AY, Shiao S, Kobald SA, et al. PEARL: a phase Ib/II biomarker study of adding radiation therapy to pembrolizumab before neoadjuvant chemotherapy in human epidermal growth factor receptor 2-negative breast cancer. J Clin Oncol. 2024;42(36):4282–93. https://doi.org/10.1200/jco.24.00003.
38. Huppert LA, Mariotti V, Chien AJ, Soliman HH. Emerging immunotherapeutic strategies for the treatment of breast cancer. Breast Cancer Res Treat. 2022;191(2):243–55. https://doi.org/10.1007/s10549-021-06406-1.
39. Jacob SL, Huppert LA, Rugo HS. Role of immunotherapy in breast cancer. JCO Oncol Pract. 2023;19(4):167–79.
40. Ignatiadis M, Bailey A, McArthur H, et al. Adjuvant atezolizumab for early triple-negative breast cancer: the ALEXANDRA/IMpassion030 randomized clinical trial. JAMA. 2025;333(13):1150–60. https://doi.org/10.1001/jama.2024.26886.
41. Conte PF, Dieci MV, Bisagni G, et al. A-BRAVE trial: a phase III randomized trial with avelumab in early triple-negative breast cancer with residual disease after neoadjuvant chemotherapy or at high risk after primary surgery and adjuvant chemotherapy. J Clin Oncol. 2024;42(17_suppl):LBA500. https://doi.org/10.1200/JCO.2024.42.17_suppl.LBA500.
42. Henry NL, Somerfield MR, Dayao Z, et al. Biomarkers for systemic therapy in metastatic breast cancer: ASCO guideline update. J Clin Oncol. 2022;40(27):3205–21. https://doi.org/10.1200/jco.22.01063.
43. Leon-Ferre RA, Jonas SF, Salgado R, et al. Tumor-infiltrating lymphocytes in triple-negative breast cancer. JAMA. 2024;331(13):1135–44. https://doi.org/10.1001/jama.2024.3056.

44. Criscitiello C, Bayar MA, Curigliano G, et al. A gene signature to predict high tumor-infiltrating lymphocytes after neoadjuvant chemotherapy and outcome in patients with triple-negative breast cancer. Ann Oncol. 2018;29(1):162–9. https://doi.org/10.1093/annonc/mdx691.
45. Tan Q, Yin S, Zhou D, Chi Y, Man X, Li H. Potential predictive and prognostic value of biomarkers related to immune checkpoint inhibitor therapy of triple-negative breast cancer. Front Oncol. 2022;12:779786. https://doi.org/10.3389/fonc.2022.779786.
46. Matson V, Fessler J, Bao R, et al. The commensal microbiome is associated with anti–PD-1 efficacy in metastatic melanoma patients. Science. 2018;359(6371):104–8.
47. Routy B, Le Chatelier E, Derosa L, et al. Gut microbiome influences efficacy of PD-1–based immunotherapy against epithelial tumors. Science. 2018;359(6371):91–7.
48. Derosa L, Routy B, Thomas AM, et al. Intestinal Akkermansia muciniphila predicts clinical response to PD-1 blockade in patients with advanced non-small-cell lung cancer. Nat Med. 2022;28(2):315–24.
49. Derosa L, Iebba V, Silva CAC, et al. Custom scoring based on ecological topology of gut microbiota associated with cancer immunotherapy outcome. Cell. 2024;187(13):3373–89. e16
50. LeVee AA, Egelston CA, Yost SE, et al. A phase I/II trial of palbociclib, pembrolizumab, and endocrine therapy for patients with HR+/HER2-locally advanced or metastatic breast cancer (MBC): clinical outcomes and stool microbial profiling. American Society of Clinical Oncology; 2024.
51. Sarfraz H, Czerniecki BJ, Stankiewicz K, et al. Evaluating gut microbiome as a biomarker of pathological complete response in patients with early locally advanced triple negative breast cancer (LA TNBC): a pilot study. American Society of Clinical Oncology; 2024.
52. Teng NM, Malfettone A, Dalby MJ, et al. Profiling the gut and oral microbiota of hormone receptor-positive, HER2-negative metastatic breast cancer patients receiving pembrolizumab and eribulin. Microbiome Res Rep. 2025;4(1):4.
53. Yuan Y, Highlander S, Yost SE, et al. Gut microbiome profiling of patients with metastatic breast cancer undergoing immune checkpoint inhibitor therapy. Philadelphia: The American Association for Cancer Research; 2020.
54. Iida M, Crossman BE, Kostecki KL, et al. MerTK drives proliferation and metastatic potential in triple-negative breast cancer. Int J Mol Sci. 2024;25(10):5109.
55. Wang X, Venet D, Lifrange F, et al. Spatial transcriptomics reveals substantial heterogeneity in triple-negative breast cancer with potential clinical implications. Nat Commun. 2024;15(1):10232. https://doi.org/10.1038/s41467-024-54145-w.
56. Wolf DM, Yau C, Campbell MJ, et al. Biomarkers predicting response to 5 immunotherapy arms in the neoadjuvant I-SPY2 trial for early-stage breast cancer (BC): evaluation of immune subtyping in the response predictive subtypes (RPS). J Clin Oncol. 2023;41(16_suppl):102. https://doi.org/10.1200/JCO.2023.41.16_suppl.102.
57. McArthur HL, Leal J, et al. A phase 2 study of neoadjuvant HER2-targeted therapy +/– immunotherapy with pembrolizumab (neoHIP). J Clin Oncol. 2024; https://doi.org/10.1200/JCO.2023.41.16_suppl.TPS634.
58. Hamilton E, Galsky MD, Ochsenreither S, et al. Trastuzumab deruxtecan with nivolumab in HER2-expressing metastatic breast or urothelial cancer: analysis of the phase Ib DS8201-A-U105 study. Clin Cancer Res. 2024;30(24):5548–58. https://doi.org/10.1158/1078-0432.ccr-24-1513.
59. Cardoso F, O'Shaughnessy J, Liu Z, et al. Pembrolizumab and chemotherapy in high-risk, early-stage, ER+/HER2– breast cancer: a randomized phase 3 trial. Nat Med. 2025;31(2):442–8. https://doi.org/10.1038/s41591-024-03415-7.
60. Loi S, Salgado R, Curigliano G, et al. Neoadjuvant nivolumab and chemotherapy in early estrogen receptor-positive breast cancer: a randomized phase 3 trial. Nat Med. 2025;31(2):433–41. https://doi.org/10.1038/s41591-024-03414-8.
61. Nanda R, Liu MC, Yau C, et al. Effect of pembrolizumab plus neoadjuvant chemotherapy on pathologic complete response in women with early-stage breast cancer: an analysis of the ongoing phase 2 adaptively randomized I-SPY2 trial. JAMA Oncol. 2020;6(5):676–84. https://doi.org/10.1001/jamaoncol.2019.6650.

62. Pusztai L, Yau C, Wolf DM, et al. Durvalumab with olaparib and paclitaxel for high-risk HER2-negative stage II/III breast cancer: results from the adaptively randomized I-SPY2 trial. Cancer Cell. 2021;39(7):989–998.e5. https://doi.org/10.1016/j.ccell.2021.05.009.
63. Cardoso F, van't Veer LJ, Bogaerts J, et al. 70-gene signature as an aid to treatment decisions in early-stage breast cancer. N Engl J Med. 2016;375(8):717–29. https://doi.org/10.1056/NEJMoa1602253.
64. Piccart M, van't Veer LJ, Poncet C, et al. 70-gene signature as an aid for treatment decisions in early breast cancer: updated results of the phase 3 randomised MINDACT trial with an exploratory analysis by age. Lancet Oncol. 2021;22(4):476–88. https://doi.org/10.1016/s1470-2045(21)00007-3.
65. van't Veer L, Wolf D, Yau C, et al. MammaPrint High1/High2 risk class as a pre-specified biomarker of response to nine different targeted agents plus standard neoadjuvant therapy for similar to 1000 breast cancer patients in the I-SPY 2 trial. Oxford: Elsevier; 2018. p. E15–5.
66. Dvir K, Giordano S, Leone JP. Immunotherapy in breast cancer. Int J Mol Sci. 2024;25(14):7517. https://doi.org/10.3390/ijms25147517.
67. Lan HR, Chen M, Yao SY, Chen JX, Jin KT. Bispecific antibodies revolutionizing breast cancer treatment: a comprehensive overview. Front Immunol. 2023;14:1266450. https://doi.org/10.3389/fimmu.2023.1266450.
68. Rolin C, Zimmer J, Seguin-Devaux C. Bridging the gap with multispecific immune cell engagers in cancer and infectious diseases. Cell Mol Immunol. 2024;21(7):643–61. https://doi.org/10.1038/s41423-024-01176-4.
69. Erler P, Kurcon T, Cho H, et al. Multi-armored allogeneic MUC1 CAR T cells enhance efficacy and safety in triple-negative breast cancer. Sci Adv. 2024;10(35):eadn9857. https://doi.org/10.1126/sciadv.adn9857.
70. Buono G, Capozzi M, Caputo R, et al. CAR-T cell therapy for breast cancer: current status and future perspective. Cancer Treat Rev. 2025;133:102868. https://doi.org/10.1016/j.ctrv.2024.102868.
71. Kantari-Mimoun C, Barrin S, Vimeux L, et al. CAR T-cell entry into tumor islets is a two-step process dependent on IFNγ and ICAM-1. Cancer Immunol Res. 2021;9(12):1425–38. https://doi.org/10.1158/2326-6066.cir-20-0837.
72. Gargett T, Yu W, Dotti G, et al. GD2-specific CAR T cells undergo potent activation and deletion following antigen encounter but can be protected from activation-induced cell death by PD-1 blockade. Mol Ther. 2016;24(6):1135–49. https://doi.org/10.1038/mt.2016.63.
73. Zacharakis N, Huq LM, Seitter SJ, et al. Breast cancers are immunogenic: immunologic analyses and a phase II pilot clinical trial using mutation-reactive autologous lymphocytes. J Clin Oncol. 2022;40(16):1741–54. https://doi.org/10.1200/jco.21.02170.
74. Han HS, Costa RL, Soliman HH, et al. Phase I study of adoptive T cell therapy following HER2-pulsed dendritic cell vaccine and pepinemab/trastuzumab in patients with metastatic HER2-positive breast cancer (MBC). J Clin Oncol. 2023;41(16_suppl):TPS1113. https://doi.org/10.1200/JCO.2023.41.16_suppl.TPS1113.
75. Patel S, Thompson J, Patel M, Daugherty FJ, Rimawi M. Abstract PO3-19-05: phase III study to evaluate the efficacy and safety of GLSI-100 (GP2+ GM-CSF) in breast cancer patients with residual disease or high-risk PCR after both neo-adjuvant and postoperative adjuvant anti-HER2 therapy, Flamingo-01. Cancer Res. 2024;84(9_Suppl):PO3-19-05.
76. Budd GT, Johnson JM, Esakov Rhoades E, et al. Phase I trial of an alpha-lactalbumin vaccine in patients with moderate- to high-risk operable triple-negative breast cancer (TNBC). J Clin Oncol. 2022;40(16_suppl):TPS1125. https://doi.org/10.1200/JCO.2022.40.16_suppl.TPS1125.
77. Gumusay O, Callan J, Rugo H. Immunotherapy toxicity: identification and management. Breast Cancer Res Treat. 2022;192(1):1–17.
78. Jayan A, Sukumar JS, Fangman B, et al. Real-world immune-related adverse events in patients with early triple-negative breast cancer who received pembrolizumab. JCO Oncol Pract. 2024;0(0):OP.24.00371. https://doi.org/10.1200/OP.24.00371.

# Colorectal Cancers and Immunotherapy

# 5

Farzad Teymouri and Gagandeep Brar

## Abbreviations

| | |
|---|---|
| CRC | colorectal cancer |
| DCs | dendritic cells |
| ICIs | immune checkpoint inhibitors |
| IBD | inflammatory bowel disease |
| MDSCs | myeloid-derived suppressor cells |
| TAA | tumor-associated antigens |
| TAMs | tumor-associated macrophages |
| TMB | tumor mutation burden |
| TSA | tumor-specific antigens |
| TCR | T-cell receptor |
| TILs | tumor-infiltrating lymphocytes |
| TME | tumor microenvironment |

## 5.1 Epidemiology

Colorectal cancer is a significant global health concern and a burden on society and families. CRC is the third most commonly diagnosed cancer and notably one of the leading causes of cancer-related deaths in the United States. It ranks third most common for men and fourth for women individually but is the second-leading cause of cancer death when combining both genders [1–3]. In the

F. Teymouri
Department of Internal Medicine, Eisenhower Health, Rancho Mirage, CA, USA

G. Brar (✉)
Department of Medical Oncology, City of Hope National Medical Center, Duarte, CA, USA
e-mail: gbrar@coh.org



R. Salgia, P. Kulkarni (eds.), *Immunotherapies in Solid Tumors*, Cancer Treatment and Research 129, https://doi.org/10.1007/978-3-031-97242-3_5

United States alone, an estimated 107,320 new cases of colon cancer and 46,950 new cases of rectal cancer are expected in 2025 [1]. Approximately 52,900 deaths from CRC are anticipated in the United States in 2025. While the overall incidence of CRC has been declining since the mid-1980s, mostly due to improved screening methods and lifestyle changes, the rate in younger adults under 50 years old has increased by approximately 2.4% annually between 2012 and 2021 [1, 2]. CRC prevalence is also rising in many regions, especially in middle- and high-income countries, likely linked to lifestyle factors [4] such as physical inactivity, rates of obesity, smoking, alcohol consumption, and low-fiber diets [2].

There are clear disparities in CRC incidence and outcomes related to gender. Men are more frequently diagnosed with CRC and have higher mortality rates than women [3, 4]. Biological sex differences, notably hormonal influences like estrogen, appear to offer women a protective advantage, resulting in lower CRC incidence and better survival rates compared to age-matched men [4, 5]. Furthermore, women more commonly develop tumors on the right side of the colon, whereas men more frequently develop tumors on the left side.

Understanding these epidemiological and biological variations in colorectal cancer is crucial for developing targeted preventive strategies, refining screening practices, and enhancing personalized treatment approaches, ultimately improving patient outcomes worldwide.

## 5.2 Risk Factors

Colorectal cancer risk factors can be divided into two main categories (1) modifiable risk factors: sedentary lifestyle, obesity, diet, smoking and alcohol consumption, diabetes and insulin resistance, and (2) non-modifiable risk factors: ethnicity, sex, age, hereditary mutations, inflammatory bowel disease, abdominal irradiation, cystic fibrosis, acromegaly, treatment with androgen derivatives [6].

Chronic inflammatory conditions like inflammatory bowel disease (IBD), including ulcerative colitis and Crohn's disease, significantly elevate the risk of CRC, especially with longer disease duration, extensive colonic involvement, or coexisting primary sclerosing cholangitis [6, 7].

Other conditions that can promote carcinogenesis through inflammatory pathways, hormonal imbalances, bile acid dysregulation, and oxidative stress include a history of childhood abdominal radiation, cystic fibrosis, obesity, and diabetes [6, 8, 9].

Environmental factors can play a cruel role in the development of CRC. Diets high in red meat, trans fats, and processed carbohydrates increase the risk, compared to diets rich in fiber, antioxidants, and anti-inflammatory nutrients [10]. Alcohol consumption and tobacco use are known risk factors for colorectal cancer, with studies showing a clear, dose-dependent association between these exposures and both CRC incidence and mortality [6, 11].

## 5.3 Screening

Primary screening for colorectal cancer is based on individual risk factors and can be performed using various modalities, including colonoscopy, flexible sigmoidoscopy, CT colonography, fecal immunochemical test (FIT), high-sensitivity guaiac fecal occult blood test (gFOBT), or multitarget stool DNA test (mt-sDNA) [12].

For individuals at average risk, screening should begin at the age of 45. Recommended options include a colonoscopy every 10 years, flexible sigmoidoscopy every 5–10 years, or CT colonography every 5 years. FIT or gFOBT annually, and the mt-sDNA every 3 years.

For individuals at increased risk, such as those with a family history of CRC or advanced adenomas, screening should begin at age 40 or 10 years earlier than the youngest affected relative, with a colonoscopy every 5 years. Patients with inflammatory bowel disease (IBD) should begin screening 8 years after diagnosis, followed by surveillance colonoscopies every 1–2 years. Those with a personal history of polyps should undergo follow-up colonoscopy at intervals determined by polyp type, size, and number. Additionally, individuals who had abdominal or pelvic radiation during childhood or early adulthood should begin screening at age 30 or 5 years after radiation, whichever comes later [12].

## 5.4 Colon Cancer Development

Colorectal cancer develops through a series of complex biological events that ultimately transform normal colonic epithelium into invasive carcinoma. One of the most well-established pathways of tumorigenesis is the adenoma–carcinoma sequence, which describes the gradual progression of benign polyps into malignant tumors, primarily caused by mutations in key genes such as APC, KRAS, and TP53 [6]. This sequence is commonly associated with chromosomal instability (CIN). Another major pathway is microsatellite instability (MSI), which arises from defects in the DNA mismatch repair system and is frequently seen in both sporadic CRC cases and inherited conditions like Lynch syndrome [13]. A third mechanism, known as the CpG island methylator phenotype (CIMP), involves widespread hypermethylation of gene promoter regions, leading to the silencing of tumor suppressor genes [14]. This is often observed in tumors that develop from sessile serrated polyps. While these pathways can act independently, they often overlap, reflecting the molecular heterogeneity of colorectal cancer.

## 5.5 The Immune Landscape in Colon Cancer

In normal circumstances, the immune system identifies and eliminates tumor cells before they grow and spread by identifying the abnormal antigens presented on these cells [6, 15]. When a tumor-associated mutation occurs, specific antigens known as tumor-specific antigens (TSA) and tumor-associated antigens

(TAA) are expressed and allow the immune system to recognize them. Recognition of TSA and TAA by dendritic cells (DCs) allow for presentation to CD4+ and CD8+ T-cells via major histocompatibility complexes (MHC) class II and class I, initiating the activation of the immune system [16]. To activate antigen-specific T-cells, two key stimulatory signals must occur simultaneously. First, the T-cell receptor (TCR) binds to the antigen-presenting MHC complex. Second, a costimulatory interaction takes place between CD80/CD86 on dendritic cells and CD28 on T-cells [17]. Once activated, antigen-specific T cells mature into memory T cells. Effector T cells then travel through the lymphatic system toward the tumor site, guided by chemokines such as CCL5, CX3CL1, CXCL10, and CXCL9 [18]. Upon infiltrating the tumor, CD8+ T cells release cytotoxic molecules like perforin and granzymes, inducing cancer cell death. Some CD8+ T cells differentiate into memory T cells, helping clear the tumor cells in the course of future presentation [19, 20]. Natural killer (NK) cells also provide an additional, non-specific mechanism for eliminating tumor cells [21]. Any failure in these processes can lead to immune resistance toward TSA or TAA and the growth of tumor cells. The physiological process of aging, on the other hand, causes remodeling, regression, and degeneration of immune organs, including the thymus, resulting in a reduction of the T-cell pool, which eventually reduces immune cell competency [22, 23]. This process leads to reduced resistance to infective agents, adaptability of the immune system, and increased likelihood of tumor formation. As a part of the physiologic aging process, the pro-inflammatory markers increase, which leads to low-grade inflammation often referred to as "inflammaging" [24]. This persistent inflammatory state provides an environment that can increase DNA damage and cause tumorigenesis [25]. These findings can explain the increased incidence of cancer in proportion to aging.

## 5.6 Mechanism of Immune Evasion

The interaction between immune system cells and cancer cells can end up with different results. In the initial stage, immune cells recognize and destroy cancer cells (Elimination). If some tumor cells survive the immune attack, they maintain a stable population without significant growth (Equilibrium). If the cancer cells develop resistance to immune defenses, they will proliferate, grow, or spread to different sites of the body (Escape) [5, 26]. This tumor escape phenomenon happens through different mechanisms.

### 5.6.1 Change in Immunogenicity

Cancer cells can evade immune detection by downregulating or losing antigen expression, reducing MHC complex presentation, and shedding NKG2D ligands, leading to interferon-gamma (IFN-γ) insensitivity [27].

### 5.6.2 Microenvironment Modulation and Immune Suppression

Cancer cells can develop immune tolerance by releasing chemokines and cytokines, creating an environment that suppresses the immune response (Fig. 5.1). Key immune suppressors in the tumor microenvironment (TME) include tumor-associated macrophages (TAMs), regulatory CD4+ T cells (Tregs), and myeloid-derived suppressor cells (MDSCs) [28, 29]. The balance of M1 and M2 types of macrophages in the tumor microenvironment plays a significant role in tumor growth, as M1 macrophages have anti-tumor activities by producing pro-inflammatory cytokines like tumor necrosis factor (TNF), IL-1, IL-6, and IL-23 [30]. In contrast, M2 macrophages can cause tumor growth by releasing factors like TGF-β and IL-10, further promoting tumor growth [31]. The balance between M1 and M2 macrophages can be altered by TGF-β, leading to the conversion of M1 to M2 macrophages and eventually influencing tumor progression [32]. Tumors containing more M2 macrophages in their microenvironment typically respond poorly to treatment. MDSCs also contribute to immunosuppression in the TME, helping tumors grow and spread. Similarly, tumor antigens can trigger CD4+ T cells to increase Treg cell activity, further weakening the body's immune response against the tumor [32, 33]. The tumor microenvironment (TME) significantly impacts the progression, immune response, and effectiveness of immunotherapy in colon cancer. Tumor-infiltrating lymphocytes (TILs), including CD8+ and CD3+ T cells, play key roles and have been extensively studied as biomarkers for prognosis and immunotherapy response [34, 35]. Studies show that higher TIL levels, particularly CD8+

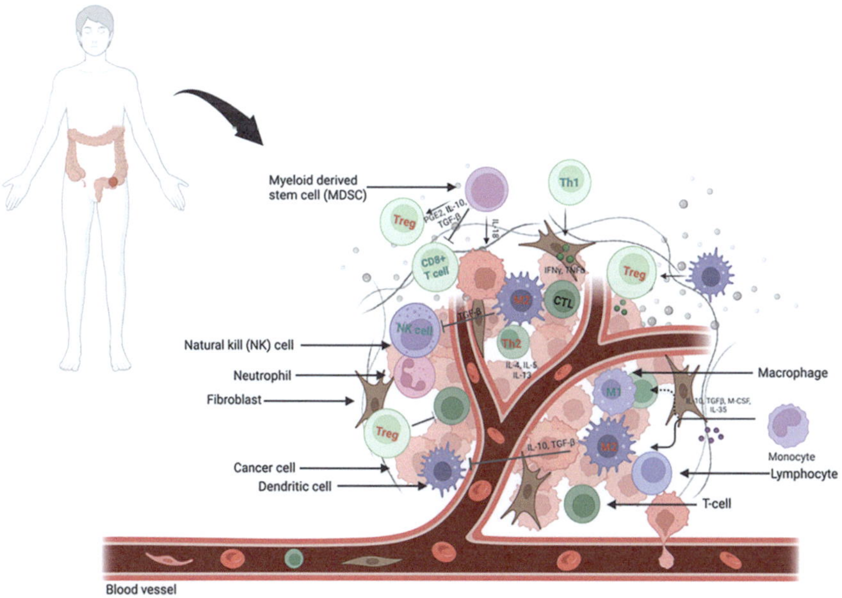


**Fig. 5.1** Tumor microenvironment in colon cancer

T cells, correlate with better outcomes and responses to treatments like immune checkpoint inhibitors (ICIs) [36].

### 5.6.3 Immune Checkpoint Manipulation

Cancer cells can develop adaptive immune resistance by manipulating the immune checkpoints to avoid detection by T cells. Immune checkpoints are part of the body's natural defense system, helping distinguish between self and foreign antigens. We will review the most commonly known checkpoint pathways.

#### 5.6.3.1 PD-1

PD-1 is one of the important checkpoint proteins found on the surface of NK cells, T cells, and B cells. Its ligands, PD-L1 and PD-L2, are present in various tumors and hematopoietic cells. When PD-1 interacts with PD-L1 or PD-L2, it initiates the process of apoptosis and converting active T cells into regulatory T cells (Tregs), leading to suppressing the immune response by reducing the number of functional T cells [37, 38]. The genetic characteristics of tumors play an important role in PD-L1 expression. PD-L1 is located on chromosome 9q24; any increase in its copy numbers, structural changes, and certain genetic polymorphisms and mutations like loss of the *PTEN* gene or mutations in *PIK3CA* can contribute to its expression [39]. It is proven that overexpression in PD-L1 can lead to more aggressive tumors and, therefore, shorter overall survival rates [40]. Environmental factors also influence PD-L1 levels. IFN-ɣ, released by tumor-infiltrating lymphocytes, increases PD-L1 expression through the JAK/STAT pathway. Another cytokine, IL-8, enhances PD-L1 expression via the STAT3/mTOR/c-Myc pathway, making tumor cells more resistant to CD8+ T cell attacks [41]. PD-L1 expression is a known predictive factor for immunotherapy response in some solid tumors, such as melanoma and renal cell cancer [42, 43], although higher PD-L1 expression is associated with a better prognosis in CRC patients [44]. PD-L1 expression alone cannot be used to predict immunotherapy response in colon cancer.

#### 5.6.3.2 Galectin-3

Galectin-3 is a small, chimeric protein found inside or outside cells, depending on the cell type and its stage of development, which plays various roles in cell survival, gene transcription, and communication between epithelial cells and extracellular matrix [45]. In tumor cells, Glectin-3 helps suppress the immune response by increasing lymphocyte activation Gene 3 (LAG-3) expression, promoting regulatory T cell (Treg) activation, and preventing T cells from maturing into effector cells [46]. Galectin-3 contributes to tumor growth by activating cancer-related genes like *MUC2, TTF-1,* and *cyclin D1* [47]. It also enhances the activity of the *K-Ras* gene, which controls cell proliferation. Mutations in *K-Ras* can lead to uncontrolled tumor growth, and the overexpression of Galectin-3 further fuels this process [47]. Additionally, Galectin-3 can trigger T cell death when present outside the cell, while inside the cell, it suppresses T cell function. It can also trap IFN-γ in the tumor's extracellular matrix, reducing T-cell infiltration [48].

#### 5.6.3.3 Galectin-9

Galectin-9 is a protein involved in immune regulation, T-cell balance, inflammation control, and nervous system stability [49]. It binds to T-cell immunoglobulin and Mucin-Domain Containing-3 (TIM-3) found on dendritic cells, CD8 + T cells, Th1 cells, and monocytes act as immune suppressor by increasing regulatory T cells while reducing helper T cells [49]. Galectin-9 binding to TIM-3 triggers T-cell apoptosis through the calcium-calpain-caspase-1 pathway [50]. The overexpression of Galectin and TIM-3 are proven to correlate with advanced tumor stage, blood vessel invasion, and worse patient survival in different kinds of cancers like gastric cancer and esophageal squamous cell carcinoma [50].

#### 5.6.3.4 Signal Regulatory Protein-α (SIRPα)

Signal regulatory protein-α (SIRPα) is a receptor found on macrophages, dendritic cells, and neutrophils [51]. The interaction of SIRPα with CD47 found on normal cells blocks phagocytosis and prevents immune response. Overexpression of CD47 on cancer cells can result in elevation of immune attack. Studies have shown the disruption of SIRPα/CD47 interaction increases immune cell activity and enhances the ability to eliminate cancer cells [52].

#### 5.6.3.5 Indoleamine-Pyrrole 2,3-Dioxygenase (IDO)

Indoleamine-pyrrole 2,3-dioxygenase (IDO) is an enzyme that normally plays a role in metabolism by breaking down the amino acid tryptophan into kynurenine. Tumor cells exploit it to support their growth and suppress the immune response [53]. The microenvironment inflammatory tumor cytokines like IFN-γ can activate IDO, leading to tryptophan depletion in T cells and suppressing the immune response [54].

#### 5.6.3.6 Sialic Acid-Binding Immunoglobulin-Type Lectins (Siglec)-15

Sialic acid-binding immunoglobulin-type lectins (Siglec)-15 can cause tumor cell immune evasion and growth via different mechanisms. Siglec-15 binding to receptors on cytotoxic T cells leads to immune suppression. Siglec-15 binding to CD44 (found in cancer cells) can promote tumor migration. Overexpressing of sialic acid in tumor cells and inflammatory cytokines in tumor microenvironment causes upregulation of Siglec-15 [55].

#### 5.6.3.7 A Disintegrin and Metalloproteinase 17 (ADAM17)

A disintegrin and metalloproteinase 17 (ADAM17), a membrane-bound sheddase enzyme, cleaves transmembrane proteins and releases their soluble domains. This process can promote tumor growth by activating Notch and Wnt signaling pathways and targeting immune checkpoint proteins such as TIM-3 and PD-L1, resulting in CD8+ cell apoptosis. The correlation between increased ADAM17 and lymph node metastasis and tumor invasion has been proven [56, 57].

#### 5.6.3.8 CD155

CD155, also known as poliovirus receptor (PVR), is an adhesion molecule that promotes tumor growth by enhancing cell proliferation and immune evasion [58]. It interacts with both activating (CD226) and inhibitory (TIGIT, CD96) receptors on immune cells, influencing their function [59]. Overexpression of CD155 in tumors can lead to increased metastasis and poor survival. In contrast, lower CD155 levels enhance T-cell activity and slow tumor progression, making it a potential target for cancer therapy [60].

#### 5.6.3.9 Carcinoembryonic Antigen-Related Cell Adhesion Molecule 1 CEACAM1 (CD66a)

Carcinoembryonic antigen-related cell adhesion molecule 1 CEACAM1 (CD66a) overexpressed on tumor cells can lead to tumors by different mechanisms. Interaction of CEACAM1 and CEACAM5 prevents the NK cell-mediated tumor cell activation and IFN-γ release inhibition [61]. CEACAM1 also supports early tumor growth and promotes angiogenesis via VEGF [61].

## 5.7 Molecular Subtypes

Different molecular characteristics of colon cancer may provide a theoretical basis to identify patients who are more likely to benefit from immunotherapy and offer potential biomarkers for future immunotherapy. But still, they are not suitable for stratifying colon cancer patients for immunotherapy. For example, POLE/POLD1 mutations impair DNA repair, contribute to cancer development, and occur in approximately 7.4% of colon cancers. Some evidence suggests POLE mutations predict favorable responses to immunotherapies [62].

Another relevant biomarker classification in colon cancer is the consensus molecular subtype (CMS) system, established through gene expression analysis into four subtypes: CMS1 (immune-activated MSI), CMS2 (canonical with WNT/MYC activation), CMS3 (metabolic dysregulation), and CMS4 (mesenchymal with high TGF-β activity). Studies indicate that CMS1 tumors respond best to immunotherapy due to high immune infiltration, whereas CMS4 shows poorer responses linked to immunosuppressive tumor environments [63]. Although informative, many questions remain unanswered, including how to incorporate this information into making treatment decisions. In clinical practice, treatment decisions are not made based on this molecular classification of a patient's tumor.

## 5.8 Rationale for Immunotherapy and Immunotherapy Effectiveness in Colon Cancer

Tumor cells develop unique capabilities to cause immune response suppression and evade the immune system. The purpose of immunotherapy is to help the immune system recognize tumor antigens and stimulate it to invade the tumor cells. Accordingly, immunotherapies currently approved in colon cancer are immune checkpoint inhibitors (ICIs). Additionally, there are many studies evaluating different modalities of immune manipulation including engineered chimeric antigen receptor T cells or CAR-T immunotherapy, T cell receptor T cells (TCR-T) immunotherapy vaccines for cancer and oncolytic viruses.

Different biomarkers and genetic alterations can potentially influence the effectiveness of immunotherapy in colon cancer and predict the potential response (Fig. 5.2).

### 5.8.1 Microsatellite Instability

Microsatellites (MS) are short, repetitive DNA sequences. Microsatellite instability (MSI) refers to a condition when the DNA mismatch repair (MMR) system fails during DNA replication, causing changes in microsatellite length [64]. This condition is associated with various cancers and can be used as an indicator of treatment response and prognosis [65]. Tumors are classified as deficient (dMMR) if there is a loss of expression in any key MMR proteins including MutS homolog 2 (MSH2), MutL homolog 1 (MLH1), MutS homolog 6 (MSH6), or postmeiotic segregation increased by 2 (PMS2), otherwise they are defined as pMMR. Based on the MSI status, tumors are categorized as MSI-high (MSI-H), MSI-low (MSI-L), or microsatellite stable (MSS). Generally, MSI-H is considered equal to dMMR [66].

### 5.8.2 Tumor Mutation Burden

Tumor mutation burden (TMB) is defined as the number of somatic mutations per million bases (muts/Mb). Patients are considered to have hypermutated tumors when the cancer cells show a markedly elevated number of somatic mutations.

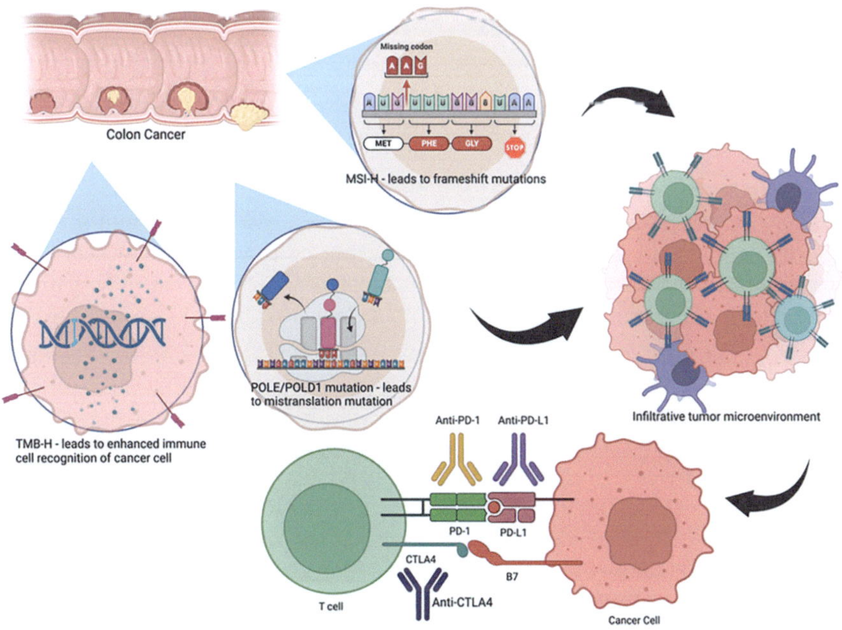


**Fig. 5.2** Alterations that suggest response to immunotherapy in colorectal cancers

Studies suggest different TMB thresholds for different cancer types in order to predict response to immunotherapy. For example, a cutoff value of 10 mut/Mb is commonly used in melanoma and non-small cell lung cancer. The National Comprehensive Cancer Network (NCCN) guidelines reference a threshold of 50 mut/Mb for patients with colorectal cancer [67–71]. Although the TMB alone may not be sufficient as an independent biomarker for predicting immunotherapy effectiveness in CRC, it remains valuable when combined with other markers like MSI or specific genetic mutations.

### 5.8.3 POLE/POLD1 Mutation

These genes are responsible for encoding the proofreading subunits of DNA polymerases. Mutations in POLE/POLD1 genes can impair the proofreading function and lead to dramatic accumulation of somatic mutations. This gives rise to an ultra-hypermutated tumor phenotype, defined by a TMB greater than 100 mut/Mb [72]. Colorectal cancers with this mutation often present in a younger age and more frequently in males and proximal colon. Studies showed patients with POLE/POLD1 mutations, associated with ultra-hypermutated tumor phenotype, have better response with immunotherapies [73].

## 5.9 Immunotherapies in Advanced Colon Cancer

There have been many studies evaluating the role of immune checkpoint inhibitors in patients with colorectal cancers (Table 5.1). We will review the practice changing studies below.

### 5.9.1 Pembrolizumab

Pembrolizumab is an anti-PD1 inhibitor that was first evaluated in the KEYNOTE-016 trial in 2015. This phase II study evaluated pembrolizumab (10 mg/kg every 14 days) in patients with advanced progressive colorectal and non-colorectal tumors, with or without mismatch-repair deficiency. In patients treated with immunotherapy, dMMR colorectal cancers showed significantly better outcomes compared to pMMR colorectal cancers. The immune-related response rate was 40% for dMMR colorectal cancer versus 0% for proficient cases. Similarly, progression-free survival rates were notably higher (78% vs 11%; HR 0.10; 95% CI, 0.03–0.37; $p < 0.001$). Median progression-free and overall survival were not reached in dMMR patients, whereas they were only 2.2 and 5.0 months (HR 0.04; 95% CI, 0.01–0.21; $P < 0.001$), respectively for pMMR patients. Non-colorectal dMMR cancers responded similarly. Genetic analysis revealed dMMR tumors had significantly higher mutation loads, which correlated with improved survival [74].

**Table 5.1** Clinical studies evaluating ICI in colorectal cancers

| Agent (s) | Pembrolizumab | Pembrolizumab | Pembrolizumab vs. SOC | Nivolumab | Dostarlimab | Tislelizumab | Cemiplimab |
|---|---|---|---|---|---|---|---|
| ORR, %(95% CI) | dMMR CRC: 40% (95% CI 12–74%)<br>pMMR CRC: 0% (95% CI 0–20%) | Cohort A: 32.8% (95% CI: 21.3–46.0%)<br>Cohort B: 34.9% (95% CI: 23.3–48.0%) | Pembrolizumab: 43.8%(95% CI: 35.8–52.0)<br>Chemotherapy: 33.1% (95% CI: 25.8–41.1) | 31.1%(95% CI: 20.8–42.9) | Overall dMMR population: 44.0% (95% CI: 38.6–49.6%)<br>dMMR CRC subgroup: 36.2% (95% CI: 25.0–48.7%) | 39.1% (95% CII: 25.1–54.6%) | – |
| mPFS, months (95% CI) | dMMR CRC: Not reached<br>pMMR CRC: 2.3 months (95% CI, 1.4–2.8) | Cohort A: 2.3 months (95% CI: 2.1–8.1)<br>Cohort B: 4.1 months (95% CI: 2.1–18.9) | Pembro: 16.5 months (95% CI: 5.4–32.4)<br>Chemotherapy: 8.2 months (95% CI: 6.1–10.2) | Not reached. 12-month PFS rate: 50% (95% CI: 38–61%) | Overall dMMR population: 6.9 months (95% CI: 4.2–13.6 months)<br>dMMR CRC subgroup: Not reached. 12-month progression-free survival 50% (95% CI: 38–61%) | Not reached | – |
| mOS, months (95% CI) | dMMR CRC: Not reached<br>pMMR CRC: 5.0 months (95% CI, 2.3–NE) | Cohort A: 31.4 months (95% CI: 21.4–58.0)<br>Cohort B: 47.0 months (95% CI: 19.2–not estimable) | Pembrolizumab: Not reached<br>Chemotherapy: 23.0 months (95% CI: 20.3–NE) | 12-month OS rate: 73% (95% CI: 61–82%) | Overall dMMR population: Not reached<br>dMMR CRC subgroup: Not reached; the 12-month overall survival rate 73% (95% CI: 61–82%) | Not reached | – |

(continued)

**Table 5.1** (continued)

| Agent (s) | Pembrolizumab | Pembrolizumab | Pembrolizumab vs. SOC | Nivolumab | Dostarlimab | Tislelizumab | Cemiplimab |
|---|---|---|---|---|---|---|---|
| Common AE | Fatigue, rash, pruritus, diarrhea | Fatigue, diarrhea, pruritus, nausea | Fatigue, diarrhea, nausea, pruritus (fewer ≥ grade 3 AEs with pembrolizumab: 22% vs. 66%) | Fatigue, diarrhea, pruritus, rash; grade ≥ 3 AEs in 20% | Fatigue, diarrhea, nausea, pruritus; grade ≥ 3 AEs in ~9.2% | Pruritus, fatigue, rash, fever; grade ≥ 3 AEs: 17.7% | Fatigue, diarrhea, rash, pruritus; grade ≥ 3 AEs: ~15% |
| References | [76] | [77] | [78] | [79] | [80] | [81, 82] | [85] |
| Agent (s) | REGN7075 + Cemiplimab | SNS-101 (monotherapy and with Cemiplimab) | Retifanlimab | Nivolumab (3 mg/kg) + ipilimumab (1 mg/kg) Q3W × 4 doses, then Nivolumab 3 mg/kg Q2W | | | |
| ORR, %(95% CI) | Not available | Not available | 51.3% (95% CI: 39.6–63.0%) | 55% | | | |
| mPFS, months (95% CI) | Not available | Not available | 12.2 months (95% CI: 6.0–33.4 months) | 9-month PFS: 76% <br> 12-month PFS: 71% | | | |
| mOS, months (95% CI) | Not available | Not available | 30.2 months (95% CI: 19.3–not estimable) | 9-month OS: 87% <br> 12-month OS: 85% | | | |
| Common AE | Not available | Grade 1 cytokine release syndrome (7%); other AEs mostly grade 1/2 | Fatigue, anemia, hypothyroidism, hyperthyroidism | Fatigue, diarrhea, pruritus, rash; grade ≥ 3 AEs: 32% | | | |
| Reference | [86] | [87] | [88] | Overman MJ et al. *J Clin Oncol*. 2018;36(8):773–779. | | | |

The KEYNOTE-164 study was a phase II trial that confirmed pembrolizumab's effectiveness in MSI-H/dMMR metastatic colorectal cancer seen in KEYNOTE-016. Patients with previously treated metastatic colorectal cancer characterized by MSI-H or dMMR were included. Patients were grouped based on one or more than one prior line of therapy. Results showed an objective response rate (ORR) of approximately 33% (HR 0.72; 95% CI, 0.51–1.00; $p = 0.048$) across both groups, with many patients experiencing durable responses. Median overall survival was not reached during the follow-up period, highlighting prolonged survival and durable clinical benefits [75].

KEYNOTE-177 was a global phase III clinical trial that led to FDA approval of pembrolizumab as a first-line treatment for metastatic MSI-H/dMMR CRC. The study compared pembrolizumab versus standard chemotherapy as a first-line treatment for patients with advanced or metastatic colorectal cancer characterized by microsatellite instability-high (MSI-H) or mismatch repair deficiency (dMMR). Pembrolizumab improved median progression-free survival (16.5 months vs. 8.2 months, HR 0.60; 95% CI, 0.45–0.80; $p = 0.0002$), with significantly more patients experiencing long-lasting responses (83% ongoing at 24 months vs. 35% with chemotherapy). The overall response rate was higher with pembrolizumab (43.8%) compared to chemotherapy (33.1%; $P = 0.027$). Grade 3 or higher treatment-related side effects occurred less frequently in the pembrolizumab group (22%) than in the chemotherapy group (66%; $P < 0.001$) [76].

Pembrolizumab was FDA-approved to treat patients with advanced colorectal cancers that harbor dMMR/MSI-H or POLE/POLD1 mutations with an ultra-hypermutated phenotype (e.g., TMB > 50 mut/Mb) in the first-line setting.

### 5.9.2 Nivolumab

Nivolumab is another PDL-1 inhibitor that was evaluated in the CheckMate-142 study. The study included patients with dMMR/MSI-H metastatic colorectal who had previously progressed on, or were intolerant of, at least one line of standard chemotherapy (including fluoropyrimidine and either oxaliplatin or irinotecan). Participants received nivolumab (3 mg/kg) every 2 weeks until disease progression, significant toxicity, withdrawal, or death. The results showed an overall response rate for nivolumab monotherapy of 31%, durable responses with responses lasting at least 12 months. Nivolumab was generally well-tolerated with manageable side effects [77].

Nivolumab was FDA-approved to treat patients with advanced dMMR/MSI-H or POLE/POLD1 colorectal cancer patients in the first-line setting, either as monotherapy or in combination with ipilimumab.

### 5.9.3 Dostarlimab

Dostarlimab is another PD-1 inhibitor which was evaluated in the GARNET study, which was a phase I, multicenter clinical trial that included 209 patients with dMMR advanced or recurrent solid tumor patients. Approximately one-third of patients enrolled had colorectal cancer. The objective response rate was 44% (95% CI, 37.3–51.3%) with durable responses lasting at least 12 months in 72.2% of responders. Median progression-free survival was 6.9 months (95% CI, 4.2–10.2), with 24-month progression-free survival rate of 41.0% (95% CI, 32.7–49.1%) The most common immune-related side effects included hypothyroidism (11.2%), elevated alanine aminotransferase (ALT) levels (5.8%), and arthralgia (5.8%), with no new safety issues reported [78].

### 5.9.4 Others in Progress

Tislelizumab is an anti-PD-1 monoclonal antibody that showed similar response in treated MSI-H/dMMR CRCs [79] In a phase II clinical trial (NCT03736889), the efficacy of tislelizumab was investigated in Chinese patients with previously treated, locally advanced, unresectable or metastatic histologically confirmed MSI-H/dMMR solid tumors; the ORR was 45.9%, and the DCR was 71.6%; the ORR was 39.1% ($n$ = 18/46) in CRC and 57.1% ($n$ = 16/28) in non-CRC patients. It is currently listed as a treatment option in NCCN guidelines [79, 80].

Cemiplimab is a PD-1 monoclonal antibody currently approved for the treatment of metastatic and unresectable locally advanced cutaneous squamous cell carcinoma (CSCC). Several ongoing clinical trials are currently exploring the efficacy of cemiplimab in colon cancer treatment. The Phoenix Trial (NCT05961709), a phase II study, evaluated the effectiveness of cemiplimab in patients with localized dMMR colon cancer, administered before surgery to assess tumor response and the potential for non-surgical management [81]. Another study (NCT04626635) evaluates REGN7075, a bispecific antibody targeting EGFR and CD28, combined with cemiplimab in patients with advanced solid tumors, including MSS Colorectal cancer [82]. Another phase I/II trial (NCT05864144) is assessing SNS-101, an anti-VISTA antibody, both alone and in combination with cemiplimab, for patients with advanced solid tumors, including colon cancer [83]. These studies aim to broaden cemiplimab's therapeutic role in colon cancer.

Retifanlimab is another PD-1 inhibitor that was evaluated in the POD1UM-101 trial, where patients with relapsed or refractory unresectable, locally advanced, or metastatic solid tumors received retifanlimab at doses ranging from 1 to 10 mg/kg every 2 or 4 weeks. The study found that retifanlimab was generally well-tolerated, with no dose-limiting toxicities observed [84]. A focused cohort reported by Berton et al. included 76 patients with MSI-H/dMMR endometrial cancer treated with 500 mg of retifanlimab every 4 weeks, showing a 51.3% response rate and a median progression-free survival of 12.2 months. Anemia was the most common grade ≥ 3 adverse event [85]. The STAR15 Trial (NCT05608044) is a phase I/II study assessing a combination immunotherapy regimen including retifanlimab in patients with metastatic colorectal cancer [86].

These are currently accepted as options for patients with advanced colorectal cancers, however, they have not yet received FDA approval specifically for a colorectal cancer indication.

### 5.9.5 Combination Therapies

The combination nivolumab and ipilimumab, an anti-CTLA-4 inhibitor, is currently approved and was evaluated in the CheckMate 142 trial. Results showed an overall response rate of 55% (HR 0.34; 95% CI, 0.20–0.56; $p < 0.0001$), with 80% experiencing disease control lasting at least 12 weeks. Progression-free survival rates were 76% at 9 months and 71% at 12 months (HR 0.21; 95% CI, 0.13–0.35; $p < 0.0001$), while overall survival was 87% and 85%, respectively (HR 0.27; 95% CI, 0.15–0.49; $p < 0.0001$). Patients reported significant improvements in quality of life and symptom management. Serious side effects (grade 3–4) occurred in 32% but were manageable. Notably, even patients who stopped treatment due to adverse effects showed a similar response rate (63%) compared to the overall group [87].

## 5.10 Conclusion

Colon cancer is a complex malignancy, and the immune system plays an important role in many aspects, including immune dysregulation and the development of cancer as well as immune modulation in the era of immune checkpoint inhibitors. A subset of patients will benefit from immunotherapies in the advanced stage setting and can maintain long-lasting durable responses over many months. Current research strategies include incorporating immunotherapy combinations in the majority of patients with colorectal cancers that do not have a targetable alteration (e.g., MSI-H).

## References

1. American Cancer Society. 2022. Available at: https://www.cancer.org/cancer/colon-rectal-cancer/about/key-statistics.html. Accessed date 06 Jan 2022.
2. Ma Z, Yang S, Yang Y, Luo J, Zhou Y, Yang H. Development and validation of prediction models for the prognosis of colon cancer with lung metastases: a population-based cohort study. Front Endocrinol (Lausanne). 2023;14:1073360. https://doi.org/10.3389/fendo.2023.1073360. PMID: 37583430; PMCID: PMC10424923.
3. Sung H, Ferlay J, Siegel RL, Laversanne M, Soerjomataram I, Jemal A, Bray F. Global cancer statistics 2020: GLOBOCAN estimates of incidence and mortality worldwide for 36 cancers in 185 countries. CA Cancer J Clin. 2021;71(3):209–49. https://doi.org/10.3322/caac.21660. Epub 2021 Feb 4. PMID: 33538338.
4. Harvey BJ, Harvey HM. Sex differences in colon cancer: genomic and nongenomic signalling of oestrogen. Genes (Basel). 2023;14(12):2225. https://doi.org/10.3390/genes14122225. PMID: 38137047; PMCID: PMC10742859.
5. Siegel RL, Miller KD, Jemal A. Cancer statistics, 2018. CA Cancer J Clin. 2018;68(1):7–30. https://doi.org/10.3322/caac.21442. Epub 2018 Jan 4. PMID: 29313949.
6. Ionescu VA, Gheorghe G, Bacalbasa N, Chiotoroiu AL, Diaconu C. Colorectal cancer: from risk factors to oncogenesis. Medicina (Kaunas). 2023;59(9):1646. https://doi.org/10.3390/medicina59091646. PMID: 37763765; PMCID: PMC10537191.
7. Olén O, Erichsen R, Sachs MC, Pedersen L, Halfvarson J, Askling J, Ekbom A, Sørensen HT, Ludvigsson JF. Colorectal cancer in ulcerative colitis: a Scandinavian population-based cohort

study. Lancet. 2020;395(10218):123–31. https://doi.org/10.1016/S0140-6736(19)32545-0. PMID: 31929014.
8. Scott P, Anderson K, Singhania M, Cormier R. Cystic fibrosis, CFTR, and colorectal cancer. Int J Mol Sci. 2020;21:2891. https://doi.org/10.3390/ijms21082891.
9. Ye P, Xi Y, Huang Z, Xu P. Linking obesity with colorectal cancer: epidemiology and mechanistic insights. Cancer. 2020;12:1408. https://doi.org/10.3390/cancers12061408.
10. Shivappa N, Godos J, Hebert JR, Wirth MD, Piuri G, Speciani AF, Grosso G. Dietary inflammatory index and colorectal cancer risk—a meta-analysis. Nutrients. 2017;9:1043. https://doi.org/10.3390/nu9091043.
11. Cai S, Li Y, Ding Y, Chen K, Jin M. Alcohol drinking and the risk of colorectal cancer death: a meta-analysis. Eur J Cancer Prev. 2014;23:532–9. https://doi.org/10.1097/CEJ.0000000000000076.
12. Benson AB, Venook AP, Adam M, Chang G, Chen YJ, Ciombor KK, Cohen SA, Cooper HS, Deming D, Garrido-Laguna I, Grem JL, Haste P, Hecht JR, Hoffe S, Hunt S, Hussan H, Johung KL, Joseph N, Kirilcuk N, Krishnamurthi S, Malla M, Maratt JK, Messersmith WA, Meyerhardt J, Miller ED, Mulcahy MF, Nurkin S, Overman MJ, Parikh A, Patel H, Pedersen K, Saltz L, Schneider C, Shibata D, Shogan B, Skibber JM, Sofocleous CT, Tavakkoli A, Willett CG, Wu C, Gurski LA, Snedeker J, Jones F. Colon cancer, version 3.2024, NCCN clinical practice guidelines in oncology. J Natl Compr Canc Netw. 2024;22(2D):e240029. https://doi.org/10.6004/jnccn.2024.0029. PMID: 38862008.
13. La Vecchia S, Sebastian C. Metabolic pathways regulating colorectal cancer initiation and progression. Semin Cell Dev Biol. 2020;98:63–70. https://doi.org/10.1016/j.semcdb.2019.05.018.
14. Limsui D, Vierkant RA, Tillmans LS, Wang AH, Weisenberg DJ, Laird PW, Lynch CF, Anderson KE, French AJ, Haile RW, et al. Cigarette smoking and colorectal cancer risk by molecularly defined subtypes. J Natl Cancer Inst. 2010;102:1012–22. https://doi.org/10.1093/jnci/djq201.
15. Burnet F. The concept of immunological surveillance. Immunol Asp Neoplasia. 1970;13:1–27.
16. Banchereau J, Steinman RM. Dendritic cells and the control of immunity. Nature. 1998;392:245–52.
17. Alberts B, Johnson A, Lewis J, Raff M, Roberts K, Walter P. Helper T cells and lymphocyte activation. In: Molecular biology of the cell. 4th ed. Garland Science; 2002.
18. Bindea G, Mlecnik B, Fridman W-H, Pages F, Galon J. Natural immunity to cancer in humans. Curr Opin Immunol. 2010;22:215–22.
19. Thiery J, Keefe D, Boulant S, Boucrot E, Walch M, Martinvalet D, Goping IS, Bleackley RC, Kirchhausen T, Lieberman J. Perforin pores in the endosomal membrane trigger the release of endocytosed granzyme B into the cytosol of target cells. Nat Immunol. 2011;12:770–7.
20. Zhang L, Conejo-Garcia JR, Katsaros D, Gimotty PA, Massobrio M, Regnani G, Makrigiannakis A, Gray H, Schlienger K, Liebman MN. Intratumoral T cells, recurrence, and survival in epithelial ovarian cancer. N Engl J Med. 2003;348:203–13.
21. Deng W, Gowen BG, Zhang L, Wang L, Lau S, Iannello A, Xu J, Rovis TL, Xiong N, Raulet DH. A shed NKG2D ligand that promotes natural killer cell activation and tumor rejection. Science. 2015;348:136–9.
22. Palmer S, Albergante L, Blackburn CC, Newman T. Thymic involution and rising disease incidence with age. Proc Natl Acad Sci. 2018;115:1883–8.
23. Thomas R, Wang W, Su D-M. Contributions of age-related thymic involution to immunosenescence and inflammaging. Immun Ageing. 2020;17:2.
24. Franceschi C, Bonafe M, Valensin S, Olivieri F, De Luca M, Ottaviani E, De Benedictis G. Inflamm-aging: an evolutionary perspective on immunosenescence. Ann N Y Acad Sci. 2000;908:244–54.
25. Yang L, Li A, Lei Q, Zhang Y. Tumor-intrinsic signaling pathways: key roles in the regulation of the immunosuppressive tumor microenvironment. J Hematol Oncol. 2019;12:125.
26. Dong D, Yu X, Liu H, Xu J, Guo J, Guo W, Li X, Wang F, Zhang D, Liu K, Sun Y. Study of immunosenescence in the occurrence and immunotherapy of gastrointestinal malignancies.

Semin Cancer Biol. 2025;111:16–35. https://doi.org/10.1016/j.semcancer.2025.01.007. Epub 2025 Feb8. PMID: 39929408.
27. Bhatia A, Kumar Y. Cancer-immune equilibrium: questions unanswered. Cancer Microenviron. 2011;4:209–17.
28. Qian B-Z, Pollard JW. Macrophage diversity enhances tumor progression and metastasis. Cell. 2010;141:39–51.
29. Murray PJ, Allen JE, Biswas SK, Fisher EA, Gilroy DW, Goerdt S, Gordon S, Hamilton JA, Ivashkiv LB, Lawrence T. Macrophage activation and polarization: nomenclature and experimental guidelines. Immunity. 2014;41:14–20.
30. Sica A, Schioppa T, Mantovani A, Allavena P. Tumour-associated macrophages are a distinct M2 polarised population promoting tumour progression: potential targets of anti-cancer therapy. Eur J Cancer. 2006;42:717–27.
31. Ramanathan S, Jagannathan N. Tumor associated macrophage: a review on the phenotypes, traits and functions. Iran J Cancer Prev. 2014;7:1.
32. Su S, Liu Q, Chen J, Chen J, Chen F, He C, Huang D, Wu W, Lin L, Huang W. A positive feedback loop between mesenchymal-like cancer cells and macrophages is essential to breast cancer metastasis. Cancer Cell. 2014;25:605–20.
33. Savage PA, Malchow S, Leventhal DS. Basic principles of tumor-associated regulatory T cell biology. Trends Immunol. 2013;34:33–40.
34. Bader JE, Voss K, Rathmell JC. Targeting metabolism to improve the tumor microenvironment for cancer immunotherapy. Mol Cell. 2020;78(6):1019–33. https://doi.org/10.1016/j.molcel.2020.05.034.
35. Zheng M, Li YM, Liu ZY, Zhang X, Zhou Y, Jiang JL, et al. Prognostic landscape of tumor-infiltrating T and b cells in human cancer. Front Immunol. 2021;12:731329. https://doi.org/10.3389/fimmu.2021.731329.
36. Bortolomeazzi M, Keddar MR, Montorsi L, Acha-Sagredo A, Benedetti L, Temelkovski D, et al. Immunogenomics of colorectal cancer response to checkpoint blockade: analysis of the KEYNOTE 177 trial and validation cohorts. Gastroenterology. 2021;161(4):1179–93. https://doi.org/10.1053/j.gastro.2021.06.064.
37. Zak KM, Grudnik P, Magiera K, Dömling A, Dubin G, Holak TA. Structural biology of the immune checkpoint receptor PD-1 and its ligands PD-L1/PD-L2. Structure. 2017;25:1163–74.
38. Dong Y, Sun Q, Zhang X. PD-1 and its ligands are important immune checkpoints in cancer. Oncotarget. 2016;8:2171.
39. Kataoka K, Shiraishi Y, Takeda Y, Sakata S, Matsumoto M, Nagano S, Maeda T, Nagata Y, Kitanaka A, Mizuno S. Aberrant PD L1 expression through 3′-UTR disruption in multiple cancers. Nature. 2016;534:402–6.
40. Zhang M, Dong Y, Liu H, Wang Y, Zhao S, Xuan Q, Wang Y, Zhang Q. The clinicopathological and prognostic significance of PD-L1 expression in gastric cancer: a meta-analysis of 10 studies with 1,901 patients. Sci Rep. 2016;6:37933.
41. Mimura K, Teh JL, Okayama H, Shiraishi K, Kua LF, Koh V, Smoot DT, Ashktorab H, Oike T, Suzuki Y. PD-L1 expression is mainly regulated by interferon gamma associated with JAK-STAT pathway in gastric cancer. Cancer Sci. 2018;109:43–53.
42. Aguilar EJ, Ricciuti B, Gainor JF, Kehl KL, Kravets S, Dahlberg S, et al. Outcomes to first-line pembrolizumab in patients with non-small-cell lung cancer and very high PD-L1 expression. Ann Oncol. 2019;30(10):1653–9. https://doi.org/10.1093/annonc/mdz288.
43. Wang X, Teng F, Kong L, Yu J. PD-L1 expression in human cancers and its association with clinical outcomes. Onco Targets Ther. 2016;9:5023–39. https://doi.org/10.2147/OTT.S105862.
44. Wang S, Yuan B, Wang Y, Li M, Liu X, Cao J, et al. Clinicopathological and prognostic significance of PD-L1 expression in colorectal cancer: a meta-analysis. Int J Color Dis. 2021;36(1):117–30. https://doi.org/10.1007/s00384-020-03734-4.
45. Sciacchitano S, Lavra L, Morgante A, Ulivieri A, Magi F, De Francesco GP, Bellotti C, Salehi LB, Ricci A. Galectin-3: one molecule for an alphabet of diseases, from A to Z. Int J Mol Sci. 2018;19:379.

46. Farhad M, Rolig AS, Redmond WL. The role of Galectin-3 in modulating tumor growth and immunosuppression within the tumor microenvironment. Onco Targets Ther. 2018;7:e1434467.
47. Nakahara S, Raz A. Regulation of cancer-related gene expression by galectin-3 and the molecular mechanism of its nuclear import pathway. Cancer Metastasis Rev. 2007;26:605–10.
48. Yashiro M, Nishioka N, Hirakawa K. K-ras mutation influences macroscopic features of gastric carcinoma. J Surg Res. 2005;124:74–8.
49. Compagno D, Tiraboschi C, Garcia JD, Rondon Y, Corapi E, Velazquez C, Laderach DJ. Galectins as checkpoints of the immune system in cancers, their clinical relevance, and implication in clinical trials. Biomol Ther. 2020;10:750.
50. Lv Y, Ma X, Ma Y, Du Y, Feng J. A new emerging target in cancer immunotherapy: Galectin-9 (LGALS9). Genes Dis. 2023;10:2366–82.
51. Yang R, Sun L, Li C-F, Wang Y-H, Yao J, Li H, Yan M, Chang W-C, Hsu J-M, Cha J-H. Galectin-9 interacts with PD-1 and TIM-3 to regulate T cell death and is a target for cancer immunotherapy. Nat Commun. 2021;12:832.
52. Zhang W, Huang Q, Xiao W, Zhao Y, Pi J, Xu H, Zhao H, Xu J, Evans CE, Jin H. Advances in anti-tumor treatments targeting the CD47/SIRPα axis. Front Immunol. 2020;11:18.
53. Zhao CL, Yu S, Wang SH, Li SG, Wang ZJ, Han SN. Characterization of cluster of differentiation 47 expression and its potential as a therapeutic target in esophageal squamous cell cancer. Oncol Lett. 2018;15:2017–23.
54. Yu C-P, Fu S-F, Chen X, Ye J, Ye Y, Kong L-D, Zhu Z. The clinicopathological and prognostic significance of IDO1 expression in human solid tumors: evidence from a systematic review and meta-analysis. Cell Physiol Biochem. 2018;49:134–43.
55. Liu M, Wang X, Wang L, Ma X, Gong Z, Zhang S, Li Y. Targeting the IDO1 pathway in cancer: from bench to bedside. J Hematol Oncol. 2018;11:1–12.
56. Angata T. Siglec-15: a potential regulator of osteoporosis, cancer, and infectious diseases. J Biomed Sci. 2020;27:10.
57. Göoz P, Göoz M, Baldys A, Hoffman S. ADAM-17 regulates endothelial cell morphology, proliferation, and in vitro angiogenesis. Biochem Biophys Res Commun. 2009;380:33–8.
58. Sun X, Wang Y, Ma R, Li W. Clinical significance of ADAM10 and ADAM17 in gastric and colorectal cancers: a systematic review and meta-analysis. Int J Clin Exp Med. 2017;10:5941–8.
59. Molfetta R, Zitti B, Lecce M, Milito ND, Stabile H, Fionda C, Cippitelli M, Gismondi A, Santoni A, Paolini R. CD155: a multi-functional molecule in tumor progression. Int J Mol Sci. 2020;21:922.
60. Deuss FA, Watson GM, Fu Z, Rossjohn J, Berry R. Structural basis for CD96 immune receptor recognition of nectin-like protein-5, CD155. Structure. 2019;27:219–228.e213.
61. Li Y-C, Zhou Q, Song Q-K, Wang R-B, Lyu S, Guan X, Zhao Y-J, Wu J-P. Overexpression of an immune checkpoint (CD155) in breast cancer associated with prognostic significance and exhausted tumor-infiltrating lymphocytes: a cohort study. J Immunol Res. 2020;2020:3948928.
62. Calinescu A, Turcu G, Nedelcu RI, Brinzea A, Hodorogea A, Antohe M, Diaconu C, Bleotu C, Pirici D, Jilaveanu LB. On the dual role of carcinoembryonic antigen-related cell adhesion molecule 1 (CEACAM1) in human malignancies. J Immunol Res. 2018;2018:7169081.
63. Mur P, García-Mulero S, Del Valle J, Magraner-Pardo L, Vidal A, Pineda M, et al. Role of POLE and POLD1 in familial cancer. Genet Med. 2020;22(12):2089–100. https://doi.org/10.1038/s41436-020-0922-2.
64. Hu F, Wang J, Zhang M, Wang S, Zhao L, Yang H, et al. Comprehensive analysis of subtype-specific molecular characteristics of colon cancer: specific genes, driver genes, signaling pathways, and immunotherapy responses. Front Cell Dev Biol. 2021;9:758776. https://doi.org/10.3389/fcell.2021.758776.
65. Li SKH, Martin A. Mismatch repair and colon cancer: mechanisms and therapies explored. Trends Mol Med. 2016;22(4):274–89. https://doi.org/10.1016/J.molmed.2016.02.003.
66. van Velzen MJM, Derks S, van Grieken NCT, Haj Mohammad N, van Laarhoven HWM. MSI as a predictive factor for treatment outcome of gastroesophageal adenocarcinoma. Cancer Treat Rev. 2020;86:102024. https://doi.org/10.1016/j.ctrv.2020.102024.

67. McCarthy AJ, Capo-Chichi JM, Spence T, Grenier S, Stockley T, Kamel- Reid S, et al. Heterogenous loss of mismatch repair (MMR) protein expression: a challenge for immunohistochemical interpretation and microsatellite instability (MSI) evaluation. J Pathol Clin Res. 2019;5(2):115–29. https://doi.org/10.1002/cjp2.120.
68. Lipson EJ, Sharfman WH, Drake CG, Wollner I, Taube JM, Anders RA, et al. Durable cancer regression off-treatment and effective reinduction therapy with an anti-PD-1 antibody. Clin Cancer Res. 2013;19(2):462–8. https://doi.org/10.1158/1078-0432.CCR-12-2625.
69. Le DT, Kim TW, Van Cutsem E, Geva R, Jäger D, Hara H, et al. Phase II open-label study of pembrolizumab in treatment-refractory, microsatellite instability-high/mismatch repair-deficient metastatic colorectal cancer: KEYNOTE-164. J Clin Oncol. 38(1):11–9.
70. Chan TA, Yarchoan M, Jaffee E, Swanton C, Quezada SA, Stenzinger A, et al. Development of tumor mutation burden as an immunotherapy biomarker: utility for the oncology clinic. Ann Oncol. 2019;30(1):44–56. https://doi.org/10.1093/annonc/mdy495.
71. Kang K, Xie F, Mao J, Bai Y, Wang X. Significance of tumor mutation burden in immune infiltration and prognosis in cutaneous melanoma. Front Oncol. 2020;10:573141. https://doi.org/10.3389/fonc.2020.573141.
72. Innocenti F, Ou FS, Qu X, Zemla TJ, Niedzwiecki D, Tam R, et al. Mutational analysis of patients with colorectal cancer in CALGB/SWOG 80405 identifies new roles of microsatellite instability and tumor mutational burden for patient outcome. J Clin Oncol. 2019;37(14):1217–27. https://doi.org/10.1200/JCO.18.01798.
73. Mosalem O, Coston TW, Imperial R, Mauer E, Thompson C, Yilma B, Bekaii-Saab TS, Stoppler MC, Starr JS. A comprehensive analysis of POLE/POLD1 genomic alterations in colorectal cancer. Oncologist. 2024;29(9):e1224–7. https://doi.org/10.1093/oncolo/oyae098. PMID: 38776551; PMCID: PMC11379631.
74. Bae JM, Yoo SY, Kim JH, Kang GH. Immune landscape and biomarkers for immuno-oncology in colorectal cancers. J Pathol Transl Med. 2020;54(5):351–60. https://doi.org/10.4132/jptm.2020.05.15. Epub 2020 Jun 26. PMID: 32580539; PMCID: PMC7483026.
75. Le DT, Uram JN, Wang H, Bartlett BR, Kemberling H, Eyring AD, Skora AD, Luber BS, Azad NS, Laheru D, Biedrzycki B, Donehower RC, Zaheer A, Fisher GA, Crocenzi TS, Lee JJ, Duffy SM, Goldberg RM, de la Chapelle A, Koshiji M, Bhaijee F, Huebner T, Hruban RH, Wood LD, Cuka N, Pardoll DM, Papadopoulos N, Kinzler KW, Zhou S, Cornish TC, Taube JM, Anders RA, Eshleman JR, Vogelstein B, Diaz LA Jr. PD-1 Blockade in tumors with mismatch-repair deficiency. N Engl J Med. 2015;372(26):2509–20. https://doi.org/10.1056/NEJMoa1500596. Epub 2015 May 30. PMID: 26028255; PMCID: PMC4481136.
76. Le DT, Diaz LA Jr, Kim TW, Van Cutsem E, Geva R, Jäger D, Hara H, Burge M, O'Neil BH, Kavan P, Yoshino T, Guimbaud R, Taniguchi H, Élez E, Al-Batran SE, Boland PM, Cui Y, Leconte P, Marinello P, André T. Pembrolizumab for previously treated, microsatellite instability-high/mismatch repair-deficient advanced colorectal cancer: final analysis of KEYNOTE-164. Eur J Cancer. 2023;186:185–95. https://doi.org/10.1016/j.ejca.2023.02.016. Epub 2023 Feb 24. PMID: 37141828.
77. André T, Shiu KK, Kim TW, Jensen BV, Jensen LH, Punt C, Smith D, Garcia-Carbonero R, Benavides M, Gibbs P, de la Fouchardiere C, Rivera F, Elez E, Bendell J, Le DT, Yoshino T, Van Cutsem E, Yang P, Farooqui MZH, Marinello P, Diaz LA Jr. KEYNOTE-177 investigators. Pembrolizumab in microsatellite-instability-high advanced colorectal cancer. N Engl J Med. 2020;383(23):2207–18. https://doi.org/10.1056/NEJMoa2017699. PMID: 33264544.
78. Overman MJ, McDermott R, Leach JL, Lonardi S, Lenz HJ, Morse MA, Desai J, Hill A, Axelson M, Moss RA, Goldberg MV, Cao ZA, Ledeine JM, Maglinte GA, Kopetz S, André T. Nivolumab in patients with metastatic DNA mismatch repair-deficient or microsatellite instability-high colorectal cancer (CheckMate 142): an open-label, multicentre, phase 2 study. Lancet Oncol. 2017;18(9):1182–1191. https://doi.org/10.1016/S1470-2045(17)30422-9. Epub 2017 Jul 19. Erratum in: Lancet Oncol. 2017;18(9):510. https://doi.org/10.1016/S1470-2045(17)30638-1. PMID: 28734759; PMCID: PMC6207072.
79. André T, Berton D, Curigliano G, Sabatier R, Tinker AV, Oaknin A, Ellard S, de Braud F, Arkenau HT, Trigo J, Gravina A, Kristeleit R, Moreno V, Abdeddaim C, Vano YA, Samouëlian

V, Miller R, Boni V, Torres AA, Gilbert L, Brown J, Dewal N, Dabrowski C, Antony G, Zografos E, Veneris J, Banerjee S. Antitumor activity and safety of dostarlimab monotherapy in patients with mismatch repair deficient solid tumors: a nonrandomized controlled trial. JAMA Netw Open. 2023;6(11):e2341165. https://doi.org/10.1001/jamanetworkopen.2023.41165. PMID: 37917058; PMCID: PMC10623195.

80. Zhang L, Geng Z, Hao B, et al. Tislelizumab: a modified anti-tumor programmed death receptor 1 antibody. Cancer Control. 2022;29:10732748221111296.
81. Li J, Xu Y, Zang A, et al. Tislelizumab in previously treated, locally advanced unresectable/metastatic microsatellite instability-high/mismatch repair-deficient solid tumors. Chin J Cancer Res. 2024;36:257–69.
82. ClinicalTrials.gov. Cemiplimab for localized dMMR colon cancer (Phoenix Trial). Available from: https://clinicaltrials.gov/ct2/show/NCT05961709
83. ClinicalTrials.gov. Study of REGN7075 in combination with cemiplimab in advanced solid tumors. Available from: https://clinicaltrials.gov/ct2/show/NCT04626635
84. ClinicalTrials.gov. SNS-101 alone and in combination with cemiplimab in advanced solid tumors. Available from: https://clinicaltrials.gov/ct2/show/NCT05864144
85. Berton D, Pautier P, Lorusso D, et al. Antitumor activity and safety of the PD-1inhibitor retifanlimab in patients with recurrent microsatellite instability high or deficient mismatch repair endometrial cancer: final safety and efficacy results from cohort H of the POD1UM-101 phase I study. Gynecol Oncol. 2024;186:191–8.
86. Lakhani N, Cosman R, Banerji U, et al. A first-in-human phase I study of the PD-1 inhibitor, retifanlimab (INCMGA00012), in patients with advanced solid tumors (POD1UM-101). ESMO Open. 2024;9:102254.
87. https://clinicaltrials.gov/ct2/show/NCT05608044/CgSASoICiMCCAf
88. Overman MJ, Lonardi S, Wong KYM, Lenz HJ, Gelsomino F, Aglietta M, Morse MA, Van Cutsem E, McDermott R, Hill A, Sawyer MB, Hendlisz A, Neyns B, Svrcek M, Moss RA, Ledeine JM, Cao ZA, Kamble S, Kopetz S, André T. Durable clinical benefit with nivolumab plus ipilimumab in DNA mismatch repair-deficient/microsatellite instability-high metastatic colorectal cancer. J Clin Oncol. 2018;36(8):773–9. https://doi.org/10.1200/JCO.2017.76.9901. Epub 2018 Jan 20. PMID: 29355075.

# Immunotherapy in Glioblastoma

# 6

Andrew Williams and Rimas V. Lukas

## 6.1 Introduction

Glioblastoma (GBM) isocitrate dehydrogenase wild type (IDHwt) is the most common primary malignant brain tumor of the central nervous system (CNS) in adults. It has an annual incidence of approximately 3 per 100,000 people [1]. Despite extensive research into various treatment options, the standard of care for management of this disease has been unchanged since the advent of temozolomide in 2005 [2] and tumor-treating fields in 2012 [3] and 2015 [4, 5]. Outcomes remain poor with median overall survival (OS) of 12–21 months [3, 4].

Given this background, there has been significant interest in developing alternate lines of treatment for GBM in the hopes of improving OS. One area of potential treatment in which there has been particular focus in recent years is that of immunotherapy. At a broad level, this is intuitive. The immune system plays a significant role in preventing the growth of malignant cells, and immunotherapeutic approaches have delivered major breakthroughs in other areas of oncology—for example, the blockade of programmed death 1 (PD-1) and cytotoxic T lymphocyte-associated protein 4 (CTLA4) initially in advanced melanoma, and subsequently across a variety of cancers, has resulted in a dramatic increase in survival with a multifold increase in median OS as well as recurrence-free survival in a large subset of patients [6]. The potential for an improvement in treatment for GBM of this magnitude has obvious appeal.

Unfortunately, the theoretical potential of immunotherapy in GBM has yet to be realized in clinical practice. Most clinical trial results in this area have thus far failed to show significant improvements in OS. In this chapter, we will explore foundational principles of the use of immunotherapy in the brain broadly and in GBM

A. Williams · R. V. Lukas (✉)
Department of Neurology, Lou & Jean Malnati Brain Tumor Institute, Northwestern University, Evanston, IL, USA
e-mail: rimas.lukas@nm.org



R. Salgia, P. Kulkarni (eds.), *Immunotherapies in Solid Tumors*, Cancer Treatment and Research 129, https://doi.org/10.1007/978-3-031-97242-3_6

specifically, review the various classes of immunotherapies that have been trialed for GBM, and consider potential future directions for research in this area.

## 6.2 The Immune System, the Brain, and GBM

To understand the landscape of clinical trials in this area, we must first highlight knowledge regarding the relationship between the immune system, the brain, and particularly GBM.

It is well established that the brain is a relatively "immunoprivileged" organ. By this we mean that there is a differentiation between immune responses occurring elsewhere in the body, and immune activity occurring in the brain. Evolutionary advantages may underpin this as the CNS is generally comprised of terminally differentiated cells with limited capacity for regeneration and innumerable physical connections which form the basis of neurologic functioning including cognition. An inflammatory response which disrupts this delicate and complex network may have catastrophic consequences. In addition, the CNS sits within the bony non-expansile confines of the skull and spinal canal, limiting the CNS's ability to tolerate substantial inflammation without additional CNS injury caused by the direct compression of its components against the bone and other fixed structures.

This immune privilege is mediated by numerous factors. These include the physical structure of the blood-brain barrier (BBB) as well as the intrinsically limited capacity of the brain's innate immune cells (microglia) to promote an immune response and for the myeloid-derived immune cells to contribute to and refine this response [7]. As an example, natural killer (NK) cells which are felt to play a critical role in the immune system's innate ability to eliminate malignant cells are known to have a very limited presence within the brain parenchyma [8, 9]. This means that the normal pathways used by the immune system to eliminate tumor cells are less active within the brain, and also pose a barrier to the use of immunotherapies for brain tumors. In addition, the negative feedback mechanisms (the "off switches") of the immune system may be more sensitive in the CNS. An example of this, the indoleamine 2,3 dioxygenase 1 (IDO) pathway will be discussed below.

This relationship between the brain and the immune system is not fixed, but evolves over the lifespan. In particular, the immunosuppressive environment of the brain becomes more harsh with age. As an example, IDO is an enzyme that is involved in the catabolic conversion of tryptophan to kynurenine. Kyneurenine plays a role in immunosuppression and may serve as a nexus for numerous processes leading to CNS dysfunction [10]. The pathway initiated by IDO is closely associated with a state of chronic inflammation and this state inhibits the activity of immune cells via numerous downstream mechanisms [11]. An age-dependent relationship exists with respect to IDO expression within the brain, with increased age associated with increased expression setting the stage for more limited immune activity in the aging brain.

Beyond the overall immunologically isolated status of the brain, GBM itself has specific features which impair the ability of immune cells to interact with the tumor.

First, tumor-infiltrating lymphocytes (TILs) tend to be present in very low density within GBM tissue [12]. It has been shown that TILs have a tendency to accumulate in the perivascular niche rather than penetrating well into the tumor parenchyma of GBM, and that TIL accretion in the perivascular niche is associated with worsened outcomes [13]. TILs are also inhibited, at least in part, by tumor-associated macrophages. In particular, M2-polarized macrophages have an immunosuppressive effect and are found in abundance within GBM tissue. Their presence is correlated with worsened survival outcomes [14, 15]. Finally, the physical microstructure of GBM with filopodia and microvilli may make it more resilient against cytotoxic damage inflicted by TILs [16]. Because TILs are a fundamental component of the immune response to malignancy, the inability of these cells to appropriately engage GBM greatly limits the impact of immunotherapeutics which heavily rely on TILs [17].

All of these factors also exist within the highly heterogenous intratumoral environment of GBM. Recent research has illustrated a great deal of genetic and epigenetic variation exists within each individual tumor. This heterogeneity directly effects treatment targets such as expression of specific protein sequences that may be targeted by therapies such as vaccines antibody-mediated approaches, and chimeric antigen receptor T cells (CAR T). This adds an additional layer of difficulty in developing treatments that successfully affect the entire tumor [18, 19]. Finally, our understanding of the dynamic immune milieu in GBM is limited by accessibility of tissue in both humans and animal models. Even at the time of initial diagnosis, certainly in humans and in most animal models, the tissue analyzed represents well-established tumors. We do not have a good glimpse at the immune milieu at the time of tumorigenesis, nor is it easy to evaluate it over the course of the disease.

In essence, the tumor cells in GBM are extremely isolated from the normal functioning immune system at large through a combination of the intrinsic immune isolated status of the CNS, increasing CNS immunosuppression with age, and the "cold" microenvironment of GBM that makes it difficult for immune cells to penetrate the tumor and actively suppresses immune cells that do manage to enter the tumor parenchyma.

It is on this challenging background that numerous clinical trials have attempted to overcome these limitations and enhance the immune response to GBM.

## 6.3 Vaccine Therapies

The concept of vaccination involves the presentation of antigens to the immune system to stimulate the production of antibodies targeting those antigens, and directly neutralizing the targeted cells or pointing the other components of both the innate and the adaptive immune system toward a specific target. While most commonly used to prevent infectious disease, vaccines have demonstrated benefit in both the prevention of virally driven malignancies as well as the treatment of other established malignancies. There are a small number of therapeutic vaccines for malignancy in active clinical use today, perhaps most notably sipuleucel-T which was approved by the FDA in 2010 for use in prostate cancer, a not overly immunogenic tumor [20].

However, in light of the tolerability and often scalability of this approach, there has been great interest in utilizing a vaccine-based method in the treatment of GBM. To date, no trials have successfully demonstrated an improved clinical outcome from vaccine-based approaches in GBM. This is likely secondary to the significant challenges of the tumor microenvironment as discussed in the previous section. However, it remains worth examining these trials as they suggest some potential avenues for future research, particularly if combined with other therapies discussed in the later sections that could modify the tumor microenvironment to improve the efficacy of vaccine-based therapies.

Vaccines for GBM can be separated into two categories, standardized vaccines (where every patient is given the exact same agent) and personalized vaccines where each patient is given a custom agent based on the unique profile of their tumor. We will first examine the standardized vaccines.

The best studied of these is rindopepimut (formerly CDX-110), a single epitope standardized vaccine containing the peptide sequence for the epidermal growth factor receptor variant III (EGFRvIII) deletion mutation. Unlike the tyrosine kinase domain EGFR mutations frequently observed in lung cancer, EGFRvIII encodes a cell surface tumor-specific epitope. This mutation is estimated to be present in ~30 percent of GBM and is correlated with worsened OS [21]. The ACT III study was a phase 2 trial using rindopepimut for EGFRVIII expressing newly diagnosed GBM patients which showed promising results with a median OS of 21.8 months [22]. Similarly, the randomized phase 2 ReACT trial for patients with recurrent GBM demonstrated improvement on secondary endpoints such as OS [23]. However, these findings were not recapitulated in the larger phase 3 trial ACT IV trial for patients with newly diagnosed GBM [24].

Another recently developed single epitope vaccine focuses on survivin (SurVaxM). Survivin is an apoptosis inhibitor protein which is highly expressed in a variety of cancers with breast cancer the most frequent but also in GBM [25]. It's expression can be induced by radiation therapy. A small phase 2a study demonstrated safety of the vaccine but it is not clear at this time if it has a benefit on outcomes [26]. Currently, a placebo-controlled trial (SURVIVE) of the survivin vaccine plus temozolomide in newly diagnosed GBM has completed accrual, and final results are awaited [27].

Given the limited results in GBM with single epitope vaccines, there has been emerging interest in vaccines which target several different epitopes rather than just one. Multi-epitope vaccines have theoretical advantages for overcoming GBM heterogeneity and have demonstrated efficacy against GBM in silico and have been demonstrated to delay tumor progression in a mouse model [28, 29]. In humans, to our knowledge only early phase trials have been completed—for example, TAS0313 which is a multi-epitope vaccine carrying three large peptide chains potentially applicable in multiple different cancers for which a phase 1/2 trial demonstrated safety in GBM patients [30].

Another avenue of investigation for GBM vaccine therapies is personalized therapy—vaccines which are customized to each patient. These can fall into two distinct categories: those derived from the individual patients' tumor tissue and those whose tumor tissue is used to select from an array of epitopes aligning with those expressed by the patient's tumor.

In GBM specifically, a phase 3 trial has been completed for an autologous tumor lysate-loaded dendritic cell vaccine (DCVax-L). This vaccine is created by harvesting dendritic cells from the patient, exposing them to antigens from the patient's tumor, and then administering them back to the patient to initiate a more robust immune response against the tumor [31]. The phase 3 trial was unable to demonstrate a survival advantage with the use of the vaccine. Cross-over study design makes it unclear if this is due to lack of efficacy [32].

Another example of an extensively studied GBM patient-specific vaccine targeted heat shock protein-peptide complex 96 (HSPPC-96). Heat shock protein complexes are expressed in tumors and can be utilized by antigen-presenting cells to trigger an immune response against the tumor. HSPPC-96 utilizes heat shock proteins from the patient's tumor to stimulate an immune response. An HSPPC-96 vaccine has been utilized safely in phase 1 and 2 trials, but efficacy has not been successfully demonstrated to date [33, 34].

Finally, an example of the patient's tumor being used to select the epitope palette specific to the patient has demonstrated the ability to promote appropriate systemic T-cell responses and evidence of infiltration of said T cells into the tumor [35].

In summary, thus far vaccine-based therapies for GBM while able to stimulate peripheral immune responses to the delineated targets have not demonstrated efficacy in terms of improved OS.

## 6.4 Immune Checkpoint Inhibitors

Immune checkpoint inhibitors have been one of the most significant breakthroughs in oncology in this century thus far by disinhibiting the immune system to increase its intrinsic anti-cancer properties. Naturally, attempts have been made to utilize this revolutionary class of therapies against GBM. Unfortunately, results have not been as successful as initially anticipated. The programmed death receptor-1 (PD-1) antibodies have been the most extensively studied and will serve as the primary focus of our discussion.

Inhibition of the PD-1 receptor on T cells prevents inactivation of the T cells by inhibiting binding of PD-1 ligands (PD-L1) on other immune cells or tumor cells. Therefore, when PD-1 is inhibited the T-cell anti-tumor response is amplified [36]. As noted earlier, PD-1 blockade has been utilized successfully in the treatment of malignancies such as metastatic melanoma.

Multiple large trials have investigated the utility of PD-1 blockade in GBM. The phase 3 CHECKMATE 143, 548, and 498 trials have utilized the PD-1 antibody nivolumab. Unfortunately, all three of these trials failed to show improvement in OS compared to standard of care. Earlier phase studies have evaluated other PD-1 antibodies as well as those targeting the respective ligand (PD-L1) [37].

Questions regarding the optimal timing of PD-1 blockade have arisen, with suggestions that pre-operative treatment may have a greater potential for efficacy. When PD-1 antibodies are given in a neoadjuvant fashion prior to surgery with continued dosing post-operatively, as compared to being given post-operatively alone an OS benefit has been observed [38]. Note here the similarity to the rindopepimut vaccine trial which showed benefit only in recurrent tumors. These data suggest that administration of immunotherapy prior to tumor resection may be more likely to confer benefit, perhaps due to increased volume of tumor antigens to help promote reaction at the time the immune system is "primed" with the immunotherapy.

Another immune checkpoint that has been explored for use in GBM is cytotoxic T lymphocyte-associated protein 4 (CTLA-4). This receptor found on T cells also triggers immunosuppression when it binds the B7 ligands (CD80 and CD86) on target cells, so blockade of CTLA-4 amplifies immune activity [37]. Ipilimumab is a monoclonal antibody targeting CTLA-4. It is often used for cancer treatment alongside a PD-1-targeting agent such as nivolumab, typically administered only at the beginning of the treatment course. This combination has been evaluated in GBM initially in cohorts of the CHECKMATE 143 trial and more recently in the definitive NRG BN007 trial [39, 40]. Unfortunately, the combination of ipilimumab and nivolumab failed to improve progression-free survival in newly diagnosed GBM and no signal toward improved OS has been observed thus far [40].

A number of additional immune checkpoint inhibitors including atezolizumab, avelumab, cemiplimab, durvalumab, relatlimab, and tislelizumab have also been investigated in trials in GBM but none have shown benefit [37]. The expression of immune checkpoint ligand proteins in GBM is known to be highly variable and this may be one of the factors contributing to the variable immune checkpoint inhibitor efficacy in GBM, in combination with the challenging tumor microenvironment as previously discussed [41]. The ability of these antibodies to adequately cross the BBB is another hypothesized reason for lack of adequate success. There are ongoing studies using focused low-intensity ultrasound to help overcome this limitation [42]. While immune checkpoint inhibitors thus far have failed to live up to the lofty expectations that they had set up for themselves based on performance outside of the CNS, there still remains the possibility of further developments in this space.

## 6.5 Modulation of the Tumor Microenvironment

As we discussed in the first section, the microenvironment of GBM is a hostile immunosuppressive space that limits the activity of the immune system in and around the tumor tissue. Recent research has begun investigating the possibility of therapies that could directly reconfigure this environment to make it a less hostile region for immune cells. These types of upstream approaches can more broadly activate the immune system potentially overcoming the difficulty related to intratumoral heterogeneity.

We discussed earlier how the enzyme IDO initiates a chronic maladaptive inflammatory state within the GBM microenvironment that helps to inhibit the immune response making this pathway a potential therapeutic target [7]. Promising results have been seen in murine studies with IDO inhibitors, typically when combined with other immunotherapeutic and non-immunotherapeutic approaches [43, 44]. Clinical trials in this area remain in the early stages. A single phase 1 trial has been completed with the IDO inhibitor PF-06840003 in patients with recurrent malignant glioma and was found to have a good safety profile, but further clinical data will be needed [45].

Another viable strategy is to either neutralize or phenotypically convert the immunosuppressive tumor-associated macrophages (TAMs) to be more immune stimulatory [46]. This has the potential for substantial impact as TAMs comprise the largest immune cell population in GBM. It is possible that the initial function of TAMs early in the disease course may be immune stimulatory, however, as noted earlier we are observing well-established tumors in our clinical samples, representing a time point after a shift to the immunosuppressive M2 phenotype has already occurred. A variety of different approaches have been and are undergoing exploration. One of these, the targeting of colony-stimulating factor 1 receptor (CSF1R) on macrophages, in turn blocking binding of the growth factors colony-stimulating factor 1 (CSF1) and interleukin-34 (IL-34) has not demonstrated efficacy as a monotherapy [47].

The microenvironment is an area of great promise in glioblastoma treatment. Therapies in this area remain in the early phases at present, but further data are likely to emerge in the coming years.

## 6.6 Stimulating the Immune System

Modulation of the microenvironment to make it "warmer" for the immune system as we just discussed is one avenue of potential treatment, but another is directly stimulating it to make the microenvironment "hot". A variety of immunostimulatory approaches have been investigated in GBM. Like immune modulation, this type of approach can be a means of addressing the intratumoral heterogeneity which limits very focused approaches such as many vaccine therapies.

The first we will discuss is a key pathway which leads to broad activation of innate and adaptive immune responses. The cyclic GMP-AMP synthase/stimulator of interferon genes (cGAS/STING) pathway detects products of DNA injury (often associated with tumor cells) and in response increases type 1 interferon (IFN) production, stimulating an immune response which leads to the production of additional immunostimulatory cytokines and the activation of innate and adaptive immune cells [48]. Signal transducer and activator of transcription 3 (STAT3) is a protein which is heavily expressed in GBM [49]. STAT3 is known to inhibit the cGAS/STING pathway which in turn decreases immune response to the tumor, serving as a "break" on this pathway [50]. One, in turn, could either inhibit the "break" (STAT3) or step on the "accelerator" (STING) to initiate and augment an immune response.

On this basis, research is currently active regarding the possibility of STAT3 inhibition. STAT3 inhibitors currently exist in an early research phase, though data is promising. The ability of STAT3 inhibitors to slow GBM growth has been shown both in vitro and in murine models [51–53]. Ongoing clinical trials of STAT3 inhibitors will be essential for evaluating the potential benefit of this approach. Research is also underway with STING agonists. In a canine model, the STING agonist IACS-8779 showed radiographic volume reduction of GBM [54]. In a mouse model, another STING agonist (8803) also showed significant increases in median survival including as monotherapy and when combined with a PD-1 inhibitor [55]. Human trials are being developed to determine safety and efficacy of this drug class.

As discussed in the introduction, part of the current standard of care for GBM is the use of tumor-treating fields (TTF) which were established to prolong OS in the phase 3 EF-14 trial [4]. This treatment was initially understood to work by using low-intensity electric fields to interfere with the mitotic spindle, resulting in apoptosis. However, recent work has shown that TTF triggers the cGAS/STING pathway discussed above, which helps to promote immune targeting of the tumor cells [56]. On this basis, the 2-THE-TOP phase 2 trial was conducted adding pembrolizumab to TTF and temozolomide for newly diagnosed GBM after resection. [57] Results appear favorable, leading to the initiation of a definitive phase 3 trial. Interestingly, more substantial improvements in patients with larger volume residual tumors (again suggesting a need for tumor volume to help stimulate a stronger immune response) [58].

Another front for enhancing the immune response to GBM is cytokine-based therapies. Cytokines are small molecules that help to regulate the inflammatory state of the tumor microenvironment. Individual cytokines can broadly be categorized as either pro or anti-inflammatory (although there is much nuance to this). There has been significant interest in utilizing cytokine-based treatments to try and encourage the immune response against tumors. Therapeutic strategies can consist of either blocking immunosuppressive or augmenting immunostimulatory cytokines. For example, multiple trials have been pursued investigating inhibitors of the cytokines TGF-β which is understood to play an immunosuppressive role in the GBM microenvironment, but these trials have failed to show clear benefit [59]. As an example of reshaping the tumor microenvironment, CSF-1 is another cytokine which promotes differentiation of macrophages into immunosuppressive M2 macrophages. CSF-1 inhibitors have also been trialed to try and ease the microenvironment and boost immune response, but were found to be ineffective [59].

In addition to cytokine inhibitors, there has also been research into utilizing anti-tumor cytokines—most prominently, IL-12 which promotes release of IFN-γ which in turn increases T-cell infiltration into tumors [59]. However, systemic activation of IL-12 carries significant adverse effects so a mechanism is needed to target the IL-12 activity to within the cancer tissue. A viral vector has been utilized to deliver IL-12 to GBM while minimizing systemic effects. This was demonstrated in phase 1 and 2 clinical trials using the viral IL-12 vector Ad-RTS-hIL-12 triggered by the oral activator veledimex which showed the safety of the delivery mechanism and increased inflammatory infiltrate within tumor tissue [60, 61]. Further research into efficacy of this treatment and other viral vector IL-12 agents is ongoing [59]. Human umbilical cord blood-derived mesenchymal stem cells have also been utilized as a delivery mechanism for modified IL-12 in animal studies with early promising results [62].

Another area which has been investigated to enhance immune activity in GBM is oncolytic viruses. These specifically engineered viruses are designed with the intent of replicating within tumor cells and producing pro-immune molecules that will result in an increased immune response to the tumor. These have been previously utilized in tumors such as melanoma with promising results [63]. There has been significant interest in applying this principle to treatment of GBM. Multiple early trials and case series have utilized oncolytic viruses in the treatment of GBM with a good safety profile and some promising results that warrant larger trials in the coming years [64–66].

An emerging area of prospective immunostimulatory therapy for GBM is the use of bi-specific T-cell engagers (BiTE). These are molecules which bind a tumor antigen on one side and cytotoxic T cells on the other side, drawing the T cells in to target the tumor. There is a long history of efficacy of such approaches in the treatment of cancer. A BiTE agent (blinatumomab) was FDA-approved for use in acute lymphoblastic anemia in 2014 [67]. There has been interest in utilizing BiTE against GBM. At this time, BiTE therapy remains in the preclinical phase but has demonstrated promise in vitro and in mouse models [68–70]. There remains concern that these agents may have difficulty penetrating the blood-brain barrier which could limit their efficacy, and this will need to be considered as potential human trials for these agents move forward [71]. One could imagine that the focused low-intensity ultrasound approach for altering BBB permeability could also be applicable here [42].

A final area of research in the immunostimulatory arena which we will highlight is phagocytic cell signaling pathways. CD47 is a protein expressed on normal healthy cells that binds with SIRPα on macrophages to inhibit phagocytosis. It is known to be overexpressed in GBM and is felt to be a contributor to the harsh tumor microenvironment by repelling phagocytic cells. Multiple agents that inhibit the CD47/SIRPα pathway have shown promise in preclinical trials but human trials have not yet been performed. CD47 is also known to inhibit the pro-phagocytotic signaling molecule CALR and there has also been interest in developing agents that may enhance the function of CALR. However, thus far no trials for any of these agents have been performed in humans [72].

## 6.7 Immune Cell-Based Therapies

The final category of GBM immunotherapy that we will touch on is cell-based therapies. These therapies seek to directly administer specially modified versions of human immune cells that have been targeted to treat cancer. While these therapies have seen great success in other areas of oncology, their utility in GBM has been more limited thus far.

The most prominent cancer treatment in this category is chimeric antigen receptor T cells (CAR-T). CAR-T utilizes T cells which are taken from the patient and reengineered to specifically target antigens associated with the patient's cancer. CAR-T has shown great success in hematologic malignancies such as B-cell lymphomas and acute lymphoblastic leukemia where there is substantial clonal homogeneity [73, 74]. In general, CAR-T has not been nearly as successful in solid tumors due to multiple factors including the tumor microenvironment and tumor heterogeneity [75]. Unsurprisingly, there has not been great success with the use of CAR-T in GBM thus far. Early phase trials utilizing CAR-T for GBM have shown that the tumor can initially respond to the CAR-T treatment quite dramatically, but that this is followed by recurrence of the tumor. Decreased expression of the sequence targeted by the CAR-T has been noted in the recurrent tumor, suggesting heterogeneity as the primary reason for the failures of CAR-T in this setting, similar to how single epitope vaccines have been inadequately effective [76, 77].

To get beyond the highly efficient, but somewhat overly focused attack of CAR-T cells, other immune cell types with less discriminatory cell-killing potential are being investigated. One such example is gamma-delta T-cell therapy. Gamma-delta T cells have recently been recognized for their anti-cancer potential in numerous subfields of oncology. They play a natural role in maintenance of the gut microbiome and also play a role in the innate anti-cancer response [78]. There has been increasing interest in utilizing engineered gamma-delta T cells to target specific cancers including colon cancer, B-cell malignancies, and breast cancer [78–80]. GBM has been identified as another potential target for this line of therapy. The INB-200 trial is an ongoing phase 1 trial evaluating the use of specifically gamma-delta T cells engineered to be resistant to the lymphocytic side effects of temozolomide chemotherapy, allowing the two approaches to be used in combination. Early trial data has shown feasibility and tolerability, as well as a possible increase in PFS when treated with the gamma-delta T cells [81].

The third and final area of current research in cell-based therapy for GBM is natural killer (NK) cell therapy. NK cells are part of the innate anti-tumor response. Very limited presence of these cells is noted in GBM tissue samples. The utilization of this cell type capable of undifferentiated tumor cell killing could prove to be effective. It could lead to direct tumor cell cytotoxicity and further stimulate the adaptive immune response for more efficient and continued tumor cell killing. There is hope since as with other cell-based approaches, positive results have been seen in other cancers, especially in hematologic malignancies [82]. One example of this approach combined the broad activity of NK cells with the targeted focus of CAR T cells. A phase 1 trial using intracranial injection of NK cells targeting the HER2 protein in patients with HER2-positive GBM. The trial demonstrated safety and showed some early evidence of immune response in the tumor triggered by the NK cell injections [83].

Cell-based therapies hold potential promise for use in GBM but questions remain about their efficacy in the face of tumor heterogeneity which has a tendency to impair treatments targeted against individual protein markers in GBM. Further research is needed as a role for these powerful therapies is determined.

## 6.8 Conclusion

The landscape of immunotherapy for GBM remains promising, particularly as we better understand the obstacles which need to be surmounted. The fundamentally limiting factors of the harsh tumor microenvironment and the great degree of heterogeneity within GBM tissue have limited the ability of many of these therapies to have significant impact on OS. In particular, therapies targeted against just a single protein or marker such as single epitope vaccines or CAR-T therapy may have greater barriers to success than therapies which enable the immune system to attack multiple different targets within the tumor and concurrently overcome the immunosuppressive milieu of the brain and brain tumor.

From this standpoint, it seems that perhaps the most useful immunotherapies for GBM will be those that, rather than directly targeting the tumor, instead alter the microenvironment around the tumor to enable the immune system to interact more closely with the tumor cells and hit multiple different markers simultaneously without having to be specifically directed at any one marker. As we gain a better understanding of the tumor microenvironment and the factors that limit the endogenous immune response, we will be able to combine the traditional therapies for GBM with therapies that can modify the microenvironment to allow the immune system to work in tandem with the traditional therapies in order to produce a more effective and durable treatment response. Much work remains to be done in this area to explore the untapped potential of the immune system to help combat this challenging disease.

## References


1. Price M, Ballard C, Benedetti J, et al. CBTRUS statistical report: primary brain and other central nervous system tumors diagnosed in the United States in 2017-2021. Neuro-Oncology. 2024;26(Suppl_6):vi1–vi85. https://doi.org/10.1093/neuonc/noae145.
2. Stupp R, Mason WP, van den Bent MJ, et al. Radiotherapy plus concomitant and adjuvant temozolomide for glioblastoma. N Engl J Med. 2005;352(10):987–96. https://doi.org/10.1056/NEJMoa043330.
3. Stupp R, Wong ET, Kanner AA, et al. NovoTTF-100A versus physician's choice chemotherapy in recurrent glioblastoma: a randomised phase III trial of a novel treatment modality. Eur J Cancer. 2012;48(14):2192–202. https://doi.org/10.1016/j.ejca.2012.04.011.
4. Stupp R, Taillibert S, Kanner A, et al. Effect of tumor-treating fields plus maintenance temozolomide vs maintenance temozolomide alone on survival in patients with glioblastoma: a randomized clinical trial [published correction appears in JAMA. 2018 May 1;319(17):1824. doi: 10.1001/jama.2018.3431.]. JAMA. 2017;318(23):2306–16. https://doi.org/10.1001/jama.2017.18718.
5. Stupp R, Taillibert S, Kanner AA, et al. Maintenance therapy with tumor-treating fields plus temozolomide vs temozolomide alone for glioblastoma: a randomized clinical trial. JAMA. 2015;314(23):2535–43. https://doi.org/10.1001/jama.2015.16669.
6. Wolchok JD, Chiarion-Sileni V, Rutkowski P, et al. Final, 10-year outcomes with nivolumab plus ipilimumab in advanced melanoma. N Engl J Med. 2025;392(1):11–22. https://doi.org/10.1056/NEJMoa2407417.

7. Muldoon LL, Alvarez JI, Begley DJ, et al. Immunologic privilege in the central nervous system and the blood-brain barrier. J Cereb Blood Flow Metab. 2013;33(1):13–21. https://doi.org/10.1038/jcbfm.2012.153.
8. Korin B, Ben-Shaanan TL, Schiller M, et al. High-dimensional, single-cell characterization of the brain's immune compartment. Nat Neurosci. 2017;20(9):1300–9. https://doi.org/10.1038/nn.4610.
9. Wolf NK, Kissiov DU, Raulet DH. Roles of natural killer cells in immunity to cancer, and applications to immunotherapy. Nat Rev Immunol. 2023;23(2):90–105. https://doi.org/10.1038/s41577-022-00732-1.
10. Heimberger AB, Lukas RV. The kynurenine pathway implicated in patient delirium: possible indications for indoleamine 2,3 dioxygenase inhibitors. J Clin Invest. 2023;133(2):e164577. https://doi.org/10.1172/JCI164577. Published 2023 Jan 17.
11. Salminen A. Role of indoleamine 2,3-dioxygenase 1 (IDO1) and kynurenine pathway in the regulation of the aging process. Ageing Res Rev. 2022;75:101573. https://doi.org/10.1016/j.arr.2022.101573.
12. Maddison K, Graves MC, Bowden NA, et al. Low tumour-infiltrating lymphocyte density in primary and recurrent glioblastoma. Oncotarget. 2021;12(21):2177–87. https://doi.org/10.18632/oncotarget.28069. Published 2021 Oct 12.
13. Mu L, Yang C, Gao Q, et al. CD4+ and perivascular Foxp3+ T cells in glioma correlate with angiogenesis and tumor progression. Front Immunol. 2017;8:1451. https://doi.org/10.3389/fimmu.2017.01451. Published 2017 Nov 7.
14. Zhang G, Tao X, Ji B, Gong J. Hypoxia-driven M2-polarized macrophages facilitate cancer aggressiveness and temozolomide resistance in glioblastoma. Oxidative Med Cell Longev. 2022;2022:1614336. https://doi.org/10.1155/2022/1614336. Published 2022 Aug 22.
15. Vidyarthi A, Agnihotri T, Khan N, et al. Predominance of M2 macrophages in gliomas leads to the suppression of local and systemic immunity. Cancer Immunol Immunother. 2019;68(12):1995–2004. https://doi.org/10.1007/s00262-019-02423-8.
16. Hoa N, Ge L, Kuznetsov Y, et al. Glioma cells display complex cell surface topographies that resist the actions of cytolytic effector lymphocytes. J Immunol. 2010;185(8):4793–803. https://doi.org/10.4049/jimmunol.1001526.
17. Yaping W, Zhe W, Zhuling C, et al. The soldiers needed to be awakened: tumor-infiltrating immune cells. Front Genet. 2022;13:988703. https://doi.org/10.3389/fgene.2022.988703. Published 2022 Sep 29.
18. Mathur R, Wang Q, Schupp PG, et al. Glioblastoma evolution and heterogeneity from a 3D whole-tumor perspective. Cell. 2024;187(2):446–463.e16. https://doi.org/10.1016/j.cell.2023.12.013.
19. Mangena V, Chanoch-Myers R, Sartore R, et al. Glioblastoma cortical organoids recapitulate cell-state heterogeneity and intercellular transfer. Cancer Discov. 2025;15(2):299–315. https://doi.org/10.1158/2159-8290.CD-23-1336.
20. Dutcher GMA, Bilen MA. Therapeutic vaccines for genitourinary malignancies. Vaccines (Basel). 2018;6(3):55. https://doi.org/10.3390/vaccines6030055. Published 2018 Aug 12.
21. Shinojima N, Tada K, Shiraishi S, et al. Prognostic value of epidermal growth factor receptor in patients with glioblastoma multiforme. Cancer Res. 2003;63(20):6962–70.
22. Schuster J, Lai RK, Recht LD, et al. A phase II, multicenter trial of rindopepimut (CDX-110) in newly diagnosed glioblastoma: the ACT III study. Neuro-Oncology. 2015;17(6):854–61. https://doi.org/10.1093/neuonc/nou348.
23. Reardon DA, Desjardins A, Vredenburgh JJ, et al. Rindopepimut with bevacizumab for patients with relapsed EGFRvIII-expressing glioblastoma (ReACT): results of a double-blind randomized phase II trial. Clin Cancer Res. 2020;26(7):1586–94. https://doi.org/10.1158/1078-0432.CCR-18-1140.
24. Weller M, Butowski N, Tran DD, et al. Rindopepimut with temozolomide for patients with newly diagnosed, EGFRvIII-expressing glioblastoma (ACT IV): a randomised, double-blind, international phase 3 trial. Lancet Oncol. 2017;18(10):1373–85. https://doi.org/10.1016/S1470-2045(17)30517-X.

25. Wheatley SP, Altieri DC. Survivin at a glance. J Cell Sci. 2019;132(7):jcs223826. https://doi.org/10.1242/jcs.223826. Published 2019 Apr 4.
26. Ahluwalia MS, Reardon DA, Abad AP, et al. Phase IIA study of SurVaxM plus adjuvant temozolomide for newly diagnosed glioblastoma. J Clin Oncol. 2023;41(7):1453–65. https://doi.org/10.1200/JCO.22.00996.
27. https://clinicaltrials.gov/study/NCT05163080
28. Salahlou R, Farajnia S, Alizadeh E, et al. Design and in silico analysis of a novel peptide-based multiepitope vaccine against glioblastoma multiforme by targeting tumor-associated macrophage. Heliyon. 2024;10(24):e40774. https://doi.org/10.1016/j.heliyon.2024.e40774. Published 2024 Nov 28.
29. Tran TA, Kim YH, Kim GE, et al. The long multi-epitope peptide vaccine combined with adjuvants improved the therapeutic effects in a glioblastoma mouse model. Front Immunol. 2022;13:1007285. https://doi.org/10.3389/fimmu.2022.1007285. Published 2022 Nov 9.
30. Narita Y, Okita Y, Arakawa Y. Evaluation of the efficacy and safety of TAS0313 in adults with recurrent glioblastoma. Cancer Immunol Immunother. 2022;71(11):2703–15. https://doi.org/10.1007/s00262-022-03184-7.
31. Yang L, Guo G, Niu XY, Liu J. Dendritic cell-based immunotherapy treatment for glioblastoma multiforme. Biomed Res Int. 2015;2015:717530. https://doi.org/10.1155/2015/717530.
32. Liau LM, Ashkan K, Brem S, et al. Association of autologous tumor lysate-loaded dendritic cell vaccination with extension of survival among patients with newly diagnosed and recurrent glioblastoma: a phase 3 prospective externally controlled cohort trial. JAMA Oncol. 2023;9(1):112–21. https://doi.org/10.1001/jamaoncol.2022.5370.
33. Ji N, Zhang Y, Liu Y, et al. Heat shock protein peptide complex-96 vaccination for newly diagnosed glioblastoma: a phase I, single-arm trial. JCI Insight. 2018;3(10):e99145. https://doi.org/10.1172/jci.insight.99145. Published 2018 May 17.
34. Bloch O, Crane CA, Fuks Y, et al. Heat-shock protein peptide complex-96 vaccination for recurrent glioblastoma: a phase II, single-arm trial. Neuro-Oncology. 2014;16(2):274–9. https://doi.org/10.1093/neuonc/not203.
35. Keskin DB, Anandappa AJ, Sun J, et al. Neoantigen vaccine generates intratumoral T cell responses in phase Ib glioblastoma trial. Nature. 2019;565(7738):234–9. https://doi.org/10.1038/s41586-018-0792-9.
36. Brahmer JR, Hammers H, Lipson EJ. Nivolumab: targeting PD-1 to bolster antitumor immunity. Future Oncol. 2015;11(9):1307–26. https://doi.org/10.2217/fon.15.52.
37. Baskaran AB, Kozel OA, Venkatesh O, et al. Immune checkpoint inhibitors in glioblastoma IDHwt treatment: a systematic review. Cancers (Basel). 2024;16(24):4148. https://doi.org/10.3390/cancers16244148. Published 2024 Dec 12.
38. Cloughesy TF, Mochizuki AY, Orpilla JR, et al. Neoadjuvant anti-PD-1 immunotherapy promotes a survival benefit with intratumoral and systemic immune responses in recurrent glioblastoma. Nat Med. 2019;25(3):477–86. https://doi.org/10.1038/s41591-018-0337-7.
39. Omuro A, Vlahovic G, Lim M, et al. Nivolumab with or without ipilimumab in patients with recurrent glioblastoma: results from exploratory phase I cohorts of CheckMate 143. Neuro-Oncology. 2018;20(5):674–86. https://doi.org/10.1093/neuonc/nox208.
40. Lassman A, Polly MY, Iwamoto F, et al. CTIM-18. NRG oncology study BN007: randomized phase II/III trial of ipilimiumab (IPI) plus nivolumab (NIVO) vs. temozolomide (TMZ) in MGMT-unmethylated (UMGMT) newly diagnosed glioblastoma (NGBM). Neuro-Oncology. 2023;25(Suppl 5):v65. https://doi.org/10.1093/neuonc/noad179.0258. Published 2023 Nov 10.
41. Nduom EK, Wei J, Yaghi NK, et al. PD-L1 expression and prognostic impact in glioblastoma. Neuro-Oncology. 2016;18(2):195–205. https://doi.org/10.1093/neuonc/nov172.
42. Gould A, Gonzales VAA, Dmello CC, et al. Advances in blood-brain barrier disruption to facilitate drug delivery for infiltrative gliomas. Adv Oncol. 2023;3(1):77–86. https://doi.org/10.1016/j.yao.2023.01.017.
43. Hanihara M, Kawataki T, Oh-Oka K, Mitsuka K, Nakao A, Kinouchi H. Synergistic antitumor effect with indoleamine 2,3-dioxygenase inhibition and temozolomide in a murine glioma model. J Neurosurg. 2016;124(6):1594–601. https://doi.org/10.3171/2015.5.JNS141901.

44. Bickerdike MJ, Nafia I, Bessede A, Chen CB, Wangpaichitr M. AT-0174, a novel dual IDO1/TDO2 enzyme inhibitor, synergises with temozolomide to improve survival in an orthotopic mouse model of glioblastoma. BMC Cancer. 2024;24(1):889. https://doi.org/10.1186/s12885-024-12631-w. Published 2024 Jul 24.
45. Reardon DA, Desjardins A, Rixe O, et al. A phase 1 study of PF-06840003, an oral indoleamine 2,3-dioxygenase 1 (IDO1) inhibitor in patients with recurrent malignant glioma. Investig New Drugs. 2020;38(6):1784–95. https://doi.org/10.1007/s10637-020-00950-1.
46. Du R, Zhang J, Lukas RV, et al. Is modulation of immune checkpoints on glioblastoma-infiltrating myeloid cells a viable therapeutic strategy? Neuro-Oncology. 2025;27(1):33–49. https://doi.org/10.1093/neuonc/noae193.
47. Butowski N, Colman H, De Groot JF, et al. Orally administered colony stimulating factor 1 receptor inhibitor PLX3397 in recurrent glioblastoma: an ivy foundation early phase clinical trials consortium phase II study. Neuro-Oncology. 2016;18(4):557–64. https://doi.org/10.1093/neuonc/nov245.
48. Low JT, Brown MC, Reitman ZJ, et al. Understanding and therapeutically exploiting cGAS/STING signaling in glioblastoma. J Clin Invest. 2024;134(2):e163452. https://doi.org/10.1172/JCI163452. Published 2024 Jan 16.
49. Fu W, Hou X, Dong L, Hou W. Roles of STAT3 in the pathogenesis and treatment of glioblastoma. Front Cell Dev Biol. 2023;11:1098482. https://doi.org/10.3389/fcell.2023.1098482. Published 2023 Feb 27.
50. Pei J, Zhang Y, Luo Q, et al. STAT3 inhibition enhances CDN-induced STING signaling and antitumor immunity. Cancer Lett. 2019;450:110–22. https://doi.org/10.1016/j.canlet.2019.02.029.
51. Ahmad N, Chen L, Yuan Z, et al. Pyrimidine compounds BY4003 and BY4008 inhibit glioblastoma cells growth via modulating JAK3/STAT3 signaling pathway. Neurotherapeutics. 2024;21(5):e00431. https://doi.org/10.1016/j.neurot.2024.e00431.
52. Kim BH, Lee H, Park CG, et al. STAT3 inhibitor ODZ10117 suppresses glioblastoma malignancy and prolongs survival in a glioblastoma xenograft model. Cells. 2020;9(3):722. https://doi.org/10.3390/cells9030722. Published 2020 Mar 15.
53. Fuh B, Sobo M, Cen L, et al. LLL-3 inhibits STAT3 activity, suppresses glioblastoma cell growth and prolongs survival in a mouse glioblastoma model. Br J Cancer. 2009;100(1):106–12. https://doi.org/10.1038/sj.bjc.6604793.
54. Boudreau CE, Najem H, Ott M, et al. Intratumoral delivery of STING agonist results in clinical responses in canine glioblastoma. Clin Cancer Res. 2021;27(20):5528–35. https://doi.org/10.1158/1078-0432.CCR-21-1914.
55. Najem H, Lea ST, Tripathi S, et al. STING agonist 8803 reprograms the immune microenvironment and increases survival in preclinical models of glioblastoma. J Clin Invest. 2024;134(12):e175033. https://doi.org/10.1172/JCI175033. Published 2024 Jun 17.
56. Chen D, Le SB, Hutchinson TE, et al. Tumor treating fields dually activate STING and AIM2 inflammasomes to induce adjuvant immunity in glioblastoma. J Clin Invest. 2022;132(8):e149258. https://doi.org/10.1172/JCI149258.
57. Chen D, Le SB, Ghiassedin AP, et al. Efficacy and safety of adjuvant TTFields plus pembrolizumab and temozolomide in newly diagnosed glioblastoma: a phase 2 study. Med. 2025. https://doi.org/10.1016/j.medj.2025.100708.
58. Tran D, Ghiaseddin A, Chen D, Le S. 581 Final analysis of 2-THE-TOP: a phase 2 study of TTFields (Optune) plus pembrolizumab plus maintenance temozolomide (TMZ) in patients with newly diagnosed glioblastoma. J Immunother Cancer. 2023;11(Suppl 1):A661. https://doi.org/10.1136/jitc-2023-SITC2023.0581.
59. Sooreshjani M, Tripathi S, Dussold C, et al. The use of targeted cytokines as cancer therapeutics in glioblastoma. Cancers (Basel). 2023;15(14):3739. https://doi.org/10.3390/cancers15143739. Published 2023 Jul 23.
60. Chiocca EA, Yu JS, Lukas RV, et al. Regulatable interleukin-12 gene therapy in patients with recurrent high-grade glioma: results of a phase 1 trial. Sci Transl Med. 2019;11(505):eaaw5680. https://doi.org/10.1126/scitranslmed.aaw5680.

61. Chiocca EA, Gelb AB, Chen CC, et al. Combined immunotherapy with controlled interleukin-12 gene therapy and immune checkpoint blockade in recurrent glioblastoma: an open-label, multi-institutional phase I trial. Neuro-Oncology. 2022;24(6):951–63. https://doi.org/10.1093/neuonc/noab271.
62. Ryu CH, Park SH, Park SA, et al. Gene therapy of intracranial glioma using interleukin 12-secreting human umbilical cord blood-derived mesenchymal stem cells. Hum Gene Ther. 2011;22(6):733–43. https://doi.org/10.1089/hum.2010.187.
63. Ribas A, Dummer R, Puzanov I, et al. Oncolytic virotherapy promotes intratumoral T cell infiltration and improves anti-PD-1 immunotherapy [published correction appears in Cell. 2018;174(4):1031–1032. doi: 10.1016/j.cell.2018.07.035]. Cell. 2017;170(6):1109–1119.e10. https://doi.org/10.1016/j.cell.2017.08.027.
64. Fares J, Ahmed AU, Ulasov IV, et al. Neural stem cell delivery of an oncolytic adenovirus in newly diagnosed malignant glioma: a first-in-human, phase 1, dose-escalation trial. Lancet Oncol. 2021;22(8):1103–14. https://doi.org/10.1016/S1470-2045(21)00245-X.
65. Todo T, Ino Y, Ohtsu H, Shibahara J, Tanaka M. A phase I/II study of triple-mutated oncolytic herpes virus G47Δ in patients with progressive glioblastoma. Nat Commun. 2022;13(1):4119. https://doi.org/10.1038/s41467-022-31262-y. Published 2022 Jul 21.
66. Gesundheit B, Ben-David E, Posen Y, et al. Effective treatment of glioblastoma multiforme with oncolytic virotherapy: a case-series. Front Oncol. 2020;10:702. https://doi.org/10.3389/fonc.2020.00702. Published 2020 May 14.
67. Klinger M, Benjamin J, Kischel R, Stienen S, Zugmaier G. Harnessing T cells to fight cancer with BiTE® antibody constructs—past developments and future directions. Immunol Rev. 2016;270(1):193–208. https://doi.org/10.1111/imr.12393.
68. Sternjak A, Lee F, Thomas O, et al. Preclinical assessment of AMG 596, a bispecific T-cell engager (BiTE) immunotherapy targeting the tumor-specific antigen EGFRvIII. Mol Cancer Ther. 2021;20(5):925–33. https://doi.org/10.1158/1535-7163.MCT-20-0508.
69. Pituch KC, Zannikou M, Ilut L, et al. Neural stem cells secreting bispecific T cell engager to induce selective antiglioma activity. Proc Natl Acad Sci USA. 2021;118(9):e2015800118. https://doi.org/10.1073/pnas.2015800118.
70. Gedeon PC, Schaller TH, Chitneni SK, et al. A rationally designed fully human EGFRvIII:CD3-targeted bispecific antibody redirects human T cells to treat patient-derived intracerebral malignant glioma. Clin Cancer Res. 2018;24(15):3611–31. https://doi.org/10.1158/1078-0432.CCR-17-0126.
71. Singh K, Hotchkiss KM, Mohan AA, Reedy JL, Sampson JH, Khasraw M. For whom the T cells troll? Bispecific T-cell engagers in glioblastoma. J Immunother Cancer. 2021;9(11):e003679. https://doi.org/10.1136/jitc-2021-003679.
72. Du R, Tripathi S, Najem H, et al. Glioblastoma phagocytic cell death: balancing the opportunities for therapeutic manipulation. Cells. 2024;13(10):823. https://doi.org/10.3390/cells13100823. Published 2024 May 11.
73. Neelapu SS, Locke FL, Bartlett NL, et al. Axicabtagene ciloleucel CAR T-cell therapy in refractory large B-cell lymphoma. N Engl J Med. 2017;377(26):2531–44. https://doi.org/10.1056/NEJMoa1707447.
74. Mahadeo KM, Khazal SJ, Abdel-Azim H, et al. Management guidelines for paediatric patients receiving chimeric antigen receptor T cell therapy. Nat Rev Clin Oncol. 2019;16(1):45–63. https://doi.org/10.1038/s41571-018-0075-2.
75. Du B, Qin J, Lin B, Zhang J, Li D, Liu M. CAR-T therapy in solid tumors. Cancer Cell. 2025;43(4):665–79. https://doi.org/10.1016/j.ccell.2025.03.019.
76. Brown CE, Alizadeh D, Starr R, et al. Regression of glioblastoma after chimeric antigen receptor T-cell therapy. N Engl J Med. 2016;375(26):2561–9. https://doi.org/10.1056/NEJMoa1610497.
77. Choi BD, Gerstner ER, Frigault MJ, et al. Intraventricular CARv3-TEAM-E T cells in recurrent glioblastoma. N Engl J Med. 2024;390(14):1290–8. https://doi.org/10.1056/NEJMoa2314390.

78. Corsale AM, Di Simone M, Lo Presti E, Dieli F, Meraviglia S. γδ T cells and their clinical application in colon cancer. Front Immunol. 2023;14:1098847. https://doi.org/10.3389/fimmu.2023.1098847. Published 2023 Jan 30.
79. Rimailho L, Faria C, Domagala M, Laurent C, Bezombes C, Poupot M. γδ T cells in immunotherapies for B-cell malignancies. Front Immunol. 2023;14:1200003. https://doi.org/10.3389/fimmu.2023.1200003. Published 2023 Jun 22.
80. Wang G, Wang S, Song W, et al. Integrating multi-omics data reveals the antitumor role and clinical benefits of gamma-delta T cells in triple-negative breast cancer. BMC Cancer. 2025;25(1):623. https://doi.org/10.1186/s12885-025-14029-8. Published 2025 Apr 7.
81. Lobbous M, Goswami T, Lamb LS, et al. INB-200: fully enrolled phase 1 study of gene-modified autologous gamma-delta (γδ) T cells in patients with newly diagnosed glioblastoma multiforme (GBM) receiving maintenance temozolomide (TMZ). JCO. 2024;42(16_suppl):2042. https://doi.org/10.1200/JCO.2024.42.16_suppl.2042.
82. Liu E, Marin D, Banerjee P, et al. Use of CAR-transduced natural killer cells in CD19-positive lymphoid tumors. N Engl J Med. 2020;382(6):545–53. https://doi.org/10.1056/NEJMoa1910607.
83. Burger MC, Forster MT, Romanski A, et al. Intracranial injection of natural killer cells engineered with a HER2-targeted chimeric antigen receptor in patients with recurrent glioblastoma. Neuro-Oncology. 2023;25(11):2058–71. https://doi.org/10.1093/neuonc/noad087.

# Immunotherapy in Head and Neck Cancer

# 7

Bridget E. Crossman, Regan L. Harmon, Mari Iida, Candie Y. Lin, Jennifer Yoon, Evan P. Pisick, Ravi Salgia, Tiffany Glazer, Randall Kimple, Justine Yang Bruce, and Deric Wheeler

## 7.1 Background

Head and neck cancer (HNC) is the seventh most common cancer worldwide, with approximately 890,000 new cases and over 450,000 deaths [1]. The incidence of HNCs has been steadily increasing, with projections suggesting a 30% rise by 2030 [2]. These malignancies arise from the mucosal surfaces of the aerodigestive tract [3], with head and neck squamous cell carcinoma (HNSCC) comprising around 90% of cases. HNSCC originates from the squamous cells lining the oral cavity, pharynx, larynx, nasal cavity, and paranasal sinuses.

B. E. Crossman · R. L. Harmon · M. Iida · C. Y. Lin · J. Yoon
Department of Human Oncology, University of Wisconsin, Madison, WI, USA

E. P. Pisick
City of Hope Chicago, Zion, IL, USA

R. Salgia
Department of Medical Oncology and Therapeutics Research, City of Hope National Medical Center, Duarte, CA, USA

T. Glazer
Department of Surgery, School of Medicine and Public Health, University of Wisconsin, Madison, WI, USA

Carbone Cancer Center, University of Wisconsin, Madison, WI, USA

R. Kimple · D. Wheeler (✉)
Department of Human Oncology, University of Wisconsin, Madison, WI, USA

Carbone Cancer Center, University of Wisconsin, Madison, WI, USA
e-mail: dlwheeler@wisc.edu

J. Y. Bruce
Carbone Cancer Center, University of Wisconsin, Madison, WI, USA

Department of Medicine, School of Medicine and Public Health, University of Wisconsin, Madison, WI, USA



R. Salgia, P. Kulkarni (eds.), *Immunotherapies in Solid Tumors*, Cancer Treatment and Research 129, https://doi.org/10.1007/978-3-031-97242-3_7

The incidence and mortality rates of HNC vary significantly by region, influenced by genetic and environmental factors [1]. For example, nasopharyngeal carcinoma is more prevalent in Southeast Asia [4]. The most well-established risk factors include tobacco use (both smoking and smokeless forms) and excessive alcohol consumption [1]. Additionally, infection with oncogenic strains of human papillomavirus (HPV), particularly HPV-16 and HPV-18, has emerged as a major etiological factor for oropharyngeal cancers, with cases rising annually [5, 6]. HPV-positive HNSCC differs significantly from HPV-negative HNSCC in terms of prognosis and response to therapy [7–9]. Other contributing factors include prolonged exposure to occupational hazards (asbestos, wood dust, and chemicals), poor oral hygiene, Epstein-Barr virus (EBV) infection (linked to nasopharyngeal carcinoma), and genetic predisposition [10].

The treatment of HNC is determined by tumor location, disease stage, and patient health status [2]. Most patients present with locally advanced disease at diagnosis, which carries a high risk of recurrence. About 10% of cases are diagnosed with metastatic disease. Standard treatment modalities include surgery, radiation therapy [11, 12], chemotherapy [13], and molecular targeted therapies [14].

Surgery: Typically, the first-line treatment for early-stage HNC, aiming to remove the tumor while preserving function. However, extensive resections can result in significant morbidity, impacting speech and swallowing.

Radiation Therapy: Used alone for early-stage disease or in combination with surgery and chemotherapy for locally advanced cases. Advances in radiation techniques have improved precision and reduced toxicity.

Chemotherapy: Primarily used for locally advanced or metastatic disease and often combined with radiation therapy (chemoradiotherapy) [15] to enhance treatment efficacy. Common agents include platinums, 5-fluorouracil, and taxanes.

Molecular Targeted Therapy: The first significant study on cetuximab, a monoclonal antibody targeting the epidermal growth factor receptor (EGFR) for HNSCC demonstrated that adding cetuximab to radiotherapy improved locoregional control and overall survival in patients with locoregionally advanced HNSCC [16–18]. These findings led to FDA approval of cetuximab in March 2006. Cetuximab, in combination with platinum-based chemotherapy, is currently used as the standard first-line treatment in patients with recurrent or metastatic HNC [19].

Immune Checkpoint Inhibitors: There are three FDA-approved targeted antibodies against immune checkpoints: nivolumab, pembrolizumab, and toripalimab-tpzi. These immune checkpoint inhibitors will be described in a later section.

Despite advancements in chemoradiotherapy and targeted treatments, 5-year survival rates for HNC remain suboptimal—35% for locally advanced disease and 4% for metastatic cases [20]. Additionally, treatment-related toxicities and long-term morbidity pose significant challenges. Furthermore, resistance to targeted therapy is a major hurdle, necessitating a deeper understanding of resistance mechanisms. Recent research has identified immune evasion as a hallmark of HNC, with the tumor immune microenvironment (TIME) playing a crucial role in treatment resistance [21]. These insights suggest that immunotherapy, which modulates the immune system, represents a promising strategy for improving patient outcomes.

This chapter focuses on immunotherapy in HNC summarizing the current understanding of the HNC immune landscape, immunomodulators, cancer vaccines, adoptive cell therapies, oncolytic viruses, combination immunotherapy approaches, and predictive biomarkers. Additionally, we highlight areas where further research is needed. As our knowledge of tumor immunology grows, immunotherapy is expected to become an increasingly integral component of HNC management, offering hope for better patient outcomes in the future.

## 7.2 The Head and Neck Cancer Immune Landscape

### 7.2.1 The Tumor Immune Microenvironment

The tumor immune microenvironment (TIME) is comprised of a complex network of immune cells, fibroblasts, mesenchymal cells, vascular endothelial cells, and signaling molecules, including cytokines, chemokines, growth factors, and enzymes. These components interact within the tumor and its surrounding stroma, facilitating crosstalk between the tumor and immune system that ultimately promotes immunosuppression and uncontrolled tumor proliferation [21]. HNC is characterized by a relatively "cold" TIME, meaning it often lacks a robust anti-tumor response while being enriched with immunosuppressive elements. Among the primary immune cells modulating the development and progression of HNC are T cells, natural killer (NK) cells, macrophages, and myeloid-derived suppressor cells (MDSCs) [22].

T cells play a central role in tumor immunity and can be broadly classified into $CD8^+$ cytotoxic T cells and $CD4^+$ helper T cells. $CD8^+$ T cells are essential for anti-tumor immunity due to their ability to recognize tumor antigens presented by major histocompatibility complex class I (MHC I) molecules, leading to the release of cytotoxic granules such as perforin and granzyme B that induce tumor cell death [23, 24]. In addition to their direct cytotoxic effects, activated $CD8^+$ T cells secrete various cytokines and chemokines, such as IFN-γ, TNF-α, CCL5, and CXCL10 which help recruit and activate other cytotoxic immune cells [23]. However, HNC tumors frequently employ various immune evasion strategies to evade $CD8^+$ cytotoxic T cell recruitment, recognition, and cytotoxicity which will be discussed in later sections. This evasion typically results in an HNC TIME characterized by reduced $CD8^+$ T cell infiltration and functionality [25].

$CD4^+$ helper T cells differentiate into various subsets that influence the tumor immune response: helper T1 (Th1), helper T2 (Th2), helper T17 (Th17), and regulatory T cells (Tregs). Differentiation of $CD4^+$ T cells is dictated by the cytokine milieu secreted by both immune cells and tumor cells in the TIME. Th1 cells are differentiated due to IL-12 signaling, typically released by antigen-presenting cells (APCs), which leads to the release of cytokines such as IFN-γ, TNF-α, and IL-2 [26]. These cytokines in turn promote the activation of cytotoxic $CD8^+$ T cells and typically support an anti-tumor immune response [27]. Conversely, Th2 cells, which differentiate in response to IL-4, are considered to promote tumor progression due to their anti-inflammatory functions. Th2 cells express IL-4, IL-10, and IL-13 which inhibit cytotoxic $CD8^+$ T cells [28]. The Th1/Th2 balance in HNC is associated with disease progression, as advanced cases tend to exhibit a dominant Th2 response [29, 30]. Th17 cells, driven by IL-1β, IL-6, and IL-23, secrete IL-17 and play a dual role in tumor immunity, sometimes enhancing anti-tumor responses while at other times fostering tumor progression [26, 31, 32]. Tregs, which are characterized by their expression of Foxp3, strongly suppress anti-tumor immunity through IL-10 and TGF-β secretion and cytotoxic T-lymphocyte antigen (CTLA-4) [33]. Increased levels of peripheral and tumor-infiltrating Tregs have been associated with a worse prognosis in HNC patients due to their immunosuppressive properties [34, 35].

The differentiation and response of $CD4^+$ T cells in the TIME are largely influenced by the phenotypes of tumor-associated macrophages (TAMs) [36]. TAMs can display two distinct phenotypes: M1 TAMs or M2 TAMs [36]. M1 TAMs, driven by IFN-γ and GM-CSF, promote anti-tumor immune responses by producing pro-inflammatory cytokines and enhancing Th1-mediated immunity [37]. In contrast, M2 TAMs are described to have pro-tumor, immunosuppressive properties due to their ability to induce a Th2 response. Additionally, activated M2 TAMs, induced by IL-4 and IL-13, secrete immunosuppressive cytokines such as IL-10, IL-1Ra, and TGF-β [38]. HNC patients frequently exhibit high levels of M2 TAMs, which correlate with metastasis and poor survival outcomes [39, 40].

MDSCs are a heterogenous population of highly immunosuppressive cells that accumulate in the HNC TIME and contribute to immune evasion [41]. These cells are recruited by tumor-secreted factors like GM-CSF, CCL2, and IL-8 [42]. Once in the TIME, MDSCs suppress T cell activity through various mechanisms, including competition with APCs for antigen presentation, depletion of essential metabolites, and secretion of nitric oxide and reactive oxygen species, which disrupt T cell receptor signaling [43, 44]. Further, membrane-bound TGF-β on MDSCs has been shown to impair NK cell functionality and cytotoxicity by reducing NKG2D expression, which is essential for tumor recognition, and IFN-γ production [45]. Studies have linked the accumulation of MDSCs in HNC tumors to poor survival and tumor progression [46, 47].

NK cells are innate immune effectors that contribute to tumor surveillance through cytotoxic activity and cytokine production. In humans, NK cells are classified into two main subgroups depending on their surface expression of CD56 and CD16. NK cells classified as $CD56^{dim}/CD16^{bright}$ are responsible for their cytotoxicity given their ability to directly kill cancer cells by releasing cytotoxic granules, such as Granzyme B [48, 49]. On the other hand, $CD56^{bright}/CD16^{dim}$ NK cells exhibit their anti-tumor properties through the release of cytokines such as IFN-γ and TNF-α to regulate other anti-tumor immune responses. Tumor cells, including those in HNC, often evade NK cell-mediated cytotoxicity by downregulating or shedding NKG2D ligands (NKG2DLs), leading to impaired NK cell recognition and function [50]. High levels of circulating soluble NKG2DLs in HNC patients have been associated with poor prognosis due to NK cell dysfunction [51].

The TIME of HNC is shaped by a complex interplay of immune cells that either promote or suppress tumor progression. While CD8$^+$ T cells and NK cells have the potential to mount effective anti-tumor responses, their activity is often impaired by immunosuppressive cells such as Tregs, M2 TAMs, and MDSCs. The predominance of Th2 and immunosuppressive signals contribute to the "cold" nature of the HNC TIME. A deeper understanding of these immune interactions may lead to the development of novel immunotherapeutic strategies aimed at re-programming the TIME to enhance anti-tumor immunity and improve patient outcomes.

### 7.2.2 Immunoediting to Evade Immunosurveillance

The TIME of HNC is shaped by complex interactions between malignant cells and various immune cell populations. While innate and adaptive immune responses initially work to eliminate transformed cells, tumors can develop mechanisms to escape immune control. This process, known as cancer immunoediting consists of three phases—elimination, equilibrium, and escape—which collectively modulate the immune landscape of HNC [52]. In the elimination phase, immune cells such as cytotoxic T cells and NK cells recognize and destroy nascent tumor cells. However, selective pressures can drive the survival of tumor variants that resist immune attack, leading to an equilibrium phase where immune surveillance restricts but does not fully eradicate tumor growth. Eventually, tumor cells acquire immune-evasive properties, enabling them to escape immunosurveillance and establish a progressively immunosuppressive TIME [53]. HNC employs a diverse array of immunosuppressive strategies, such as suppression of antigen presentation, immune checkpoint activation, and modulation of the recruitment and activity of immune cell populations, to disrupt effective anti-tumor immunity, ultimately fostering disease progression [54].

Antigen presentation (AP) is a critical process for initiating an effective anti-tumor immune response, yet HNC cells manipulate this pathway to evade immune recognition. HNC cells have been found to downregulate, mutate, or hinder AP components [55, 56]. One of the most common mechanisms by which HNC disrupts AP is through the modulation of MHC I expression. MHC I molecules present tumor-associated antigens (TAA) to cytotoxic T cells, facilitating immune-mediated tumor cell elimination [57]. However, diminished MHC I expression in HNC—caused by genomic defects, epigenetic changes, or dysregulation of oncogenic pathways such as EGFR—prevents efficient antigen presentation and T cell activation [58–60]. Partial or total loss of MHC I expression has been detected in 30–80% of HNC tumors and is associated with an increased risk of lymph node metastasis and poor prognosis [54, 61]. Furthermore, other essential components of the antigen processing machinery, such as transporter associated with antigen processing 1 (TAP1), and TAP2, and tapasin, are commonly downregulated in HNC, further impairing antigen presentation and immune detection [62]. MHC II expression in HNC is pivotal for presenting antigens to CD4$^+$ T cells, thereby initiating adaptive immune responses [63]. Interestingly, HPV+ HNC tumors exhibit significantly higher MHC II expression compared to HPV-tumors [64, 65]. This differential expression may partly explain the improved immune responsiveness and better outcomes observed in HPV+ HNC compared to HPV-HNC.

HNC tumors also evade immune destruction by leveraging immune checkpoint pathways to suppress the activation and function of infiltrating T cells. One of the most well-characterized immune checkpoints in HNC is the PD-1/PD-L1 axis, which plays a crucial role in T cell exhaustion. Over 50–60% of HNCs overexpress PD-L1, which binds to the PD-1 receptor on T cells, leading to T cell inactivation, dysfunction, and apoptosis [66–68]. PD-L1 overexpression in HNC cells is driven by oncogenic pathways, including JAK2/STAT1 and PI3K/Akt signaling and can be further upregulated by inflammatory signals within the TIME [66, 69]. In addition to PD-L1, HNC tumors also overexpress PD-L2, another inhibitory ligand for PD-1 that contributes to immune suppression, often via EGFR-driven upregulation [70, 71]. Beyond the PD-1 axis, cytotoxic T-lymphocyte-associated protein 4 (CTLA-4) is another key immune checkpoint molecule that is expressed in HNC. By binding to dendritic cells (DCs) and outcompeting co-stimulatory signals necessary for T cell activation, CTLA-4 further dampens the anti-tumor immune response [72].

Beyond antigen presentation defects and checkpoint activation, HNC cells actively shape the TIME by secreting immunosuppressive cytokines and chemokines that modulate immune cell recruitment and function. These secreted factors suppress effector immune cells while promoting accumulation of regulatory and suppressive immune populations that facilitate tumor progression. Overexpression of TGF-β [73, 74], IL-1Rα [75, 76], IL-6 [77, 78], and IL-8 [72] by HNC tumors impair the maturation, activation, and cytotoxicity of T cells and NK cells while inhibiting antigen-presenting functions of DCs. Additionally, these secreted factors promote the recruitment of immunosuppressive cells that in turn further inhibit the activity of cytotoxic immune cells. Macrophages are recruited by HNC cells secreting factors such as CCL3, CCL4, CCL5, MCSF, and MCP-1 [79, 80]. Once recruited to the TIME, HNC cells promote the polarization of macrophages to the pro-tumor M2 phenotype through the release of IL-4, IL-13, macrophage colony-stimulating factor (MCSF), IL-10, and TGF-β [81, 82]. Tregs are recruited to the HNC TIME through several secreted factors such as CCL2, CCL28, and CXCL12 [83–85]. The secreted cytokine milieu from HNC cells can also promote differentiation of naïve $CD4^+$ T cells into Tregs once inside the tumor [86]. Myeloid-derived suppressor cells (MDSCs) are also recruited to the TIME in response to HNC cells releasing factors such as IL-10, granulocyte-macrophage colony-stimulating factor (GM-CSF), IL-8, and monocyte chemoattractant protein-1 (MCP-1), further suppressing T cell and NK cell function [80, 87, 88]. Hypoxic conditions typically found in HNC tumors enhance the recruitment and accumulation of MDSCs within the TIME.

HNC tumors employ a multifaceted array of immunoreactive strategies to subvert immune surveillance and promote disease progression. While this section highlights key immune evasion mechanisms, numerous additional factors contribute to immune suppression in HNC, including metabolic reprogramming, extracellular vesicle-mediated immune modulation, and regulatory RNA signaling [21, 54, 55]. Understanding these complex interactions is crucial for developing immunotherapeutic strategies to restore anti-tumor immunity in HNC patients.

### 7.2.3 Tumor Mutational Burden and Neoantigens

Tumor mutational burden (TMB) plays a critical role in shaping the immune landscape of HNC by influencing the generation of neoantigens that can be recognized by the immune system. Generally, a higher TMB correlates with increased neoantigen load capable of eliciting T cell responses and enhancing the potential for immune-mediated tumor destruction [89]. Neoantigens are non-self-peptides derived from tumor mutations, and their presence on the tumor surface can make the cancer cells recognizable to the immune system [90]. Although the complex interplay between TMB and neoantigen load is still being investigated, their ability to modulate tumor immune responses has led to studies evaluating their potential as novel immunotherapy targets and biomarkers to predict immune checkpoint inhibitor (ICI) responses in HNC [91].

TMB, defined as the total number of mutations per megabase (Mb) of sequenced DNA, has emerged as a key biomarker for predicting response to immunotherapy across various cancer types [92–96]. High TMB has been associated with greater neoantigen expression, which in turn increases the likelihood of immune recognition and T cell-mediated tumor destruction [91]. A recent study identified TMB as a predictive biomarker for ICI response in HNC, observing that patients with a higher TMB demonstrated improved responses and clinical benefits from ICI therapy [71]. This improved response to ICIs is attributed to the fact that TMB directly correlates with the number of neoantigens expressed and presented by MHC molecules on tumor cells, promoting immune recognition and enhanced immune responses [90, 91].

However, the relationship between TMB and immunogenicity in HNC is complex and varies between HPV+ and HPV- tumors. HPV-HNCs, often associated with chronic tobacco and alcohol use, typically exhibit higher TMB due to accumulated somatic mutations from environmental carcinogen exposure [58]. These tumors are more likely to produce a diverse range of neoantigens, as a result of these mutations, increasing their immunogenicity. In contrast, HPV+ tumors, despite a lower TMB, can still generate strong immune responses. This is largely due to the expression of viral antigens, including E6 and E7, which are recognized as foreign by the immune system and can activate both innate and adaptive immune responses [97, 98]. These viral proteins, despite overall lower mutational burden, offer a distinct immunogenic profile that can still promote effective immune surveillance and response to immunotherapies.

While high TMB and neoantigen expression in HNC provide a promising therapeutic target for immunotherapies, challenges remain. Tumor-induced immune evasion mechanisms often limit the effectiveness of therapies despite the enhanced presentation of neoantigens [99]. A better understanding of how the immune system recognizes and responds to HNC neoantigens, combined with strategies to overcome immune suppression within the TIME, will be essential for improving patient outcomes with immunotherapies.

## 7.3 Immunomodulatory Agents

With more evidence emerging on the impact of the immune system on cancer progression, hundreds of strategies are being developed to harness patients' immune systems against their tumors. HNCs have become excellent candidates for immunomodulatory therapies due to their modest response to standard treatment and immunosuppressive TIME. ICIs were the first immunomodulators to take hold in HNC, with monoclonal antibodies against the PD-1/PD-L1 axis already approved, and even more in clinical trial. Other immune checkpoints are also showing promise, including CTLA-4, lectin-like transcript 1 (LLT-1), CD39, V-domain immunoglobulin suppressor of T cell activation (VISTA), and lymphocyte activation gene 3 (LAG3) (Fig. 7.1a). Beyond monospecific antibodies, bispecific compounds have gained popularity due to their diverse applications, including T cell engagement, NK cell engagement, and targeted cytokine delivery (Fig. 7.1b). Cytokine delivery,

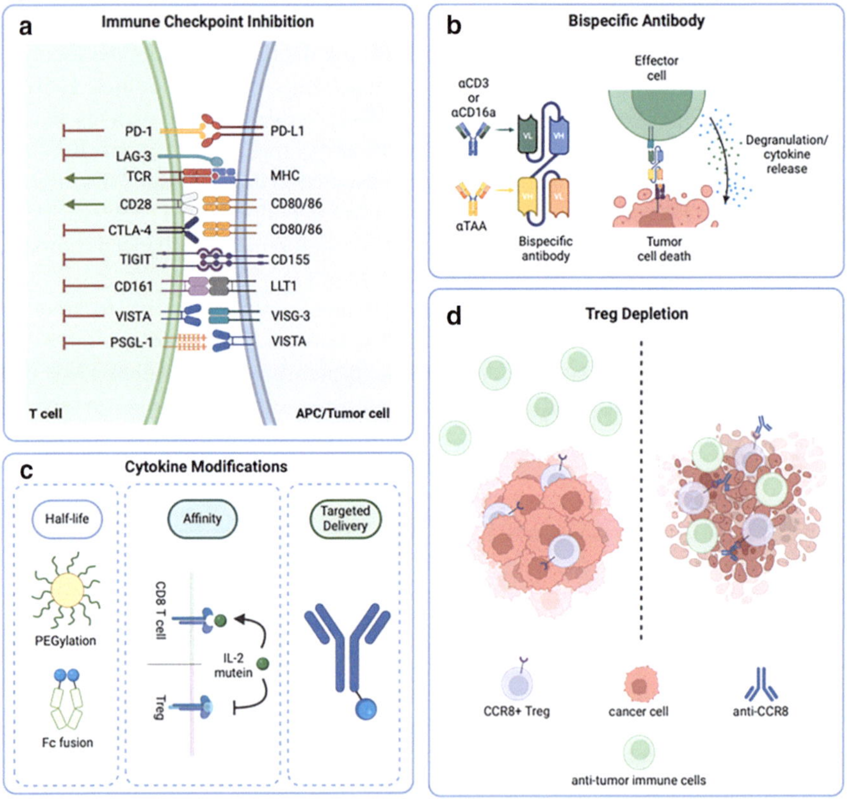


**Fig. 7.1** Immunomodulatory strategies in clinical trial for HNSCC. (**a**) Immune checkpoint inhibitors. (**b**) Example of bispecific compound targeting a TAA and NK or T cell receptor. (**c**) Cytokine modifications to improve half-life, modulate receptor affinity, or target delivery. (**d**) Treg depletion using anti-CCR8

which has been investigated as a monotherapy since the 1990s with little success, has regained potential as a therapeutic option with the introduction of modifications to enhance specificity and improve half-life in circulation, thus improving safety and efficacy (Fig. 7.1c). Finally, monoclonal antibodies targeting the cytokine receptor CCR8, expressed only on tumor-infiltrating Tregs, are being studied as Treg inhibitors in HNC (Fig. 7.1d). In this section, we will discuss in detail the landmark clinical trials that have led to FDA approval of PD-1/PD-L1 inhibitors, mechanisms of action for key immunomodulatory agents, and an overview of immunomodulators currently in clinical trial to treat HNC.

### 7.3.1 PD-1/PD-L1 Inhibitors

In normal tissues, the programmed death 1/programmed death ligand 1(PD-1/PD-L1) axis plays a critical role as an immune checkpoint in maintaining immune homeostasis and reducing autoimmune attacks by limiting T cell activation [100]. For a T cell to become activated, APCs process antigens and present them to the T cell receptor (TCR) on an MHC molecule. This initiates the first of two T cell-activating signaling cascades. The TCR/MHC complex is highly specific, and once formed, a co-stimulatory signal is required to complete T cell activation. When a co-stimulatory molecule on the APC, CD80 or CD86 for example, binds CD28 on the T cell, the T cell will become activated and licensed to kill infected cells or cells deemed to be non-self [101]. PD-1 serves as a much-needed "brake" on the immune system under normal circumstances to mediate self-tolerance. PD-1 expression is upregulated during antigen presentation when the T cell is activated, and again at the immunological synapse. The PD-1 ligand, PD-L1, is expressed by APCs and some nonlymphoid tissues, including the heart and lung [102]. When PD-1 engages PD-L1, TCR-mediated T cell proliferation and cytokine secretion are downregulated to avoid excessive T cell responses that could harm healthy tissue [103, 104]. Manipulating the PD-1/PD-L1 axis is one method that tumor cells employ to evade the immune system. When tumor cells upregulate PD-L1 on their surface, CD8 T cell activity is inhibited and tumor cells are spared from immune-mediated death, making PD-1/PD-L1 blockade a promising modality to restore anti-tumor immunity [105].

To date, three anti-PD-1 monoclonal antibodies have been FDA-approved for use in HNC: pembrolizumab, nivolumab, and toripalimab (Table 7.1). The landmark clinical trials that led to FDA approval of these agents are detailed in the following subsections.

#### 7.3.1.1 KEYNOTE-012

The KEYNOTE-012 trial (NCT01848834) was the first trial of pembrolizumab, a high-affinity, humanized monoclonal PD-1 antibody, in patients with recurrent or metastatic (R/M) HNSCC. The phase 1b trial aimed to evaluate safety and efficacy of pembrolizumab in patients with R/M PD-L1-positive HNSCC regardless of previous treatments. Sixty patients were enrolled in the study and evaluated for safety

**Table 7.1** FDA-approved ICIs in HNC

| Trial | Treatment | Phase | Enrolled patients | FDA approval |
|---|---|---|---|---|
| KEYNOTE-012 (NCT01848834) | Pembrolizumab for R/M HNSCC | 1b | 60 | Accelerated approval: August 2016 |
| KEYNOTE-048 (NCT02358031) | Pembrolizumab as first-line for R/M HNSCC | 3 | 191 | June 2019 |
| CheckMate 141 (NCT02105636) | Nivolumab for platinum-refractory R/M HNSCC | 3 | 361 | November 2016 |
| POLARIS-02 (NCT02915432) | Toripalimab for previously treated R/M nasopharyngeal carcinoma | 2 | 191 | October 2023 |
| JUPITER-02 (NCT03581786) | Toripalimab plus gemcitabine and cisplatin as first-line for R/M nasopharyngeal | 3 | 289 | October 2023 |

(56 of these patients were eligible for efficacy analysis); 37 were HPV-negative and 23 were HPV-positive. Sixty-eight percent of patients experienced drug-related adverse effects of any grade with 17% experiencing grade-3 adverse effects. In terms of response rate, 18% of patients exhibited confirmed overall response, and one patient exhibited complete response. Median progression-free survival was 2 months for the full analysis population (56 patients), and median overall survival was 13 months in the intention-to-treat population (61 patients). Of note, the proportions of patients who experienced overall response were comparable regardless of HPV status. Overall, this study found pembrolizumab to be safe, while further evaluation of efficacy would be required as survival data was comparable to that of patients receiving first-line combination of platinum-based chemotherapy plus cetuximab [106]. Based on these results, the FDA granted accelerated approval to pembrolizumab in patients with R/M HNSCC who progressed after platinum-based chemotherapy. This landmark clinical trial brought a new therapeutic agent to the clinic for HNSCC patients for the first time since the approval of cetuximab in 2006 [107].

#### 7.3.1.2 KEYNOTE-048

The KEYNOTE-048 trial (NCT02358031) was a phase 3 study of treatment-naïve participants with locally incurable R/M HNSCC regardless of PD-L1 status. 882 total participants received either pembrolizumab monotherapy (n=301), pembrolizumab plus chemotherapy ($n$ = 281) or cetuximab plus chemotherapy ($n$ = 300). Patients were evaluated for the PD-L1 combined positive score; 43% of participants had a score ≥20, and 85% participants had a PD-L1 CPS ≥1. Platinum and 5-fluorouracil (FU) were the chemotherapy agents used in the study. Participants who experienced grade 3 or worse adverse events were the highest in the pembrolizumab plus chemotherapy arm (85%), followed by cetuximab plus chemotherapy (83%) and pembrolizumab monotherapy (55%). Median overall survival for pembrolizumab plus chemotherapy and cetuximab plus chemotherapy arms were 13.0 months and 10.7 months, respectively and were similar in both PD-L1 CPS ≥ 20 and PD-L1

CPS ≥ 1 groups. For participants with PD-L1 CPS of 1 or more, median overall survival for the pembrolizumab monotherapy and cetuximab plus chemotherapy arms was 12.3 months and 10.3 months, respectively. For participants with PD-L1 CPS of 20 or more, median overall survival for the pembrolizumab monotherapy and cetuximab plus chemotherapy arms was 14.9 months and 10.7 months, respectively [108]. As a result of this landmark trial, the FDA approved pembrolizumab as a first-line treatment, either in combination with platinum and FU for all patients regardless of the PD-L1 status, or as a monotherapy for patients with a PD-L1 CPS ≥ 1.

#### 7.3.1.3 CheckMate-141

The CheckMate-141 trial (NCT02105636) was a randomized, open-label, phase 3 trial of the anti-PD-1 monoclonal antibody nivolumab to assess overall survival of platinum-refractory R/M HNSCC. Two hundred forty patients received nivolumab and 121 patients received standard single-agent systemic therapy (investigator's choice of docetaxel, cetuximab, or methotrexate). Nivolumab was deemed to be well tolerated as 13.1% of patients in the nivolumab group and 35.1% of patients in the standard therapy group experienced grade 3 or 4 adverse events. Median overall survival for the nivolumab group was longer than that for the standard therapy group, at 7.5 months and 5.1 months, respectively however there was no difference between the two groups in progression-free survival. Of the patients treated with nivolumab, 13.3% responded to treatment (6 complete responses, 26 partial responses), compared to 5.8% of patients treated with standard therapy. This trial found treatment of platinum-refractory HNSCC with nivolumab to be both safe and effective as a monotherapy regardless of PD-L1 status compared to standard systemic therapy [109]. As a result, the FDA approved nivolumab to treat patients with HNSCC who had progressed during platinum-based chemotherapy or had recurred or metastasized after platinum-based chemotherapy. Nivolumab was the second PD-1 inhibitor to be approved for use in HNSCC.

#### 7.3.1.4 POLARIS-02

The POLARIS-02 trial (NCT02915432) was a phase 2 study of toripalimab, a monoclonal PD-1 antibody, aimed at evaluating safety and efficacy. Eligible participants had nasopharyngeal carcinoma (NPC) who did not previously respond to standard chemotherapy or whose disease progressed within 6 months of completing standard therapy. 95.8% of participants had nonkeratinizing and 4.2% of participants had keratinizing disease according to histological subtyping. 191 participants received toripalimab, with four discontinuations occurring due to treatment-related adverse effects. 14.5% of participants experienced grade 3–5 adverse effects. For 190 participants assessed, the median overall survival was 17.4 months. Participants with EBV DNA titer <10,000 IU/mL exhibited higher overall response than participants with Epstein-Barr Virus (EBV) DNA titer ≤10,000 IU/mL (26.7% and 15.4%, respectively), though the difference did not reach statistical significance. 25.3% of participants were PD-L1-positive and 70.5% of participants were negative for PD-L1 according to SP142 IHC staining. 4.2% of participants had unknown PD-L1 status. While statistical significance was not reached, participants with high PD-L1 expression experienced higher overall response (38.1% vs 19.3%), progression-free survival (7.2 months vs. 1.9 months), and overall survival (unreached vs. 15.1 months) compared to patients with low PD-L1 expression. This study found toripalimab to be safe and effective in participants with R/M NPC who did not respond to standard chemotherapy. Additionally, this trial identified potential biomarkers to predict patient response, including plasma EBV DNA copy number and PD-L1 status. This landmark clinical trial led to the first FDA approval for a PD-1 inhibitor in NPC [110]. Toripalimab was approved in 2023 as a single agent for the treatment of recurrent or metastatic NPC with disease progression following standard chemotherapy.

#### 7.3.1.5 JUPITER-02

The JUPITER-02 trial (NCT03581786) was a randomized double-blind phase 3 trial of first-line toripalimab in combination with chemotherapy aimed at evaluating efficacy of the combination versus gemcitabine-cisplatin alone. 289 patients were enrolled, with 146 receiving toripalimab and 143 receiving placebo in combination with gemcitabine-cisplatin for six cycles followed by toripalimab or placebo as maintenance until disease progression. Median progression-free survival was extended for participants receiving toripalimab (21.4 vs 8.2 months). At the 36-month median survival follow-up, median overall survival was not reached in the toripalimab group and was 33.7 months in the placebo group, with a significant improvement in overall survival noted for toripalimab over placebo. Of note, the overall survival improvement for the toripalimab group over the placebo group was consistent across all PD-L1 expression and EBV DNA copy number subgroups. Treatment-related adverse events were similar for both treatment groups, with the most common TRAEs attributable to chemotherapy-induced toxicity. Overall, this study found that addition of troipalimab to first-line chemotherapy improved survival benefit over chemotherapy alone with a favorable safety profile [111]. This study led to FDA approval of toripalimab with gemcitabine and cisplatin for the first-line treatment of patients with metastatic or recurrent, locally advanced NPC in 2023.

Ongoing work is still being done to expand the repertoire of PD-1/PD-L1 inhibitors available for many solid tumors, including HNSCC. The anti-PD-1 antibody Penpulimab has been granted breakthrough therapy and fast-track designations as a third-line treatment for nasopharyngeal carcinoma and is currently in phase three trial for first-line treatment (NCT04974398) [112]. Details on PD-1 inhibitors currently in clinical trial for HNC are outlined in Table 7.2.

### 7.3.2 CTLA-4 Inhibitors

Cytotoxic T-lymphocyte-associated antigen 4 (CTLA-4) is an immune checkpoint molecule and T cell co-receptor that negatively regulates activation of T cells. In the event of a weak TCR signal, CTLA-4 is internalized for storage in the T cell and the co-stimulatory CD28:CD80/86 signal is transduced, allowing the T cell to enter an

**Table 7.2** PD-1 inhibitors in clinical trial

| Drug | Trial | Treatment | Phase | Enrollment | Status |
|---|---|---|---|---|---|
| Cemiplimab | NCT04988074 | Neoadjuvant cemiplimab with or without carboplatin/paclitaxel | 2 | 32 | Recruiting |
| Dostarlimab | NCT06256588 | Dostarlimab following chemoradiation | 3 | 864 | Recruiting |
| Penpulimab | NCT04974398 | Penpulimab plus chemotherapy for first-line treatment | 3 | 296 | Active – not recruiting |

activated state. However, in the presence of a strong TCR signal, CTLA-4 expression is upregulated on the T cell surface before the co-stimulatory signal is initiated. In this case, CTLA-4 outcompetes CD28 for CD80/86 binding and produces inhibitory signals through a mechanism that is not yet well understood. This in turn causes the T cell to cease effector activity and reduce proliferation and production of IL-2 [113]. In addition to its role on effector T cells, CTLA-4 is constitutively expressed on Tregs. Tregs that express CTLA-4 are thought to impair effector T cell function by downregulating CD80/86 ligands on APCs, making CD28 co-stimulation less likely [114, 115]. It is thought that blocking CTLA-4 enhances the immune priming phase where effector T cell proliferation and activation are enhanced, and Treg-mediated suppression of effector T cell responses is dampened [116]. Further, it has been reported that the T cell repertoire following CTLA-4 inhibition in melanoma exhibited increased diversity [117].

Two humanized anti-CTLA-4 monoclonal antibodies, ipilimumab and tremelimumab, are currently used either in monotherapy or combination with nivolumab to treat melanoma, renal cell carcinoma, hepatocellular carcinoma, non-small cell lung cancer, and colorectal cancer [118]. These regimens have so far been unsuccessful in HNC. The CheckMate 651 trial (NCT02741570) comparing the EXTREME regimen to nivolumab plus ipilimumab showed no overall survival benefit and was considered a negative trial [119]. The CheckMate 714 trial (NCT02823574) comparing nivolumab alone to nivolumab plus ipilimumab was also considered negative as the primary endpoint of objective response rate was not met [120]. The EAGLE study (NCT02369874) comparing durvalumab alone to durvalumab plus tremelimumab did not meet its primary endpoint of objective response [121]. There are not yet any FDA-approved uses for CTLA-4 inhibitors in HNSCC, though one new agent, ONC-392 (NCT04140526), is in early-stage clinical trial (Table 7.3).

### 7.3.3 Other Immune Checkpoint Inhibitors

While PD-1/PD-L1 and CTLA-4 were the first immune checkpoint inhibitors to take hold in solid tumors, many other immune checkpoint molecules have been identified in recent years as promising targets. Lectin-like transcript 1 (LLT1) expressed on cancer cells is known to bind its receptor CD161 on NK cells to facilitate immune evasion [122]. The ectonucleotidase CD39 is a newly discovered

**Table 7.3** CTLA-4 inhibitor in clinical trial

| Drug | Trial | Treatment | Phase | Enrollment | Status |
|---|---|---|---|---|---|
| ONC-392 | NCT04140526 | ONC-392 single agent or combined with pembrolizumab | 1/2 | 733 | Recruiting |

**Table 7.4** Other immune checkpoint inhibitors in clinical trial

| Drug (Target) | Trial | Treatment | Phase | Enrollment | Status |
|---|---|---|---|---|---|
| ZM008 (LLT1) | NCT06451497 | ZM008 single agent followed by combination with pembrolizumab f | 1 | 33 | Recruiting |
| AB598 (CD39) | NCT05891171 | AB598 single agent or combined with zimberelimab | 1 | 87 | Recruiting |
| COM902 (TIGIT) | NCT04354246 | COM902 single agent or combined with COM701 | 1 | 110 | Recruiting |
| SNS-101 (VISTA) | NCT05864144 | SNS-101 single agent or combined with cemiplimab | 1/2 | 169 | Recruiting |
| KVA12123 (VISTA) | NCT05708950 | KVA12123 single agent or combined with pembrolizumab | 1/2 | 314 | Recruiting |
| Relatlimab (LAG-3) | NCT06029270 | Addition of relatlimab to standard of care nivolumab | 2 | 156 | Recruiting |

immunological "switch" that converts ATP to adenosine, the accumulation of which has been linked to an immunosuppressive TIME [123]. T cell immunoglobulin and immunoreceptor tyrosine-based inhibitory motif (TIGIT) is widely expressed on many cell types, including $CD4^+$ and $CD8^+$ T cells, NK cells, endothelial cells, fibroblasts, and tumor cells. When TIGIT on NK cells and T cells is bound by its ligand CD155 expressed on tumor cells, IL-10 secretion is increased, and the anti-tumor immune response is dampened [124, 125]. V-domain Ig suppressor of T cell activation (VISTA) plays a similar role in inhibiting T cell activation as PD-L1, though the pathways are non-redundant. VISTA, highly expressed on tumor-infiltrating leukocytes, is known to play a role in promoting an anti-inflammatory TIME by enhancing maturation of regulatory T cells and inhibiting T cell activation, proliferation, and cytokine production [125, 126]. Lymphocyte-activated gene-3 (LAG3) plays a similar role as PD-L1 and CTLA-4 in maintaining inhibitory functions of regulatory T cells and is highly expressed on Tregs in HNSCC [125, 127]. Current clinical trials of agents targeting LLT1 (NCT06451497), CD39 (NCT05891171), TIGIT (NCT04354246), VISTA (NCT05864144, NCT05708950), and LAG-3 (NCT06029270) are detailed in Table 7.4.

### 7.3.4 Immune Cell Engagers

#### 7.3.4.1 Bispecific T Cell Engagers (BiTEs)

BiTEs are small antibodies composed of two single chain variable fragments (scFvs) that selectively bind to distinct antigens. One scFv is specific for a T cell receptor (TCR) molecule, which allows for T cell activation. The other scFV is specific for a tumor antigen that is not expressed in normal tissues, limiting off-target effects. For the BiTE to be effective, both scFVs must bind their respective antigens. A unique feature of BiTEs compared to other types of bispecific antibodies is their ability to induce formation of the cytotoxic synapse and T cell cytotoxic activity without costimulation [128]. EGFR is highly expressed and has been widely studied in HNC, making it a popular tumor antigen target for BiTE development (NCT05983133, NCT05783622, NCT04844073) [129, 130]. Other tumor antigen targets being applied to BiTEs in HNC include B7-H3 (NCT05585034), MET, and TROP2 (NCT06239194) [131–133]. Clinical trials of these agents in HNC are outlined in Table 7.5.

#### 7.3.4.2 NK Cell Engagers

Like BiTEs, NK cell engagers act by bridging an NK cell and tumor cell to promote tumor cell lysis and can be either bi- or trispecific. Bispecific NK cell engagers consist of two scFvs, one targeting an NK activating receptor and the other binding a tumor-associated antigen (TAA), linked by a short peptide. Trispecific NK cell engagers employ the same basic structure as bispecific engagers but feature the NK-activating cytokine IL-15 as a linker [134]. NK cell engagers are unique over other types of NK cell therapies like therapeutic antibodies or CAR-NK cells, as they do not compete with endogenous IgG1 for binding of the activating receptor CD16a. There are multiple platforms to develop NK cell engagers based on different activating receptors, including CD16a, NKG2D, Nkp30, Nkp46, Nkp80, and NKG2C [135]. Currently, there is one NK cell engager, PBA-0405, in clinical trial for HNC (NCT06273852). PBA-0405 targets the NK cell activating receptor CD16a and the TAA ROR1 (Table 7.5).

### 7.3.5 Bispecific Compounds

Like immune cell engagers, bispecific compounds are engineered to target two different antigens to improve immunotherapy efficacy by modulating immune checkpoints, blocking certain signaling pathways, or facilitating targeted cytokine

**Table 7.5** Immune cell engagers in clinical trial

| Drug (Target) | Trial | Treatment | Phase | Enrollment | Status |
|---|---|---|---|---|---|
| SGN-EGFRd2 (EGFR/VγVδ2) | NCT05983133 | SGN-EGFRd2 single agent | 1 | 275 | Recruiting |
| JANX008 (EGFR/ CD3) | NCT05783622 | JANX008 single agent | 1 | 130 | Recruiting |
| XmAb808 (B7-H3/CD28) | NCT05585034 | XmAb808 plus pembrolizumab | 1 | 220 | Recruiting |
| PBA-0405 (ROR1/ CD16) | NCT06273852 | Intratumoral microdose of PBA-0405 | 1 | 15 | Recruiting |
| TAK-186 (EGFR/ CD3) | NCT04844073 | TAK-186 single agent | 1/2 | 258 | Active, not recruiting |
| MDX2001 (CD3/ CD28/MET/ TROP2) | NCT06239194 | MDX2001 single agent | 1/2 | 115 | Recruiting |

delivery [136]. Bispecific antibodies targeting immune checkpoints may enhance efficacy and reduce acquired resistance by targeting more than one checkpoint at the same time to prevent compensatory signaling, and several are in clinical trial for HNC. Further, co-expression of immune checkpoint molecules is uncommon in peripheral lymphocytes, so these agents may also be more specific for tumor-infiltrating lymphocytes [137]. In addition to bispecific antibodies, bispecific fusion proteins are also promising candidates to treat HNC. These compounds can deliver cytokines to preferentially activate some immune cells but not others. One example is CD8 or CD80 fusions to a modified IL-2. The CD8-IL-2 fusion allows for highly selective delivery of IL-2 only to $CD8^+$ T cells, while the CD80-IL-2 fusion plays a dual role in blocking CTLA-4 and delivering a modified IL-2 that preferentially binds the medium-affinity IL-2Rβ [138, 139]. Clinical trials testing bispecific compounds in HNC are outlined in Table 7.6.

### 7.3.6 Modified Cytokines

Cytokines are small molecules that bind receptors with high affinity and can have pleiotropic effects on the immune system. Once bound, cytokine receptors signal through the target cell to modulate proliferation, differentiation, and different effector functions. Two highly potent anti-tumor cytokines, interferon-alpha (IFN-α) and IL-2, were studied as monotherapies in the 1990s but showed only modest efficacy due to their short half-life and high levels of toxicity [140, 141]. There are currently three modified cytokines in clinical trial for HNSCC: IL-12 (NCT06580938), IL-2 (NCT05098132), and IL-18 (NCT04787042; Table 7.7).

#### 7.3.6.1 IL-12

IL-12 is produced by APCs in response to activation of pattern recognition receptors (PRRs) or binding of CD40-CD40L on two immune cells. In cancer, the majority of IL-12 is produced by contact between two immune cells and binds the high-affinity

**Table 7.6** Bispecific compounds in clinical trial

| Drug (Target) | Trial | Treatment | Phase | Enrollment | Status |
|---|---|---|---|---|---|
| SPX-303 (LILRB2/PD-L1) | NCT06259552 | SPX-303 as single agent | 1 | 232 | Recruiting |
| CTX-8371 (PD-1/PD-L1) | NCT06150664 | CTX-8371 as single agent | 1 | 55 | Recruiting |
| AB248 (CD8/IL-2) | NCT05653882 | AB248 as single agent or combined with pembrolizumab | 1 | 552 | Recruiting |
| GI-101 (CD80/IL-2) | NCT04977453 | GI-101 as single agent or combined with ICI or RT | 1/2 | 430 | Recruiting |
| AZD2936 (TIGIT/PD-1) | NCT05414032 | AZD2936 as single agent | 2 | 200 | Recruiting |
| Volrustomig (PD-1/ CTLA-4) | NCT06129864 | Volrustomig as single agent | 3 | 1145 | Recruiting |

**Table 7.7** Modified cytokines in clinical trial

| Drug | Trial | Treatment | Phase | Enrollment | Status |
|---|---|---|---|---|---|
| PF-07921585 | NCT06580938 | IL-12 mutein as single agent | 1 | 190 | Recruiting |
| STK-012 | NCT05098132 | IL-2 mutein as single agent | 1 | 202 | Recruiting |
| ST-067 | NCT04787042 | Decoy-resistant IL-18 as single agent or combined with pembrolizumab | 1/2 | 316 | Recruiting |

IL-12 receptor (IL-12R) on T cells and NK cells. Activation of the IL-12R leads to downstream activation of JAK2, Tyk2, and STAT4, resulting in production of interferon-gamma (IFN-γ). Increases in IFN-γ levels promote differentiation of T cells to the Th1 type, maturation of NK cells, and M1 macrophage polarization, leading to a potent anti-tumor environment [140]. Different delivery methods have been explored to overcome toxicity seen in early clinical trials including local IL-12 gene delivery in viral vectors, liposomes, or in vivo electroporation and modifications to the IL-12 protein itself [142]. One such modified IL-12 has been developed as a fusion of low-potency IL-12 and PD1. This design is unique in that it drives IL-12 only to PD-1-positive T cells, potentially lowering toxicity with the added benefit of PD-1 checkpoint blockade and is currently in clinical trial for HNSCC (NCT06580938; Table 7.7).

#### 7.3.6.2 IL-2

IL-2 is a critical cytokine for promoting expansion of NK and T cell populations, and while FDA-approved for use in renal cell carcinoma, utility in the clinic has been largely thwarted by high occurrence of grade 3 and 4 adverse effects [140]. Several strategies to improve the safety and efficacy profile of IL-2 administration have been developed, including PEGylation or mutation of IL-2 itself to improve half-life and modify interactions of IL-2 with its receptors [143–145]. One such strategy being used in HNSCC is generation of an IL-2 mutein. The modified IL-2 lacks the ability to bind to the IL-2Rα present in the high-affinity receptor, which skews IL-2 activity toward Treg expansion, and preferentially binds to the medium-affinity receptor containing IL2-Rβ and the common γ chain to promote proliferation of activated T cells (NCT05098132; Table 7.7) [146].

#### 7.3.6.3 IL-18

IL-18 is a potent inflammatory cytokine that binds to the high-affinity IL-18BP, which acts as a decoy receptor sequestering free IL-18 and inhibiting its activity in the TIME [147]. As a result of a yeast display screen, a mutant was identified that was able to bind the IL-18Rα, but not the decoy IL-18BP. The authors of this study found that IL-18 signaling through the IL-18Rα in combination with PD-1 blockade resulted in expansion of memory T cells and minimized levels of T cell exhaustion coupled with lower levels of TOX, a regulator of T cell exhaustion downstream of nuclear factor of activated T cells (NFAT). Beyond its combinatorial role on effector T cell expansion with anti-PD-1, decoy-resistant IL-18 can help overcome one

**Table 7.8** Treg inhibitors in clinical trial

| Drug | Trial | Treatment | Phase | Enrollment | Status |
|---|---|---|---|---|---|
| CHS-114 | NCT05635643 | CHS-114 as single agent | 1 | 47 | Recruiting |
| RO7502175 | NCT05581004 | RO7502175 as single agent or combined with ICI | 1 | 450 | Recruiting |
| ABBV-514 | NCT05005403 | ABBV-514 as single agent or combined with budigalimab | 1 | 268 | Recruiting |
| BMS-986340 | NCT04895709 | BMS-986340 as single agent or combined with ICI | 1/2 | 905 | Recruiting |

aspect of resistance to checkpoint therapy associated with MHC I-deficiency on tumors by licensing NK cells. A modified cytokine therapy utilizing the decoy-resistant IL-18 as a single agent is currently in clinical trial for HNSCC (NCT04787042; Table 7.7) [148].

### 7.3.7 Treg Inhibitors

Regulatory T cells (Tregs) play a critical inhibitory role in anti-tumor immunity by inducing T cell anergy and immunosuppression. In normal tissues, Tregs protect the host against autoimmunity and help maintain self-tolerance by secreting inhibitory cytokines, cytolytic activity, disrupting cellular metabolism, or modulating dendritic cell (DC) function [149]. However, in the TIME, the inhibitory activity of these cells can have detrimental effects on anti-tumor immunity by sequestering IL-2, expressing checkpoint molecules (e.g., CTLA-4, PD-1, LAG3), secreting anti-inflammatory cytokines (e.g., TGF-β, IL-10, IL-35), and mediating conversion of ATP to adenosine among many other functions [150]. An emerging target to inhibit Tregs is the chemokine receptor CCR8. CCR8 is a unique target, as it is expressed almost exclusively on tumor-infiltrating Tregs as opposed to peripheral Tregs, a feature which could overcome toxicity seen when depleting Tregs in previous studies [151]. Preclinical studies of anti-CCR8 antibodies revealed delayed tumor growth, decreased Treg/CD8 T cell ratio, and low levels of Treg functional markers and exhaustion markers on T cells in lymph nodes [152]. There are currently four different CCR8-targeting agents in clinical trial for HNSCC, outlined in Table 7.8.

## 7.4 Therapeutic Cancer Vaccines

Immunosurveillance, a process in which the immune system searches for foreign antigens, is the central tenet of the anti-tumor activity of therapeutic cancer vaccines. The therapeutic effect is achieved by targeting one or more TAAs to trigger immune-mediated cytotoxic activity, dampen immunosuppressive activity, and reinvigorate existing anti-tumor immunity [153]. While therapeutic vaccines to treat cancer have been studied since the early 2000s, the initial clinical trials failed to meet their primary endpoints. Further understanding of the TIME and how to modulate it and when patients should receive therapeutic vaccines has led to promising new avenues in their development. In this section, we will discuss three categories of therapeutic vaccines aimed at improving antigen delivery and enhancing tumor specificity including autophagosome vaccines (Fig. 7.2a), DNA and RNA-based vaccines (Fig. 7.2b), peptide vaccines (Fig. 7.2c) and viral vector vaccines (Fig. 7.2d).

### 7.4.1 Autophagosome Vaccines

Autophagosomes are vesicles that engulf a wide array of cellular material and fuse with lysosomes to degrade and recycle cellular debris through a process called autophagy. When autophagy takes place in the dendritic cell (DC) or any other MHC II-expressing cell, products of lysosomal degradation are presented on MHC II molecules to CD4 T cells [154]. In tumor cells, autophagy has been shown to play a critical role in cross-presentation of TAAs to CD8 T cells on MHC I [155]. The group that discovered autophagosomes as the TAA carriers responsible for this cross-presentation, which is critical for effective cancer vaccines, developed an autophagosome-based tumor vaccine called DPV-001 that carries 25 TAAs. They generated autophagosome-enriched defective ribosomal product (DRiP) blebs (DRibbles) that can be internalized by APCs

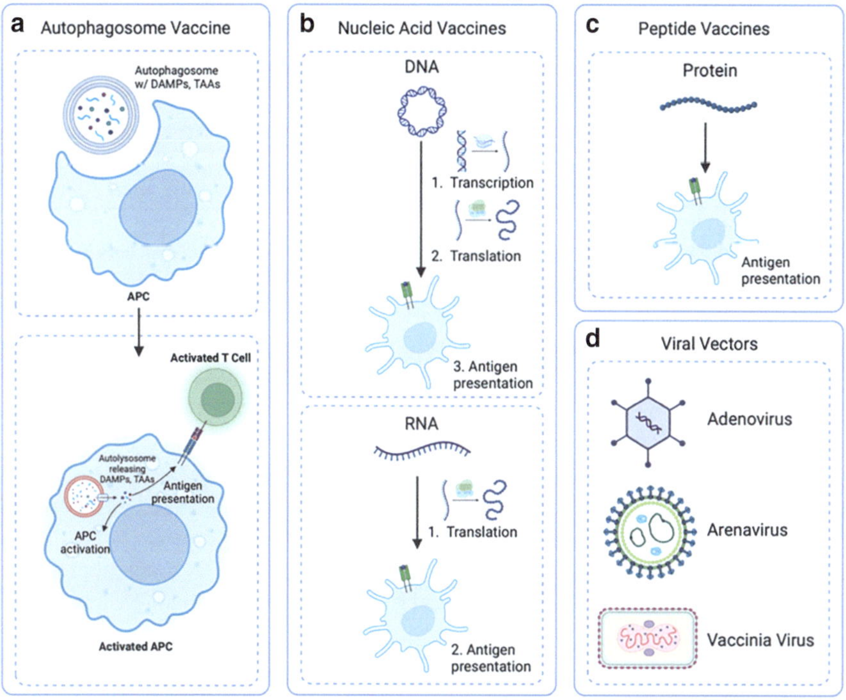


**Fig. 7.2** Types of therapeutic vaccines. (**a**) Autophagosome vaccines, (**b**) DNA and RNA vaccines, (**c**) peptide vaccines, and (**d**) viral vector-based vaccines

to activate target cells and have their cargo processed for antigen-cross presentation and subsequent T cell activation [156]. DPV-001 was initially developed utilizing non-small cell lung cancer (NSCLC) cell lines and is currently the only autophagosome vaccine in clinical trial for HNSCC (NCT04470025; Table 7.9).

### 7.4.2 Antigen-Specific Vaccines

Antigen vaccines, which directly deliver a concentrated bolus of antigen by injection, work by introducing antigens to processing pathways of APCs to induce an anti-tumor immune response. The main platforms for antigen vaccine development are DNA, RNA, peptide, and viral vector-based vaccines. DNA vaccines, when administered in high doses, can induce CD4 and CD8 T cell responses, but not DC responses. Since RNA vaccines don't require the transcriptional steps the DNA vaccines do, they are more easily able to be processed by APCs and presented on APC molecules as antigens. The benefits of DNA and RNA vaccines are the ability to build in adjuvants, or helper molecules to boost immune response. Unlike DNA and RNA vaccines, peptide vaccines can easily be presented on MHC directly, but responses could be transient due to rapid degradation and acquired tolerance [153, 157]. Three major vectors are used as backbones for viral vector-based vaccines in clinical trial for HNSCC: adenovirus, arenavirus, and vaccinia virus. Adenoviral vectors are good candidates for vaccine development as they do not integrate into the host genome but have strong immunogenic activity, however anti-vector immunity is common after inoculation [158]. Arenaviruses, such as lymphocytic choriomeningitis virus (LCMV), infect APCs, facilitate co-stimulation and antigen presentation, and promote CD8 T cell activity. Further, arenaviruses are not typically subject to pre-existing immunity like adenoviruses are, potentially increasing their long-term efficacy and ability to be re-administered as boosters [159]. Vaccinia viruses have been studied as platforms for vaccine development since the 1980s, following the success of the smallpox vaccine. Vaccinia virus backbones are promising candidates to develop therapeutic cancer vaccines due to their quick replication time and spread as well as their large genome. One concern with developing a vaccinia virus-based vaccine is the unknown activity of about half of its viral genes [160].

Beyond optimizing the delivery platform, selecting the right antigens to deliver is a critical facet of therapeutic vaccine development. HPV-related disease comprises about 25% of HNSCCs, with HPV16 and HPV18 being the cause of more than 80% of HPV-associated HNSCCs. The high rate of HPV-related disease makes targeting HPV-related antigens, especially E6 and E7, a logical choice [153]. Elevated expression of EGFR in HNSCC makes its ligand, EGF, a potential target. The CIMAvax vaccine currently in clinical trial aims to promote anti-EGF antibody

**Table 7.9** Autophagosome vaccine in clinical trial

| Drug | Trial | Treatment | Phase | Enrollment | Status |
|---|---|---|---|---|---|
| DPV-001 | NCT04470025 | DPV-001 plus anti-PD-1 with or without anti-GITR | 1 | 56 | Recruiting |

**Table 7.10** Antigen-specific vaccines in clinical trial

| Drug (Target) | Trial | Treatment | Phase | Enrollment | Status |
|---|---|---|---|---|---|
| IBRX-042 (HPV-16) | NCT05976828 | IBRX-042 as single agent | 1 | 12 | Recruiting |
| HB-202, 203 (HPV E6/E7) | NCT05108870 | HB202,203 plus neoadjuvant chemotherapy | 1/2 | 98 | Recruiting |
| TG4050 (neoantigen) | NCT04183166 | TG4050 as single agent | 1/2 | 80 | Recruiting |
| CIMAvax (EGF) | NCT02955290 | CIMAvax plus with nivolumab | 1/2 | 242 | Recruiting |
| PNeoVCA (neoantigen) | NCT05269381 | PNeoVCA as single agent or combined with pembrolizumab | 1/2 | 36 | Recruiting |
| BNT-113 (HPV E6/E7) | NCT04534205 | BNT-113 plus pembrolizumab as first line | 2 | 285 | Recruiting |
| pBI-11/TA-HPV (HPV 16/17 E6/E7) | NCT05799144 | pBI-11/TA-HPV plus pembrolizumab | 2 | 54 | Recruiting |
| IO102- IO103 (IDO1/PD-L1) | NCT05977907 | Adjuvant IO102-IO103 plus pembrolizumab | 2 | 15 | Recruiting |
| PRGN-2009 (HPV-16,18) | NCT06223568 | PRGN-2009 as single agent or combined with neoadjuvant chemotherapy | 2 | 70 | Recruiting |

production to prevent ligand-receptor engagement [161]. One challenge of therapeutic vaccines targeting TAAs is the lack of tumor specificity. Neoantigens, unique proteins or peptides that arise from tumor cells as the result of mutations that are not present in normal cells, may help overcome this challenge by improving immunogenicity, tumor specificity, and efficacy of therapeutic vaccines [162]. Clinical trials of antigen-specific therapeutic vaccines in HNC are detailed in Table 7.10.

## 7.5 Adoptive Cell Therapy

Adoptive cell therapy, pioneered for treatment of hematological malignancies, involves isolating a patient's immune cells, expanding and modifying them *ex vivo,* and infusing them back into the patient. Cells are typically modified to enhance their ability to target and kill malignant cells. Two forms of adoptive cell therapy are currently being studied to treat HNSCCs: chimeric antigen receptor (CAR)-T cell (Fig. 7.3a) and natural killer (NK) cell therapy (Fig. 7.3b).

### 7.5.1 CAR-T Cell Therapy

Chimeric antigen receptor (CAR)-T cell therapy involves development of a synthetic receptor, the CAR, to reprogram T cells to recognize and respond to a particular antigen. The CAR protein is made up of a genetically engineered extracellular recognition domain that recognizes the tumor antigen and an intracellular signaling

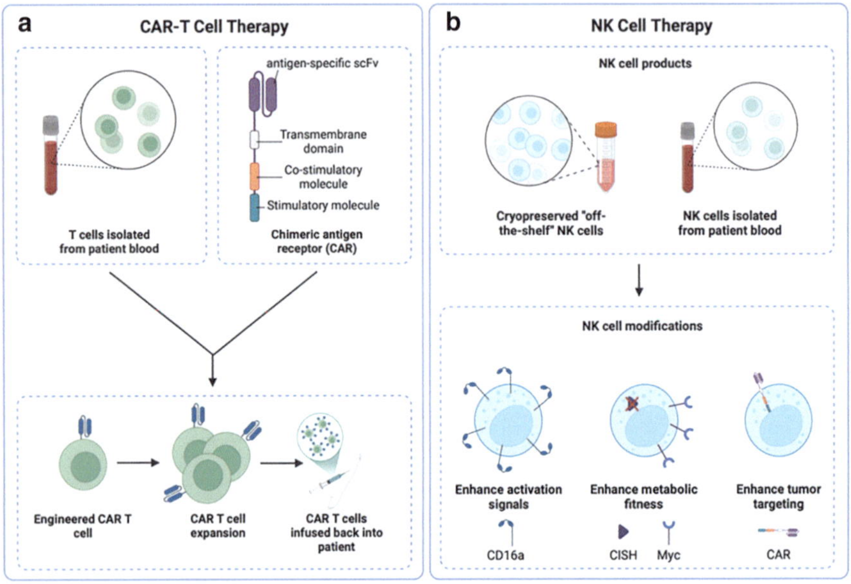


**Fig. 7.3** Adoptive cell therapy modalities. (**a**) CAR-T cell therapy and (**b**) NK cell therapy

region to activate the T cell. The extracellular domain is made up of a scFv that recognizes and binds the antigen and a structural TCR domain such as CD3, CD28, 4-1BB, or OX40. The scFv can be modified with variable heavy and light chain regions to ensure specificity for the target antigen. The intracellular domain, typically the CD3 domain, facilitates signaling to initiate T cell activation. Co-stimulation is required for the CAR-T cell to survive and proliferate, and this is achieved utilizing CD28, 4-1BB, or OX40 as co-stimulatory factors. Although CAR-T therapy has shown outstanding success in treating hematological malignancy, many challenges remain in their application toward solid tumors. Toxicity associated with cytokine release syndrome (CRS) because of tonic signaling, and off-target binding of CAR-T cells are major hurdles for patients receiving therapy. Further, efficacy is limited by selection and heterogeneity of target antigens, tumor antigen loss, and the makeup of the TIME in solid tumors [163]. Table 7.11 outlines CAR-T cell therapies currently in clinical trial for HNC.

### 7.5.2 NK Cell Therapy

NK cells pose a unique option for adoptive cell therapy over T cells as they are not antigen-specific and do not require priming to recognize tumor cells. Further, NK cell functionality increases as tumors downregulate MHC I expression, which is a common mechanism of T cell evasion. Beyond their cytotoxic activity, NK cells are also known to produce IFNγ and induce immunogenic cell death which aids in controlling metastatic spread. Further, they secrete FLT-3L, XCL1, and CCL5 to

**Table 7.11** CAR-T cell therapies in clinical trial

| Drug | Trial | Treatment | Phase | Enrollment | Status |
|---|---|---|---|---|---|
| P-MUC1-ALLO1 (MUC1) | NCT05239143 | P-MUC1-ALLO1 as single agent | 1 | 180 | Active, not recruiting |
| NT-175 (TP53 R175H) | NCT05877599 | NT-175 as single agent | 1 | 162 | Recruiting |
| ADP-A2M4CD8 (MAGE-A4) | NCT04044859 | ADP-A2M4CD8 as single agent or combined with anti-PD-1 | 1 | 120 | Active, not recruiting |
| iC9.CAR-CSPG4 T Cells (CSPG4) | NCT06096038 | iC9.CAR-CSPG4 as single agent | 1/2 | 33 | Suspended |
| E7 TCR T Cells (HPV 16 E7) | NCT05686226 | E7 TCR T Cells as single agent | 2 | 20 | Recruiting |

**Table 7.12** NK cell therapies in clinical trial

| Drug (Target) | Trial | Treatment | Phase | Enrollment | Status |
|---|---|---|---|---|---|
| WU-NK-101 | NCT05674526 | WU-NK-101 plus cetuximab | 1 | 30 | Recruiting |
| PD-LL1 t-haNK (PD-L1) | NCT06239220 | PD-L1 t-haNK plus cetuximab | 2 | 25 | Recruiting |

promote anti-tumor activity of other immune cells, including dendritic cells. Their safety profile also shows potential over CAR-T cells as they do not mediate graft-versus-host disease with allogenic grafts. NK cells are typically stimulated with cytokines *ex vivo* to enhance activation and expansion before being cryo-preserved for use as off-the-shelf infusion products. One common challenge between CAR-T and NK cell therapy in solid tumors is often the presence of an immunosuppressive TIME. Genetic engineering of NK cells can help to enhance their function. Expressing high affinity activating receptors to enhance tolerance to hypoxic conditions or reducing cytokine-inducible SH2-containing protein (CISH) or inducing MYC expression to enhance metabolic fitness and cell survival. The two NK cell therapies in clinical trial in HNSCC are being tested in combination with the EGFR inhibitor cetuximab with the goal of reducing the presence of immunosuppressive cells in the TIME to foster greater NK cell activity (Table 7.12) [164].

## 7.6 Oncolytic Viruses

Oncolytic viruses (OVs) harness the ability of viruses to replicate in and selectively lyse cancer cells while also inducing an immune response. One major draw to utilizing OVs in HNSCC is their ability to turn immunologically cold tumors hot [165]. There are several mechanisms by which OVs can alter a cold microenvironment: (1) Oncolytic lysis of tumors can promote release of TAAs and enhance antigen cross-presentation, (2) OVs can induce immunogenic tumor cell death, (3) OVs can directly interact with APCs to enhance their antigen priming activity, (4) OVs can

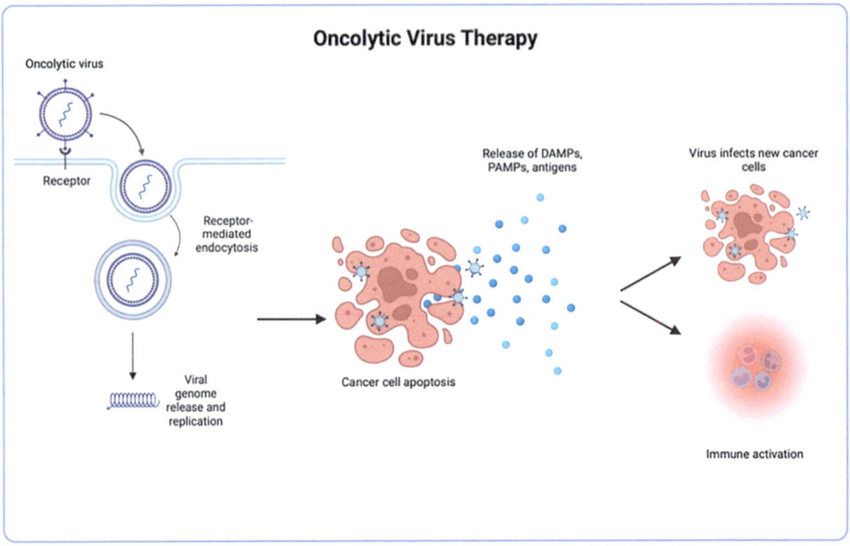


**Fig. 7.4** Oncolytic virus therapy

promote retreat of Tregs and MDSCs from the microenvironment, and (5) OVs can modulate the cytokine profile in the TIME [166] (Fig. 7.4). There are several different types of oncolytic viruses, with adenovirus, herpes simplex virus (HSV), and vesicular stomatitis virus (VSV) making up the therapeutics being tested in HNSCC.

### 7.6.1 Adenovirus

Oncolytic adenoviruses are naked viruses that are taken up by the cell via receptor-mediated endocytosis. Once viral particles are disassembled in the cytoplasm, they are transported to the nucleus where viral genes initiate progression into S-phase of the cell cycle, prevent cell death, and prolong viral replication time. Adenoviruses have very potent lytic activity and can be manufactured at high viral titers, but readily infect many cell types, so tumor targeting is an ongoing area to address [167]. Two adenovirus-based OVs are currently in clinical trial for HNC: TILT123 (NCT05222932) and MEM-228 (NCT05076760; Table 7.13).

### 7.6.2 Herpes Simplex Virus (HSV)

HSV is an enveloped virus with four viral glycoproteins expressed on its surface to facilitate binding to the target cell. The viral envelope fuses with the cell's membrane, releasing its genome into the cytoplasm which will make its way to the nucleus. HSVs are good candidates as oncolytic agents as their large genome allows for insertion of larger fragments. Pathogenicity of HSV and presence of neutralizing

**Table 7.13** Therapeutic vaccines in clinical trial

| Drug | Trial | Treatment | Phase | Enrollment | Status |
|---|---|---|---|---|---|
| TILT-123 | NCT05222932 | TILT-123 plus avelumab | 1 | 15 | Recruiting |
| MEM-288 | NCT05076760 | MEM-288 as single agent | 1 | 61 | Recruiting |
| MVR-T3011 | NCT04370587 | MVR-T3011 as single agent or combined with pembrolizumab | 1/2 | 64 | Recruiting |
| Voyager V1 | NCT04291105 | Voyager V1 plus cemiplimab | 2 | 87 | Recruiting |

antibodies in most subjects pose potential downsides to its use, however there is a drug available to shut off activity of the oncolytic HSV. One oncolytic HSV in clinical trial for HNSCC, MVR-T3011 has been granted fast-track designation for intratumoral injection for patients with recurrent or metastatic HNSCC who have received immune checkpoint therapy and are platinum-refractory (NCT04370587; Table 7.13) [167].

### 7.6.3 Vesicular Stomatitis Virus (VSV)

VSVs are enveloped viruses expressing glycoproteins that bind the low-density lipoprotein (LDL) receptor on host cells. VSVs enter the host cell via receptor-mediated endocytosis and replicate in the cytoplasm. While the interferon response mounted by normal cells against viruses does not allow VSVs to replicate, cancerous cells typically have lower interferon responses and are susceptible to viral replication and subsequent apoptosis. There is only one VSV FDA-approved currently as an Ebola virus vaccine, with questions around safety still prominent [168]. The VSV glycoprotein that binds the LDL receptor has high affinity for those receptors on neurons, leading to possible neurotoxicity. To address this, VSVs are being engineered with mutated G proteins to avoid neuronal targeting [169]. The Voyager V1 agent is a VSV-based OV currently in clinical trial in HNC (NCT04291105; Table 7.13).

## 7.7 Combination Strategies

The wide variety of immunotherapeutics making their way into the HNSCC space usher in an exciting new era of treatment options for patients. However, even with the early successes of the immune checkpoint inhibitors not all patients benefit from these strategies. HNSCCs exhibit high levels of oncogenic signaling, making the combination of targeted therapies to slow oncogenic progression and immune suppression and immune checkpoint inhibition to activate the immune system a rational strategy [170]. EGFR, receptor tyrosine kinase (RTK), PI3K, and JAK/STAT signaling all contribute to progression of HNSCC and inhibitors targeting these pathways are being studied in combination with pembrolizumab and nivolumab in an effort to improve patient response [171–176]. To take advantage of the varying immunomodulatory properties of different immune checkpoint inhibitors, combinations of ICIs with each other are being explored. CTLA-4 inhibition combined with PD-1/PD-L1 inhibition aims to target both T cell priming as well as T cell exhaustion and Treg activity. These combinations have been successful in melanoma and NSCLC but have yet to show any improvement over single-agent checkpoint inhibitor treatment in HNSCC [177–179]. A recent window trial evaluating CD8 T cell dynamics following different ICI regimens in HNSCC reported that tumors treated with the combination of anti-PD-1 and anti-LAG-3 exhibited significantly higher abundance of CD8 T cells that correlated with pathologic response compared to tumors treated with the combination of anti-PD-1 and anti-CTLA-4 [180].

Radiation therapy is a mainstay in the treatment of HNSCC, and studies have shown increased immunogenicity in irradiated tumors [181, 182]. A preclinical model of HNSCC showed that PD-L1-resistant murine tumors could be sensitized by combining radiation and PD-L1 inhibition [183]. The NRG-HN004 trial aimed to evaluate whether radioimmunotherapy could be used as an alternative to chemoradiotherapy in patients unable to tolerate cisplatin. The results of this study were negative, with the durvalumab (anti-PD-L1) plus radiotherapy group exhibiting no improvement in outcomes versus the cetuximab plus radiotherapy group [184]. While immunotherapy combinations still hold promise, much more investigation into the right combinations, timing, dosage, and selection of optimal patient populations needs to be done.

## 7.8 Biomarkers

Despite the advances made in a variety of immunotherapy categories and combinatorial strategies, only about 18% of HNSCC patients experience clinical benefit. Discovery of new biomarkers to identify the optimal populations of patients to receive immunotherapy is critical to improving outcomes. PD-L1 expression is the most widely used biomarker in HNSCC, but it is not perfect. Results from the KEYNOTE 012, KEYOTE 055, and CHECKMATE 141 trials show that while PD-L1-positive patients respond well to checkpoint therapy as expected, some PD-L1-negative patients also exhibit remarkable response [106, 109, 185]. Tumor mutational load was also evaluated in the KEYNOTE 012 trial. Total mutational load of greater than 102 mutations per exome was found to correlate positively with response to pembrolizumab. Specifically, patients with *NOTCH1* and *SMARCA4* mutations were found to respond better to checkpoint therapy [186]. An interferon-gamma gene signature was also evaluated in the KEYNOTE 012 trial in pre-treatment biopsies and was associated with improved overall response [106]. The TIME may also serve as a source of predictive biomarkers for checkpoint therapy. The presence of tertiary lymphoid structures has shown to be a potential predictor of sensitivity to ICIs in many tumor types, including HNSCC [187]. HNSCC tumors may also be stratified based on the composition of their TIME into two classes:

activated and exhausted. The activated class is associated with ICI sensitivity and contains high levels of B cell and M1 macrophage infiltration. The exhausted class, associated with ICI resistance, exhibits M2 macrophage enrichment and increased WNT/TGF-β activation [188].

## 7.9 Conclusion

Head and neck cancers (HNCs) are the seventh most common type of cancer worldwide with incidence increasing steadily each year. While surgery, chemotherapy, radiation, and systemic therapy are all options for these patients, 5-year survival for locally advanced and metastatic disease remains low, around 35% and 4%, respectively. Immune therapies have shown remarkable efficacy in hotter tumor types, such as melanoma and NSCLC, however response remains low in cold tumors like HNC. The HNC TIME is highly immunosuppressive, with low infiltration of pro-inflammatory factors and high infiltration of anti-inflammatory cells and signaling molecules.

Currently, three immune checkpoint inhibitors, pembrolizumab nivolumab, and toripalimab are approved for HNC as the result of the KEYNOTE-012, KEYNOTE-048, CheckMate 141, POLARIS-02, and JUPITER-02 trials, however resistance to therapy is a persistent problem. To address this, many other immunotherapeutic modalities are being tested in HNC. Additional ICIs targeting CTLA-4, TIGIT, VISTA, LLT1, CD39, and LAG-3 are in early-stage clinical trials. Beyond immune checkpoints, other immunomodulatory agents including immune cell engagers, bispecific compounds, modified cytokines, and Treg inhibitors are in the early stages of development with promising preclinical results in murine models of HNC. Following the success of adoptive cell therapy in hematological malignancy, CAR-T and NK cell therapies have gained traction in solid tumors, specifically HNSCC. Viral therapies, including therapeutic vaccines and oncolytic viruses, are in early stages of investigation for HNC, and while there remains some uncertainty about their efficacy at this point, they appear to be well-tolerated.

To combat the low rates of sensitivity to ICI in HNC, combinatorial strategies to improve tumor immunogenicity are becoming more popular lines of preclinical study. Some success in combining two ICIs with one another, ICIs with molecular targeted therapies, and ICIs with radiotherapy has been seen in murine models of HNC and pose exciting alternatives to monotherapy. In addition to development of new therapeutic options, additional biomarkers to pinpoint the most likely populations to respond to specific therapies are critically needed. These biomarkers can be tumor-specific, such as PD-L1 expression, tumor mutational burden or IFN-γ signatures, or specific to the TIME including factors such as tertiary lymphoid structures and relative immune infiltration. As these new therapeutic modalities and biomarkers start to enter the clinic, we are stepping into an optimistic new area of HNC treatment and groundbreaking advances to improve outcomes for HNC patients in the future.

## References


1. Barsouk A, Aluru JS, Rawla P, Saginala K, Barsouk A. Epidemiology, risk factors, and prevention of head and neck squamous cell carcinoma. Med Sci (Basel). 2023;11(2):42. https://doi.org/10.3390/medsci11020042.
2. Wierzbicka M, Pietruszewska W, Maciejczyk A, Markowski J. Trends in incidence and mortality of head and neck cancer subsites among elderly patients: a population-based analysis. Cancers (Basel). 2025;17(3):548. https://doi.org/10.3390/cancers17030548.
3. Klein JD, Grandis JR. The molecular pathogenesis of head and neck cancer. Cancer Biol Ther. 2010;9(1):1–7. https://doi.org/10.4161/cbt.9.1.10905.
4. Chang ET, Ye W, Zeng YX, Adami HO. The evolving epidemiology of nasopharyngeal carcinoma. Cancer Epidemiol Biomarkers Prev. 2021;30(6):1035–47. https://doi.org/10.1158/1055-9965.EPI-20-1702.
5. Mahal BA, Catalano PJ, Haddad RI, Hanna GJ, Kass JI, Schoenfeld JD, et al. Incidence and demographic burden of HPV-associated oropharyngeal head and neck cancers in the united states. Cancer Epidemiol Biomarkers Prev. 2019;28(10):1660–7. https://doi.org/10.1158/1055-9965.EPI-19-0038.
6. Yan F, Knochelmann HM, Morgan PF, Kaczmar JM, Neskey DM, Graboyes EM, et al. The evolution of care of cancers of the head and neck region: state of the science in 2020. Cancers (Basel). 2020;12(6):1543. https://doi.org/10.3390/cancers12061543.
7. Mehanna H, Taberna M, von Buchwald C, Tous S, Brooks J, Mena M, et al. Prognostic implications of p16 and HPV discordance in oropharyngeal cancer (HNCIG-EPIC-OPC): a multicentre, multinational, individual patient data analysis. Lancet Oncol. 2023;24(3):239–51. https://doi.org/10.1016/S1470-2045(23)00013-X.
8. Rischin D, Young RJ, Fisher R, Fox SB, Le QT, Peters LJ, et al. Prognostic significance of p16 and human papillomavirus in patients with oropharyngeal cancer treated on TROG 02.02 phase III trial. J Clin Oncol. 2010;28(27):4142–8. https://doi.org/10.1200/Jco.2010.29.2904.
9. Dayyani F, Etzel CJ, Liu M, Ho CH, Lippman SM, Tsao AS. Meta-analysis of the impact of human papillomavirus (HPV) on cancer risk and overall survival in head and neck squamous cell carcinomas (HNSCC). Head Neck Oncol. 2010;2:15. https://doi.org/10.1186/1758-3284-2-15.
10. Khetan P, Boffetta P, Luce D, Stucker I, Curado MP, Menezes A, et al. Occupations and the risk of head and neck cancer: a pooled analysis of the international head and neck cancer epidemiology (INHANCE) consortium. J Occup Environ Med. 2019;61(5):397–404. https://doi.org/10.1097/JOM.0000000000001563.
11. Anderson G, Ebadi M, Vo K, Novak J, Govindarajan A, Amini A. An updated review on head and neck cancer treatment with radiation therapy. Cancers (Basel). 2021;13(19) https://doi.org/10.3390/cancers13194912.
12. Zhang S, Zeng N, Yang J, He J, Zhu F, Liao W, et al. Advancements of radiotherapy for recurrent head and neck cancer in modern era. Radiat Oncol. 2023;18(1):166. https://doi.org/10.1186/s13014-023-02342-0.
13. Chow LQM. Head and neck cancer. N Engl J Med. 2020;382(1):60–72. https://doi.org/10.1056/NEJMra1715715.
14. Li Q, Tie Y, Alu A, Ma X, Shi H. Targeted therapy for head and neck cancer: signaling pathways and clinical studies. Signal Transduct Target Ther. 2023;8(1):31. https://doi.org/10.1038/s41392-022-01297-0.
15. Li Y, Jiang Y, Qiu B, Sun H, Wang J. Current radiotherapy for recurrent head and neck cancer in the modern era: a state-of-the-art review. J Transl Med. 2022;20(1):566. https://doi.org/10.1186/s12967-022-03774-0.
16. Bonner JA, Harari PM, Giralt J, Azarnia N, Shin DM, Cohen RB, et al. Radiotherapy plus cetuximab for squamous-cell carcinoma of the head and neck. New Engl J Med. 2006;354(6):567–78. https://doi.org/10.1056/NEJMoa053422.

17. Sato JD, Kawamoto T, Le AD, Mendelsohn J, Polikoff J, Sato GH. Biological effects in vitro of monoclonal antibodies to human epidermal growth factor receptors. Mol Biol Med. 1983;1(5):511–29.
18. Kawamoto T, Sato JD, Le A, Polikoff J, Sato GH, Mendelsohn J. Growth-Stimulation of A431 cells by epidermal growth-factor—identification of high-affinity receptors for epidermal growth-factor by an anti-receptor monoclonal-antibody. Proc Nat Acad Sci Biol. 1983;80(5):1337–41. https://doi.org/10.1073/pnas.80.5.1337.
19. Vermorken JB, Mesia R, Rivera F, Remenar E, Kawecki A, Rottey S, et al. Platinum-based chemotherapy plus cetuximab in head and neck cancer. N Engl J Med. 2008;359(11):1116–27. https://doi.org/10.1056/NEJMoa0802656.
20. Beckham TH, Leeman JE, Xie P, Li X, Goldman DA, Zhang Z, et al. Long-term survival in patients with metastatic head and neck squamous cell carcinoma treated with metastasis-directed therapy. Br J Cancer. 2019;121(11):897–903. https://doi.org/10.1038/s41416-019-0601-8.
21. Elmusrati A, Wang J, Wang CY. Tumor microenvironment and immune evasion in head and neck squamous cell carcinoma. Int J Oral Sci. 2021;13(1) https://doi.org/10.1038/s41368-021-00131-7.
22. Wang G, Zhang M, Cheng M, Wang X, Li K, Chen J, et al. Tumor microenvironment in head and neck squamous cell carcinoma: functions and regulatory mechanisms. Cancer Lett. 2021;507:55–69. https://doi.org/10.1016/j.canlet.2021.03.009.
23. Damasio MPS, Nascimento CS, Andrade LM, de Oliveira VL, Calzavara-Silva CE. The role of T-cells in head and neck squamous cell carcinoma: from immunity to immunotherapy. Front Oncol. 2022;12:1021609. https://doi.org/10.3389/fonc.2022.1021609.
24. Raskov H, Orhan A, Christensen JP, Gögenur I. Cytotoxic CD8+ T cells in cancer and cancer immunotherapy. Br J Cancer. 2021;124(2):359–67. https://doi.org/10.1038/s41416-020-01048-4.
25. Wang H-C, Chan L-P, Cho S-F. Targeting the immune microenvironment in the treatment of head and neck squamous cell carcinoma. Front Oncol. 2019;9:1084.
26. Zhu J, Yamane H, Paul WE. Differentiation of effector CD4 T cell populations (*). Annu Rev Immunol. 2010;28:445–89. https://doi.org/10.1146/annurev-immunol-030409-101212.
27. Janssen EM, Lemmens EE, Gour N, Reboulet RA, Green DR, Schoenberger SP, et al. Distinct roles of cytolytic effector molecules for antigen-restricted killing by CTL in vivo. Immunol Cell Biol. 2010;88(7):761–5.
28. Olver S, Groves P, Buttigieg K, Morris ES, Janas ML, Kelso A, et al. Tumor-derived interleukin-4 reduces tumor clearance and deviates the cytokine and granzyme profile of tumor-induced CD8+ T cells. Cancer Res. 2006;66(1):571–80.
29. Sparano A, Lathers DMR, Achille N, Petruzzelli GJ, Young MRI. Modulation of Th1 and Th2 cytokine profiles and their association with advanced head and neck squamous cell carcinoma. Otolaryngol Head Neck Surg. 2004;131(5):573–6. https://doi.org/10.1016/j.otohns.2004.03.016.
30. Wang R, Yin G, Guo W, Li N, Zhang Y, Chen X, et al. Analysis of Th1/Th2 cytokine profile and clinical characteristics of patients with head and neck squamous cell carcinoma. Biomol Biomed. 2024;24(6):1776–84. https://doi.org/10.17305/bb.2024.10783.
31. Bailey SR, Nelson MH, Himes RA, Li Z, Mehrotra S, Paulos CM. Th17 cells in cancer: the ultimate identity crisis. Front Immunol. 2014;5:276. https://doi.org/10.3389/fimmu.2014.00276.
32. Kesselring R, Thiel A, Pries R, Trenkle T, Wollenberg B. Human Th17 cells can be induced through head and neck cancer and have a functional impact on HNSCC development. Br J Cancer. 2010;103(8):1245–54. https://doi.org/10.1038/sj.bjc.6605891.
33. Strauss L, Bergmann C, Szczepanski M, Gooding W, Johnson JT, Whiteside TL. A unique subset of CD4+ CD25highFoxp3+ T cells secreting interleukin-10 and transforming growth factor-β1 mediates suppression in the tumor microenvironment. Clin Cancer Res. 2007;13(15):4345–54.

34. Weed DT, Vella JL, Reis IM, De la Fuente AC, Gomez C, Sargi Z, et al. Tadalafil reduces myeloid-derived suppressor cells and regulatory T cells and promotes tumor immunity in patients with head and neck squamous cell carcinoma. Clin Cancer Res. 2015;21(1):39–48.
35. Weed DT, Walker G, De La Fuente AC, Nazarian R, Vella JL, Gomez-Fernandez CR, et al. FOXP3 subcellular localization predicts recurrence in oral squamous cell carcinoma. PLoS One. 2013;8(8):e71908.
36. Murray PJ, Allen JE, Biswas SK, Fisher EA, Gilroy DW, Goerdt S, et al. Macrophage activation and polarization: nomenclature and experimental guidelines. Immunity. 2014;41(1):14–20.
37. Weagel E, Smith C, Liu P, Robison R, O'neill K. Macrophage polarization and its role in cancer. J Clin Cell Immunol. 2015;6(4):338.
38. Sica A, Mantovani A. Macrophage plasticity and polarization: in vivo veritas. J Clin Invest. 2012;122(3):787–95.
39. Costa NL, Valadares MC, Souza PPC, Mendonça EF, Oliveira JC, Silva TA, et al. Tumor-associated macrophages and the profile of inflammatory cytokines in oral squamous cell carcinoma. Oral Oncol. 2013;49(3):216–23.
40. Wolf GT, Chepeha DB, Bellile E, Nguyen A, Thomas D, McHugh J. Tumor infiltrating lymphocytes (TIL) and prognosis in oral cavity squamous carcinoma: a preliminary study. Oral Oncol. 2015;51(1):90–5.
41. Ribechini E, Greifenberg V, Sandwick S, Lutz MB. Subsets, expansion and activation of myeloid-derived suppressor cells. Med Microbiol Immunol. 2010;199:273–81.
42. Lesokhin AM, Hohl TM, Kitano S, Cortez C, Hirschhorn-Cymerman D, Avogadri F, et al. Monocytic CCR2+ myeloid-derived suppressor cells promote immune escape by limiting activated CD8 T-cell infiltration into the tumor microenvironment. Cancer Res. 2012;72(4):876–86.
43. Corzo CA, Cotter MJ, Cheng P, Cheng F, Kusmartsev S, Sotomayor E, et al. Mechanism regulating reactive oxygen species in tumor-induced myeloid-derived suppressor cells. J Immunol. 2009;182(9):5693–701.
44. Veglia F, Perego M, Gabrilovich D. Myeloid-derived suppressor cells coming of age. Nat Immunol. 2018;19(2):108–19.
45. Li H, Han Y, Guo Q, Zhang M, Cao X. Cancer-expanded myeloid-derived suppressor cells induce anergy of NK cells through membrane-bound TGF-β1. J Immunol. 2009;182(1):240–9.
46. Lang S, Bruderek K, Kaspar C, Höing B, Kanaan O, Dominas N, et al. Clinical relevance and suppressive capacity of human myeloid-derived suppressor cell subsets. Clin Cancer Res. 2018;24(19):4834–44.
47. Chen W-C, Lai C-H, Chuang H-C, Lin P-Y, Chen M-F. Inflammation-induced myeloid-derived suppressor cells associated with squamous cell carcinoma of the head and neck. Head Neck. 2017;39(2):347–55. https://doi.org/10.1002/hed.24595.
48. Cooper MA, Fehniger TA, Caligiuri MA. The biology of human natural killer-cell subsets. Trends Immunol. 2001;22(11):633–40.
49. Martínez-Lostao L, Anel A, Pardo J. How do cytotoxic lymphocytes kill cancer cells? Clin Cancer Res. 2015;21(22):5047–56.
50. Dhar P, Wu JD. NKG2D and its ligands in cancer. Curr Opin Immunol. 2018;51:55–61. https://doi.org/10.1016/j.coi.2018.02.004.
51. Weil S, Memmer S, Lechner A, Huppert V, Giannattasio A, Becker T, et al. Natural killer group 2D ligand depletion reconstitutes natural killer cell immunosurveillance of head and neck squamous cell carcinoma. Front Immunol. 2017;8:387.
52. O'Donnell JS, Teng MWL, Smyth MJ. Cancer immunoediting and resistance to T cell-based immunotherapy. Nat Rev Clin Oncol. 2019;16(3):151–67. https://doi.org/10.1038/s41571-018-0142-8.
53. Wilczynski JR, Nowak M. Cancer immunoediting: elimination, equilibrium, and immune escape in solid tumors. In: Interaction of immune and cancer cells; 2014. p. 143–205. https://doi.org/10.1007/978-3-030-91311-3_1.
54. Kostecki KL, Iida M, Crossman BE, Salgia R, Harari PM, Bruce JY, et al. Immune escape strategies in head and neck cancer: evade, resist, inhibit. Recruit Cancer. 2024;16(2):312.

55. Duray A, Demoulin S, Hubert P, Delvenne P, Saussez S. Immune suppression in head and neck cancers: a review. J Immunol Res. 2010;2010(1):701657. https://doi.org/10.1155/2010/701657.
56. Moy JD, Moskovitz JM, Ferris RL. Biological mechanisms of immune escape and implications for immunotherapy in head and neck squamous cell carcinoma. Eur J Cancer. 2017;76:152–66.
57. Luo X, Qiu Y, Fitzsimonds ZR, Wang Q, Chen Q, Lei YL. Immune escape of head and neck cancer mediated by the impaired MHC-I antigen presentation pathway. Oncogene. 2024;43(6):388–94. https://doi.org/10.1038/s41388-023-02912-2.
58. Network CGA. Comprehensive genomic characterization of head and neck squamous cell carcinomas. Nature. 2015;517(7536):576.
59. Grandis JR, Falkner DM, Melhem MF, Gooding WE, Drenning SD, Morel PA. Human leukocyte antigen class I allelic and haplotype loss in squamous cell carcinoma of the head and neck: clinical and immunogenetic consequences. Clin Cancer Res. 2000;6(7):2794–802.
60. Ferris RL, Hunt JL, Ferrone S. Human leukocyte antigen (HLA) class I defects in head and neck cancer: molecular mechanisms and clinical significance. Immunol Res. 2005;33:113–33.
61. Bandoh N, Ogino T, Katayama A, Takahara M, Katada A, Hayashi T, et al. HLA class I antigen and transporter associated with antigen processing downregulation in metastatic lesions of head and neck squamous cell carcinoma as a marker of poor prognosis. Oncol Rep. 2010;23(4):933–9.
62. Ferris RL, Whiteside TL, Ferrone S. Immune escape associated with functional defects in antigen-processing machinery in head and neck cancer. Clin Cancer Res. 2006;12(13):3890–5.
63. Pishesha N, Harmand TJ, Ploegh HL. A guide to antigen processing and presentation. Nat Rev Immunol. 2022;22(12):751–64.
64. Yan S, Zhang X, Lin Q, Du M, Li Y, He S, et al. Deciphering the interplay of HPV infection, MHC-II expression, and CXCL13+ CD4+ T cell activation in oropharyngeal cancer: implications for immunotherapy. Cancer Immunol Immunother. 2024;73(10):206.
65. Tosi A, Parisatto B, Menegaldo A, Spinato G, Guido M, Del Mistro A, et al. The immune microenvironment of HPV-positive and HPV-negative oropharyngeal squamous cell carcinoma: a multiparametric quantitative and spatial analysis unveils a rationale to target treatment-naïve tumors with immune checkpoint inhibitors. J Exp Clin Cancer Res. 2022;41(1):279. https://doi.org/10.1186/s13046-022-02481-4.
66. Concha-Benavente F, Srivastava RM, Trivedi S, Lei Y, Chandran U, Seethala RR, et al. Identification of the cell-intrinsic and-extrinsic pathways downstream of EGFR and IFNγ that induce PD-L1 expression in head and neck cancer. Cancer Res. 2016;76(5):1031–43.
67. Ishida Y, Agata Y, Shibahara K, Honjo T. Induced expression of PD-1, a novel member of the immunoglobulin gene superfamily, upon programmed cell death. EMBO J. 1992;11(11):3887–95.
68. Ludwig S, Floros T, Theodoraki M-N, Hong C-S, Jackson EK, Lang S, et al. Suppression of lymphocyte functions by plasma exosomes correlates with disease activity in patients with head and neck cancer. Clin Cancer Res. 2017;23(16):4843–54.
69. Skinner HD, Giri U, Yang LP, Kumar M, Liu Y, Story MD, et al. Integrative analysis identifies a novel AXL–PI3 Kinase–PD-L1 signaling axis associated with radiation resistance in head and neck cancer. Clin Cancer Res. 2017;23(11):2713–22.
70. Latchman Y, Wood CR, Chernova T, Chaudhary D, Borde M, Chernova I, et al. PD-L2 is a second ligand for PD-1 and inhibits T cell activation. Nat Immunol. 2001;2(3):261–8.
71. Yearley JH, Gibson C, Yu N, Moon C, Murphy E, Juco J, et al. PD-L2 expression in human tumors: relevance to anti-PD-1 therapy in cancer. Clin Cancer Res. 2017;23(12):3158–67.
72. Wu J, Gao F-x, Wang C, Qin M, Han F, Xu T, et al. IL-6 and IL-8 secreted by tumour cells impair the function of NK cells via the STAT3 pathway in oesophageal squamous cell carcinoma. J Exp Clin Cancer Res. 2019;38:1–15.
73. Chen Y, Di C, Zhang X, Wang J, Wang F, Yan JF, et al. Transforming growth factor β signaling pathway: a promising therapeutic target for cancer. J Cell Physiol. 2020;235(3):1903–14.

74. Moutsopoulos NM, Wen J, Wahl SM. TGF-β and tumors—an ill-fated alliance. Curr Opin Immunol. 2008;20(2):234–40.
75. Wolf J, Chen Z, Dong G, Sunwoo J, Bancroft C, Capo D, et al. 1alpha promotes nuclear factor-kappaB and AP-1-induced IL-8 expression, cell survival, and proliferation in head and neck squamous cell carcinomas. Clin Cancer Res. 2001;7(6):1812–20.
76. Woods KV, Adler-Storthz K, Clayman GL, Francis GM, Grimm EA. Interleukin-1 regulates interleukin-6 secretion in human oral squamous cell carcinoma in vitro: possible influence of p53 but not human papillomavirus E6/E7. Cancer Res. 1998;58(14):3142–9.
77. Hargadon KM. Tumor-altered dendritic cell function: implications for anti-tumor immunity. Front Immunol. 2013;4:192.
78. Park S-J, Nakagawa T, Kitamura H, Atsumi T, Kamon H, Sawa S-i, et al. IL-6 regulates in vivo dendritic cell differentiation through STAT3 activation. J Immunol. 2004;173(6):3844–54.
79. Coffelt SB, Hughes R, Lewis CE. Tumor-associated macrophages: effectors of angiogenesis and tumor progression. Biochim Biophys Acta Rev Cancer. 2009;1796(1):11–8.
80. Liss C, Fekete MJ, Hasina R, Lam CD, Lingen MW. Paracrine angiogenic loop between head-and-neck squamous-cell carcinomas and macrophages. Int J Cancer. 2001;93(6):781–5.
81. Mantovani A, Sica A, Sozzani S, Allavena P, Vecchi A, Locati M. The chemokine system in diverse forms of macrophage activation and polarization. Trends Immunol. 2004;25(12):677–86.
82. Van Overmeire E, Stijlemans B, Heymann F, Keirsse J, Morias Y, Elkrim Y, et al. M-CSF and GM-CSF receptor signaling differentially regulate monocyte maturation and macrophage polarization in the tumor microenvironment. Cancer Res. 2016;76(1):35–42.
83. Facciabene A, Peng X, Hagemann IS, Balint K, Barchetti A, Wang L-P, et al. Tumour hypoxia promotes tolerance and angiogenesis via CCL28 and Treg cells. Nature. 2011;475(7355):226–30.
84. Nishikawa H, Sakaguchi S. Regulatory T cells in cancer immunotherapy. Curr Opin Immunol. 2014;27:1–7.
85. Zou L, Barnett B, Safah H, LaRussa VF, Evdemon-Hogan M, Mottram P, et al. Bone marrow is a reservoir for CD4+ CD25+ regulatory T cells that traffic through CXCL12/CXCR4 signals. Cancer Res. 2004;64(22):8451–5.
86. Valzasina B, Piconese S, Guiducci C, Colombo MP. Tumor-induced expansion of regulatory T cells by conversion of CD4+ CD25− lymphocytes is thymus and proliferation independent. Cancer Res. 2006;66(8):4488–95.
87. Thomas GR, Chen Z, Leukinova E, Van Waes C, Wen J. Cytokines IL-1α, IL-6, and GM-CSF constitutively secreted by oral squamous carcinoma induce down-regulation of CD80 costimulatory molecule expression: restoration by interferon γ. Cancer Immunol Immunother. 2004;53:33–40.
88. Lathers DM, Young MRI. Increased aberrance of cytokine expression in plasma of patients with more advanced squamous cell carcinoma of the head and neck. Cytokine. 2004;25(5):220–8.
89. Chalmers ZR, Connelly CF, Fabrizio D, Gay L, Ali SM, Ennis R, et al. Analysis of 100,000 human cancer genomes reveals the landscape of tumor mutational burden. Genome Med. 2017;9:1–14.
90. Schumacher TN, Scheper W, Kvistborg P. Cancer neoantigens. Annu Rev Immunol. 2019;37(1):173–200.
91. Schumacher TN, Schreiber RD. Neoantigens in cancer immunotherapy. Science. 2015;348(6230):69–74.
92. Rodrigo JP, Sánchez-Canteli M, Otero-Rosales M, Martínez-Camblor P, Hermida-Prado F, García-Pedrero JM. Tumor mutational burden predictability in head and neck squamous cell carcinoma patients treated with immunotherapy: systematic review and meta-analysis. J Transl Med. 2024;22(1):135. https://doi.org/10.1186/s12967-024-04937-x.
93. Klempner SJ, Fabrizio D, Bane S, Reinhart M, Peoples T, Ali SM, et al. Tumor mutational burden as a predictive biomarker for response to immune checkpoint inhibitors: a

review of current evidence. Oncologist. 2020;25(1):e147–e59. https://doi.org/10.1634/theoncologist.2019-0244.
94. Li Y, Ma Y, Wu Z, Zeng F, Song B, Zhang Y, et al. Tumor mutational burden predicting the efficacy of immune checkpoint inhibitors in colorectal cancer: a systematic review and meta-analysis. Front Immunol. 2021;12:751407.
95. Cao D, Xu H, Xu X, Guo T, Ge W. High tumor mutation burden predicts better efficacy of immunotherapy: a pooled analysis of 103078 cancer patients. Onco Targets Ther. 2019;8(9):e1629258.
96. Gandara DR, Paul SM, Kowanetz M, Schleifman E, Zou W, Li Y, et al. Blood-based tumor mutational burden as a predictor of clinical benefit in non-small-cell lung cancer patients treated with atezolizumab. Nat Med. 2018;24(9):1441–8.
97. Gameiro SF, Evans AM, Mymryk JS. The tumor immune microenvironments of HPV+ and HPV− head and neck cancers. WIREs Mech Dis. 2022;14(2):e1539.
98. Qureshi HA, Zhu X, Yang GH, Steadele M, Pierce RH, Futran ND, et al. Impact of HPV status on immune responses in head and neck squamous cell carcinoma. Oral Oncol. 2022;127:105774.
99. Xie N, Shen G, Gao W, Huang Z, Huang C, Fu L. Neoantigens: promising targets for cancer therapy. Signal Transduct Target Ther. 2023;8(1):9. https://doi.org/10.1038/s41392-022-01270-x.
100. Liu J, Chen Z, Li Y, Zhao W, Wu J, Zhang Z. PD-1/PD-l1 checkpoint inhibitors in tumor immunotherapy. Front Pharmacol. 2021;12:731798. https://doi.org/10.3389/fphar.2021.731798.
101. Smith-Garvin JE, Koretzky GA, Jordan MS. T cell activation. Annu Rev Immunol. 2009;27:591–619. https://doi.org/10.1146/annurev.immunol.021908.132706.
102. Freeman GJ, Long AJ, Iwai Y, Bourque K, Chernova T, Nishimura H, et al. Engagement of the PD-1 immunoinhibitory receptor by a novel B7 family member leads to negative regulation of lymphocyte activation. J Exp Med. 2000;192(7):1027–34. https://doi.org/10.1084/jem.192.7.1027.
103. Karwacz K, Bricogne C, MacDonald D, Arce F, Bennett CL, Collins M, et al. PD-L1 co-stimulation contributes to ligand-induced T cell receptor down-modulation on CD8+ T cells. EMBO Mol Med. 2011;3(10):581–92. https://doi.org/10.1002/emmm.201100165.
104. Escors D, Bricogne C, Arce F, Kochan G, Karwacz K. On the mechanism of T cell receptor down-modulation and its physiological significance. J Biosci Med. 2011;1(1):2011.5.
105. Juneja VR, McGuire KA, Manguso RT, LaFleur MW, Collins N, Haining WN, et al. PD-L1 on tumor cells is sufficient for immune evasion in immunogenic tumors and inhibits CD8 T cell cytotoxicity. J Exp Med. 2017;214(4):895–904. https://doi.org/10.1084/jem.20160801.
106. Seiwert TY, Burtness B, Mehra R, Weiss J, Berger R, Eder JP, et al. Safety and clinical activity of pembrolizumab for treatment of recurrent or metastatic squamous cell carcinoma of the head and neck (KEYNOTE-012): an open-label, multicentre, phase 1b trial. Lancet Oncol. 2016;17(7):956–65. https://doi.org/10.1016/S1470-2045(16)30066-3.
107. Larkins E, Blumenthal GM, Yuan W, He K, Sridhara R, Subramaniam S, et al. FDA approval summary: pembrolizumab for the treatment of recurrent or metastatic head and neck squamous cell carcinoma with disease progression on or after platinum-containing chemotherapy. Oncologist. 2017;22(7):873–8. https://doi.org/10.1634/theoncologist.2016-0496.
108. Burtness B, Harrington KJ, Greil R, Soulieres D, Tahara M, de Castro G Jr, et al. Pembrolizumab alone or with chemotherapy versus cetuximab with chemotherapy for recurrent or metastatic squamous cell carcinoma of the head and neck (KEYNOTE-048): a randomised, open-label, phase 3 study. Lancet. 2019;394(10212):1915–28. https://doi.org/10.1016/S0140-6736(19)32591-7.
109. Ferris RL, Blumenschein G Jr, Fayette J, Guigay J, Colevas AD, Licitra L, et al. Nivolumab for recurrent squamous-cell carcinoma of the head and neck. N Engl J Med. 2016;375(19):1856–67. https://doi.org/10.1056/NEJMoa1602252.
110. Wang FH, Wei XL, Feng J, Li Q, Xu N, Hu XC, et al. Efficacy, safety, and correlative biomarkers of toripalimab in previously treated recurrent or metastatic nasopharyngeal

carcinoma: a phase II clinical trial (POLARIS-02). J Clin Oncol. 2021;39(7):704–12. https://doi.org/10.1200/JCO.20.02712.
111. Mai HQ, Chen QY, Chen D, Hu C, Yang K, Wen J, et al. Toripalimab plus chemotherapy for recurrent or metastatic nasopharyngeal carcinoma: the JUPITER-02 randomized clinical trial. JAMA. 2023;330(20):1961–70. https://doi.org/10.1001/jama.2023.20181.
112. Chen XZ, Wang W, Zou QF, Li JG, Hu CS, Hu CS, et al. A phase II study of the anti-programmed cell death-1 (Pd-1) antibody penpulimab in patients with metastatic nasopharyngeal carcinoma (Npc) who had progressed after two or more lines of chemotherapy. J Immunother Cancer. 2020;8:A481–A. https://doi.org/10.1136/jitc-2020-SITC2020.0804.
113. Buchbinder EI, Desai A. CTLA-4 and PD-1 pathways: similarities, differences, and implications of their inhibition. Am J Clin Oncol. 2016;39(1):98–106. https://doi.org/10.1097/COC.0000000000000239.
114. Wing K, Onishi Y, Prieto-Martin P, Yamaguchi T, Miyara M, Fehervari Z, et al. CTLA-4 control over Foxp3+ regulatory T cell function. Science. 2008;322(5899):271–5. https://doi.org/10.1126/science.1160062.
115. Qureshi OS, Zheng Y, Nakamura K, Attridge K, Manzotti C, Schmidt EM, et al. Trans-endocytosis of CD80 and CD86: a molecular basis for the cell-extrinsic function of CTLA-4. Science. 2011;332(6029):600–3. https://doi.org/10.1126/science.1202947.
116. Fife BT, Bluestone JA. Control of peripheral T-cell tolerance and autoimmunity via the CTLA-4 and PD-1 pathways. Immunol Rev. 2008;224:166–82. https://doi.org/10.1111/j.1600-065X.2008.00662.x.
117. Robert L, Tsoi J, Wang X, Emerson R, Homet B, Chodon T, et al. CTLA4 blockade broadens the peripheral T-cell receptor repertoire. Clin Cancer Res. 2014;20(9):2424–32. https://doi.org/10.1158/1078-0432.CCR-13-2648.
118. Vaddepally RK, Kharel P, Pandey R, Garje R, Chandra AB. Review of indications of FDA-approved immune checkpoint inhibitors per NCCN guidelines with the level of evidence. Cancers (Basel). 2020;12(3) https://doi.org/10.3390/cancers12030738.
119. Haddad RI, Harrington K, Tahara M, Ferris RL, Gillison M, Fayette J, et al. Nivolumab plus ipilimumab versus EXTREME regimen as first-line treatment for recurrent/metastatic squamous cell carcinoma of the head and neck: the final results of checkmate 651. J Clin Oncol. 2023;41(12):2166–80. https://doi.org/10.1200/JCO.22.00332.
120. Harrington KJ, Ferris RL, Gillison M, Tahara M, Argiris A, Fayette J, et al. Efficacy and safety of nivolumab plus ipilimumab vs nivolumab alone for treatment of recurrent or metastatic squamous cell carcinoma of the head and neck: the phase 2 checkmate 714 randomized clinical trial. JAMA Oncol. 2023;9(6):779–89. https://doi.org/10.1001/jamaoncol.2023.0147.
121. Ferris RL, Haddad R, Even C, Tahara M, Dvorkin M, Ciuleanu TE, et al. Durvalumab with or without tremelimumab in patients with recurrent or metastatic head and neck squamous cell carcinoma: EAGLE, a randomized, open-label phase III study. Ann Oncol. 2020;31(7):942–50. https://doi.org/10.1016/j.annonc.2020.04.001.
122. Mandal T, Gnanasegaran S, Rodrigues G, Kashipathi S, Tiwari A, Dubey AK, et al. Targeting LLT1 as a potential immunotherapy option for cancer patients non-responsive to existing checkpoint therapies in multiple solid tumors. BMC Cancer. 2024;24(1):1365. https://doi.org/10.1186/s12885-024-13074-z.
123. Guo S, Han F, Zhu W. CD39—a bright target for cancer immunotherapy. Biomed Pharmacother. 2022;151:113066. https://doi.org/10.1016/j.biopha.2022.113066.
124. Hansen K, Kumar S, Logronio K, Whelan S, Qurashi S, Cheng HY, et al. COM902, a novel therapeutic antibody targeting TIGIT augments anti-tumor T cell function in combination with PVRIG or PD-1 pathway blockade. Cancer Immunol Immunother. 2021;70(12):3525–40. https://doi.org/10.1007/s00262-021-02921-8.
125. Mei Z, Huang J, Qiao B, Lam AK. Immune checkpoint pathways in immunotherapy for head and neck squamous cell carcinoma. Int J Oral Sci. 2020;12(1):16. https://doi.org/10.1038/s41368-020-0084-8.

126. Huang X, Zhang X, Li E, Zhang G, Wang X, Tang T, et al. VISTA: an immune regulatory protein checking tumor and immune cells in cancer immunotherapy. J Hematol Oncol. 2020;13(1):83. https://doi.org/10.1186/s13045-020-00917-y.
127. Long L, Zhang X, Chen F, Pan Q, Phiphatwatchara P, Zeng Y, et al. The promising immune checkpoint LAG-3: from tumor microenvironment to cancer immunotherapy. Genes Cancer. 2018;9(5-6):176–89. https://doi.org/10.18632/genesandcancer.180.
128. Huehls AM, Coupet TA, Sentman CL. Bispecific T-cell engagers for cancer immunotherapy. Immunol Cell Biol. 2015;93(3):290–6. https://doi.org/10.1038/icb.2014.93.
129. Psyrri A, Seiwert TY, Jimeno A. Molecular pathways in head and neck cancer: EGFR, PI3K, and more. Am Soc Clin Oncol Educ Book. 2013:246–55. https://doi.org/10.14694/EdBook_AM.2013.33.246.
130. Harari PM, Wheeler DL, Grandis JR. Molecular target approaches in head and neck cancer: epidermal growth factor receptor and beyond. Semin Radiat Oncol. 2009;19(1):63–8. https://doi.org/10.1016/j.semradonc.2008.09.009.
131. Wang C, Li Y, Jia L, Kim JK, Li J, Deng P, et al. CD276 expression enables squamous cell carcinoma stem cells to evade immune surveillance. Cell Stem Cell. 2021;28(9):1597–613.e7. https://doi.org/10.1016/j.stem.2021.04.011.
132. Centuori SM, Bauman JE. c-Met signaling as a therapeutic target in head and neck cancer. Cancer J. 2022;28(5):346–53. https://doi.org/10.1097/PPO.0000000000000619.
133. Shvartsur A, Bonavida B. Trop2 and its overexpression in cancers: regulation and clinical/therapeutic implications. Genes Cancer. 2015;6(3-4):84–105. https://doi.org/10.18632/genesandcancer.40.
134. Huan T, Guan B, Li H, Tu X, Zhang C, Tang B. Principles and current clinical landscape of NK cell engaging bispecific antibody against cancer. Hum Vaccin Immunother. 2023;19(2):2256904. https://doi.org/10.1080/21645515.2023.2256904.
135. Zhang M, Lam KP, Xu S. Natural Killer Cell Engagers (NKCEs): a new frontier in cancer immunotherapy. Front Immunol. 2023;14:1207276. https://doi.org/10.3389/fimmu.2023.1207276.
136. Klein C, Brinkmann U, Reichert JM, Kontermann RE. The present and future of bispecific antibodies for cancer therapy. Nat Rev Drug Discov. 2024;23(4):301–19. https://doi.org/10.1038/s41573-024-00896-6.
137. Herrera M, Pretelli G, Desai J, Garralda E, Siu LL, Steiner TM, et al. Bispecific antibodies: advancing precision oncology. Trends Cancer. 2024;10(10):893–919. https://doi.org/10.1016/j.trecan.2024.07.002.
138. Pyo KH, Koh YJ, Synn CB, Kim JH, Byeon Y, Jo HN, et al. Comprehensive preclinical study on GI-101, a novel CD80-IgG4-IL2 variant protein, as a therapeutic antibody candidate with bispecific immuno-oncology target. Cancer Res. 2021;81(13):1826.
139. Moynihan KD, Pappas D, Park T, Chen W, Ni I, Bessette P, et al. AB248 is a CD8+T cell selective IL-2 designed for superior safety and anti-tumor efficacy. Cancer Res. 2022;82(12):3518.
140. Berraondo P, Sanmamed MF, Ochoa MC, Etxeberria I, Aznar MA, Perez-Gracia JL, et al. Cytokines in clinical cancer immunotherapy. Br J Cancer. 2019;120(1):6–15. https://doi.org/10.1038/s41416-018-0328-y.
141. Waldmann TA. Cytokines in cancer immunotherapy. Cold Spring Harb Perspect Biol. 2018;10(12):a028472. https://doi.org/10.1101/cshperspect.a028472.
142. Jia Z, Ragoonanan D, Mahadeo KM, Gill J, Gorlick R, Shpal E, et al. IL12 immune therapy clinical trial review: novel strategies for avoiding CRS-associated cytokines. Front Immunol. 2022;13:952231. https://doi.org/10.3389/fimmu.2022.952231.
143. Charych D, Khalili S, Dixit V, Kirk P, Chang T, Langowski J, et al. Modeling the receptor pharmacology, pharmacokinetics, and pharmacodynamics of NKTR-214, a kinetically-controlled interleukin-2 (IL2) receptor agonist for cancer immunotherapy. PLoS One. 2017;12(7):e0179431. https://doi.org/10.1371/journal.pone.0179431.
144. Klein C, Waldhauer I, Nicolini VG, Freimoser-Grundschober A, Nayak T, Vugts DJ, et al. Cergutuzumab amunaleukin (CEA-IL2v), a CEA-targeted IL-2 variant-based immunocytokine for combination cancer immunotherapy: overcoming limitations of aldesleukin and

conventional IL-2-based immunocytokines. Onco Targets Ther. 2017;6(3):e1277306. https://doi.org/10.1080/2162402X.2016.1277306.
145. Levin AM, Bates DL, Ring AM, Krieg C, Lin JT, Su L, et al. Exploiting a natural conformational switch to engineer an interleukin-2 'superkine'. Nature. 2012;484(7395):529–33. https://doi.org/10.1038/nature10975.
146. Izar B, Zamarin D, Spigel DR, Hoimes CJ, McDermott DF, Sehgal K, et al. Initial results from a phase 1a/1b study of STK-012, a first-in-class α/β IL-2 receptor biased partial agonist in advanced solid tumors (NCT05098132). Cancer Res. 2024;84(7) https://doi.org/10.1158/1538-7445.Am2024-Ct183.
147. Biet F, Locht C, Kremer L. Immunoregulatory functions of interleukin 18 and its role in defense against bacterial pathogens. J Mol Med (Berl). 2002;80(3):147–62. https://doi.org/10.1007/s00109-001-0307-1.
148. Dixon KO, Kuchroo VK. IL-18: throwing off the shackles to boost anti-tumor immunity. Cell Res. 2020;30(10):831–2. https://doi.org/10.1038/s41422-020-00396-3.
149. Vignali DA, Collison LW, Workman CJ. How regulatory T cells work. Nat Rev Immunol. 2008;8(7):523–32. https://doi.org/10.1038/nri2343.
150. Chen BJ, Zhao JW, Zhang DH, Zheng AH, Wu GQ. Immunotherapy of cancer by targeting regulatory T cells. Int Immunopharmacol. 2022;104:108469. https://doi.org/10.1016/j.intimp.2021.108469.
151. Wen Y, Xia Y, Yang X, Li H, Gao Q. CCR8: a promising therapeutic target against tumor-infiltrating regulatory T cells. Trends Immunol. 2025;46(2):153–65. https://doi.org/10.1016/j.it.2025.01.001.
152. Chen Q, Shen M, Yan M, Han X, Mu S, Li Y, et al. Targeting tumor-infiltrating CCR8(+) regulatory T cells induces antitumor immunity through functional restoration of CD4(+) T(convs) and CD8(+) T cells in colorectal cancer. J Transl Med. 2024;22(1):709. https://doi.org/10.1186/s12967-024-05518-8.
153. Devaraja K, Aggarwal S, Singh M. Therapeutic vaccination in head and neck squamous cell carcinoma—a review. Vaccines (Basel). 2023;11(3) https://doi.org/10.3390/vaccines11030634.
154. Germic N, Frangez Z, Yousefi S, Simon HU. Regulation of the innate immune system by autophagy: monocytes, macrophages, dendritic cells and antigen presentation. Cell Death Differ. 2019;26(4):715–27. https://doi.org/10.1038/s41418-019-0297-6.
155. Li Y, Wang LX, Yang G, Hao F, Urba WJ, Hu HM. Efficient cross-presentation depends on autophagy in tumor cells. Cancer Res. 2008;68(17):6889–95. https://doi.org/10.1158/0008-5472.CAN-08-0161.
156. Li Y, Wang LX, Pang P, Cui Z, Aung S, Haley D, et al. Tumor-derived autophagosome vaccine: mechanism of cross-presentation and therapeutic efficacy. Clin Cancer Res. 2011;17(22):7047–57. https://doi.org/10.1158/1078-0432.CCR-11-0951.
157. Saxena M, van der Burg SH, Melief CJM, Bhardwaj N. Therapeutic cancer vaccines. Nat Rev Cancer. 2021;21(6):360–78. https://doi.org/10.1038/s41568-021-00346-0.
158. Travieso T, Li J, Mahesh S, Mello J, Blasi M. The use of viral vectors in vaccine development. NPJ Vaccines. 2022;7(1):75. https://doi.org/10.1038/s41541-022-00503-y.
159. Sharma B, Bekerman E, Truong H, Lee J, Gamez-Guerrero M, Boopathy A, et al. Arenavirus-based vectors generate robust SIV immunity in non-human primates. Vaccines (Basel). 2024;12(7) https://doi.org/10.3390/vaccines12070735.
160. Guo ZS, Lu B, Guo Z, Giehl E, Feist M, Dai E, et al. Vaccinia virus-mediated cancer immunotherapy: cancer vaccines and oncolytics. J Immunother Cancer. 2019;7(1):6. https://doi.org/10.1186/s40425-018-0495-7.
161. Beyaert S, Machiels JP, Schmitz S. Vaccine-based immunotherapy for head and neck cancers. Cancers (Basel). 2021;13(23) https://doi.org/10.3390/cancers13236041.
162. Wu DW, Jia SP, Xing SJ, Ma HL, Wang X, Tang QY, et al. Personalized neoantigen cancer vaccines: current progression, challenges and a bright future. Clin Exp Med. 2024;24(1):229. https://doi.org/10.1007/s10238-024-01436-7.

163. Sun D, Shi X, Li S, Wang X, Yang X, Wan M. CAR-T cell therapy: a breakthrough in traditional cancer treatment strategies (Review). Mol Med Rep. 2024;29(3) https://doi.org/10.3892/mmr.2024.13171.
164. Vivier E, Rebuffet L, Narni-Mancinelli E, Cornen S, Igarashi RY, Fantin VR. Natural killer cell therapies. Nature. 2024;626(8000):727–36. https://doi.org/10.1038/s41586-023-06945-1.
165. Sharma P, Hu-Lieskovan S, Wargo JA, Ribas A. Primary, adaptive, and acquired resistance to cancer immunotherapy. Cell. 2017;168(4):707–23. https://doi.org/10.1016/j.cell.2017.01.017.
166. Chaurasiya S, Chen NG, Fong Y. Oncolytic viruses and immunity. Curr Opin Immunol. 2018;51:83–90. https://doi.org/10.1016/j.coi.2018.03.008.
167. Lin D, Shen Y, Liang T. Oncolytic virotherapy: basic principles, recent advances and future directions. Signal Transduct Target Ther. 2023;8(1):156. https://doi.org/10.1038/s41392-023-01407-6.
168. Poetsch JH, Dahlke C, Zinser ME, Kasonta R, Lunemann S, Rechtien A, et al. Detectable vesicular stomatitis virus (VSV)-specific humoral and cellular immune responses following VSV-Ebola virus vaccination in humans. J Infect Dis. 2019;219(4):556–61. https://doi.org/10.1093/infdis/jiy565.
169. Zhang Y, Nagalo BM. Immunovirotherapy based on recombinant vesicular stomatitis virus: where are we? Front Immunol. 2022;13:898631. https://doi.org/10.3389/fimmu.2022.898631.
170. Chai AWY, Yee PS, Cheong SC. Rational combinations of targeted therapy and immune checkpoint inhibitors in head and neck cancers. Front Oncol. 2022;12:837835. https://doi.org/10.3389/fonc.2022.837835.
171. Sacco AG, Chen R, Worden FP, Wong DJL, Adkins D, Swiecicki P, et al. Pembrolizumab plus cetuximab in patients with recurrent or metastatic head and neck squamous cell carcinoma: an open-label, multi-arm, non-randomised, multicentre, phase 2 trial. Lancet Oncol. 2021;22(6):883–92. https://doi.org/10.1016/S1470-2045(21)00136-4.
172. Chung CH, Bonomi M, Steuer CE, Li J, Bhateja P, Johnson M, et al. Concurrent cetuximab and nivolumab as a second-line or beyond treatment of patients with recurrent and/or metastatic head and neck squamous cell carcinoma: results of phase I/II study. Cancers (Basel). 2021;13(5) https://doi.org/10.3390/cancers13051180.
173. Kato Y, Tabata K, Kimura T, Yachie-Kinoshita A, Ozawa Y, Yamada K, et al. Lenvatinib plus anti-PD-1 antibody combination treatment activates CD8+ T cells through reduction of tumor-associated macrophage and activation of the interferon pathway. PLoS One. 2019;14(2):e0212513. https://doi.org/10.1371/journal.pone.0212513.
174. Oliva M, Chepcha D, Araujo DV, Diaz-Mejia JJ, Olson P, Prawira A, et al. Antitumor immune effects of preoperative sitravatinib and nivolumab in oral cavity cancer: SNOW window-of-opportunity study. J Immunother Cancer. 2021;9(10):e003476. https://doi.org/10.1136/jitc-2021-003476.
175. Shayan G, Srivastava R, Li J, Schmitt N, Kane LP, Ferris RL. Adaptive resistance to anti-PD1 therapy by Tim-3 upregulation is mediated by the PI3K-Akt pathway in head and neck cancer. Onco Targets Ther. 2017;6(1):e1261779. https://doi.org/10.1080/2162402X.2016.1261779.
176. Proia TA, Singh M, Woessner R, Carnevalli L, Bommakanti G, Magiera L, et al. STAT3 antisense oligonucleotide remodels the suppressive tumor microenvironment to enhance immune activation in combination with anti-PD-L1. Clin Cancer Res. 2020;26(23):6335–49. https://doi.org/10.1158/1078-0432.CCR-20-1066.
177. Hellmann MD, Paz-Ares L, Bernabe Caro R, Zurawski B, Kim SW, Carcereny Costa E, et al. Nivolumab plus ipilimumab in advanced non-small-cell lung cancer. N Engl J Med. 2019;381(21):2020–31. https://doi.org/10.1056/NEJMoa1910231.
178. Wolchok JD, Chiarion-Sileni V, Gonzalez R, Rutkowski P, Grob JJ, Cowey CL, et al. Overall survival with combined nivolumab and ipilimumab in advanced melanoma. N Engl J Med. 2017;377(14):1345–56. https://doi.org/10.1056/NEJMoa1709684.
179. Siu LL, Even C, Mesia R, Remenar E, Daste A, Delord JP, et al. Safety and efficacy of durvalumab with or without tremelimumab in patients with PD-L1-low/negative recurrent

or metastatic HNSCC: the phase 2 CONDOR randomized clinical trial. JAMA Oncol. 2019;5(2):195–203. https://doi.org/10.1001/jamaoncol.2018.4628.
180. Li H, Zandberg DP, Kulkarni A, Chiosea SI, Santos PM, Isett BR, et al. Distinct CD8(+) T cell dynamics associate with response to neoadjuvant cancer immunotherapies. Cancer Cell. 2025; https://doi.org/10.1016/j.ccell.2025.02.026.
181. Vanpouille-Box C, Diamond JM, Pilones KA, Zavadil J, Babb JS, Formenti SC, et al. TGFbeta is a master regulator of radiation therapy-induced antitumor immunity. Cancer Res. 2015;75(11):2232–42. https://doi.org/10.1158/0008-5472.CAN-14-3511.
182. Weichselbaum RR, Liang H, Deng L, Fu YX. Radiotherapy and immunotherapy: a beneficial liaison? Nat Rev Clin Oncol. 2017;14(6):365–79. https://doi.org/10.1038/nrclinonc.2016.211.
183. Oweida A, Lennon S, Calame D, Korpela S, Bhatia S, Sharma J, et al. Ionizing radiation sensitizes tumors to PD-L1 immune checkpoint blockade in orthotopic murine head and neck squamous cell carcinoma. Onco Targets Ther. 2017;6(10):e1356153. https://doi.org/10.1080/2162402X.2017.1356153.
184. Mell LK, Torres-Saavedra PA, Wong SJ, Kish JA, Chang SS, Jordan RC, et al. Radiotherapy with cetuximab or durvalumab for locoregionally advanced head and neck cancer in patients with a contraindication to cisplatin (NRG-HN004): an open-label, multicentre, parallel-group, randomised, phase 2/3 trial. Lancet Oncol. 2024;25(12):1576–88. https://doi.org/10.1016/S1470-2045(24)00507-2.
185. Bauml J, Seiwert TY, Pfister DG, Worden F, Liu SV, Gilbert J, et al. Pembrolizumab for platinum- and cetuximab-refractory head and neck cancer: results from a single-arm, phase II study. J Clin Oncol. 2017;35(14):1542–9. https://doi.org/10.1200/JCO.2016.70.1524.
186. Hanna GJ, Lizotte P, Cavanaugh M, Kuo FC, Shivdasani P, Frieden A, et al. Frameshift events predict anti-PD-1/L1 response in head and neck cancer. JCI Insight. 2018;3(4):e98811. https://doi.org/10.1172/jci.insight.98811.
187. Sautes-Fridman C, Petitprez F, Calderaro J, Fridman WH. Tertiary lymphoid structures in the era of cancer immunotherapy. Nat Rev Cancer. 2019;19(6):307–25. https://doi.org/10.1038/s41568-019-0144-6.
188. Chen YP, Wang YQ, Lv JW, Li YQ, Chua MLK, Le QT, et al. Identification and validation of novel microenvironment-based immune molecular subgroups of head and neck squamous cell carcinoma: implications for immunotherapy. Ann Oncol. 2019;30(1):68–75. https://doi.org/10.1093/annonc/mdy470.

# Novel Immune Modulatory Agents in the Treatment of Non-small Cell Lung Cancer

8

Amanda Reyes and Matthew Lee

## 8.1 Introduction

Despite recent advances, lung cancer remains the leading cause of cancer-related mortality [1]. Non-small cell lung cancer (NSCLC), which encompasses 85% of lung cancer diagnoses, is often further designated by histology into non-squamous 78% and squamous 18% [2]. The standard of care treatment for lung cancer has evolved beyond traditional chemotherapy in the last decade after the recognition of driver mutations and utilization of immune system to target cancer cells [3, 4]. Various types of immune modulators [Immunotherapy] have been implemented, such as immune checkpoint inhibitors (ICI), oncolytic viruses, and vaccines, among others [4]. ICI, which specifically target proteins like Program Cell Death Protein 1 (PD-1), Programmed Cell Death Ligand 1 (PD-L1), and Cytotoxic T-Lymphocyte Associated Protein 4 (CTLA-4), facilitate the patient's immune system ability to kill cancer cells [5, 6].

Several ICIs demonstrated efficacy in PD-L1-positive NSCLC when utilized in the first line, including pembrolizumab, atezolizumab, and cemiplimab [7–9]. Further, combination agents targeting both PD-L1 and CTLA-4, namely nivolumab and ipilimumab [10] and durvalumab/tremelimumab [11] have shown clinical benefit and have been approved for NSCLC patients with PDL1 > 1%. The combination of traditional chemotherapy with various ICIs is now the standard of care in metastatic NSCLC after several large phase 3 clinical trials [12–15]. Combination treatment is also effective in the non-metastatic setting with curative intent, in the perioperative setting with Stage IB-IIIB and exclusion of patients with N3 disease [16–22]. Thus, with the widespread adoption of immunotherapy in the treatment

A. Reyes (✉) · M. Lee
Department of Medical Oncology and Therapeutics Research, City of Hope National Medical Center, Duarte, CA, USA
e-mail: amareyes@coh.org; matthlee@coh.org



R. Salgia, P. Kulkarni (eds.), *Immunotherapies in Solid Tumors*, Cancer Treatment and Research 129, https://doi.org/10.1007/978-3-031-97242-3_8

paradigm of NSCLC, this review seeks to explore various topics including mechanisms of resistance to immunotherapy and novel combinations.

## 8.2 Mechanisms of Resistance

Among the patients with initial response to ICI therapy both primary and secondary resistance remain a concern. The Society for Immunotherapy of Cancer (SITC) defined primary resistance to ICIs as patients who completed at least 6 weeks of treatment and have progression within less than 6 months, whereas secondary resistance includes patients who progress after the 6 months timeframe [23]. Further, intrinsic resistance refers to alterations in the genetic, transcriptional, or functional aspects of immune response while extrinsic generally refers to external factors [24]. There has been a focus on mechanisms of intrinsic resistance for some time, therefore there is substantial data on HLA antigen presenting deficiencies, mutations in beta-2 microglobulin, low mutational burden, mutations in the IFN-y pathway, and increased neoantigen intratumor heterogeneity and the development of resistance [25–31].

External factors or extrinsic resistance also plays a role, including changes in tumor microenvironment, upregulation of alternative immune checkpoint receptors, and decreased levels of circulating T lymphocytes [32–34]. Further investigation identified patient-specific characteristics such as recent antibiotic use and baseline gut microbiota can also affect response to immunotherapy, ICI in particular [35, 36]. Concurrent mutations also contribute to treatment resistance. Examples include Kelch-like ECH-associated protein 1 [KEAP1] which has a role in response to oxidative stress and therefore is associated with an unfavorable tumor microenvironment [immune cold] with fewer CD8+ T cells [37]. Mutations in serine–threonine kinase liver kinase B1 [STK11] cause the upregulation of AMP-kinase pathway, another known mechanism of resistance [38]. Given the multiple patterns of resistance, researchers have focused on developing novel combination treatments to overcome this limitation in the current treatment paradigm.

## 8.3 Combination Immunotherapy

One such novel treatment method is the combination of immune checkpoint inhibitors with targeted treatment like vascular endothelial growth factor (VEGF) receptor inhibition. Several VEGF inhibitors have been utilized, including bevacizumab in combination with atezolizumab and chemotherapy in the IMPOWER 150 trial, which improved median OS to 19.2 months, compared to 14.7 months (HR 0.78 95% CI 0.64–0.96; $p = 0.02$) with bevacizumab and chemotherapy alone [39]. Ramucirumab was also investigated in a phase 2 trial in combination with pembrolizumab in patients who had progressed on ICI; the combination improved OS to 14.5 months (80% CI 13.9–16.1) from 11.6 months (80% CI 0.9–13.0) [40]. This prompted further evaluation to validate the OS benefit in the PRAGMATICA-LUNG trial, which is currently underway [NCT05633602] [41].

Moving beyond traditional ICIs which target PD-L1/CTLA4, newer agents are being developed that target entities outside of this blockade, like T-cell receptor with immunoglobulin and immunoreceptor tyrosine-based inhibitory motif domains [TIGIT] monoclonal antibodies. An anti-TIGIT antibody, Tiragolumab, in combination with atezolizumab demonstrated improved ORR of 31.3% (95% CI 19.5–43.2) compared to 16.2% (95% CI 6.7–25.7, $p = 0.031$) with atezolizumab in NSCLC patients with PD-L1 > 1% in the CITYSCAPE trial [42]. Given the clinical benefit, the combination was evaluated in a randomized phase 3 trial in the PD-L1 high metastatic NSCLC SKYSCRAPER-01[NCT04294810] but results median OS of 22.9 months (95% CI, 17.5–not evaluable) vs 16.7 months (95% CI 14.6–20.2) with atezolizumab (HR, 0.81) [NCT04294810] [43]. Further, the phase 2/3 SKYSCRAPER-06 evaluating tiragolumab in combination with atezolizumab and chemotherapy versus pembrolizumab and chemotherapy in first-line NSCLC did not meet its primary endpoint of PFS and immature OS data [NCT04619797] [44]. It remains to be seen if anti-TIGIT antibodies will be able to demonstrate clinical efficacy in NSCLC.

From preclinical studies, lymphocyte-Activation Gene 3 (LAG-3), which has been shown to alter T helper 1 cell activation, is associated with tumor progression [45, 46]. In mouse models dual blockade of PD-1 and LAG-3 increases CD8+ T cells and decreases T regulatory cell in the tumor microenvironment, thereby improving immune-mediated tumor killing [47]. In metastatic NSCLC PD-L1 non-selected in the first line, the combination of eftilagimod alpha (LAG-3 protein) and pembrolizumab achieved an ORR of 31% and median OS of 15.5, which was expected in the PDL1 negative population [48]. In the updated results of this combination in the second-line setting of NSCLC refractory to ICI, ORR was 8.3% with disease control rate of 33.3% and median OS of 9.9 months [49].

Designed to promote and enhance the cytotoxic T-cell response, utomilumab, a human IgG2 monoclonal antibody agonist of the T-cell costimulatory receptor 4-1BB, inhibited tumor growth in xenograft models [50]. These preclinical findings led to a phase 1b study evaluating the combination of utomilumab and pembrolizumab in solid tumors including NSCLC; 6 out of 23 patients had a complete or partial response and the combination was well tolerated [51] [NCT02179918]. Utomilumab is now being evaluated in combination with avelumab and radiation in solid tumors [NCT03217747].

Another agent, CD134 also known as OX40 is a member of the tumor necrosis factor (TNF) receptor family, and has shown antitumor activity in pre-clinical models [52]. Additional studies demonstrated the presence of OX40 on infiltrating lymphocytes in NSCLC specifically and its ligand, OX40L on tumor cells [53]. High expression of OX40 correlated with a better prognosis in NSCLC [54]. Unfortunately, this did not translate to a significant clinical benefit in patients with advanced solid tumors, when GSK3174998, an OX40 monoclonal antibody agonist was evaluated in combination with Pembrolizumab [55] [NCT02528357]. Summary of combinatorial immunotherapy regimens is given in Table 8.1 and Fig. 8.1.

**Table 8.1** Clinical trials involving combination immunotherapy regimens

| Trial | Study treatment | Status | NCI | Phase | Prior ICI? | Primary endpoint |
|---|---|---|---|---|---|---|
| PRAGMATICA-LUNG[1] | Ramucirumab + Pembrolizumab | Active | NCT05633602 | III | Yes | OS |
| SKYSCRAPER-01[1] | Tiragolumab + Atezolizumab | Completed | NCT04294810 | III | No | PFS, OS, Adverse Events |
| SKYSCRAPER-06[1] | Tiragolumab + Atezolizumab + Chemotherapy | Completed | NCT04619797 | II/III | No | ORR, PFS, OS |
| | Avelumab, Utomilumab, Anti-OX40 Antibody PF-04518600, and Radiation | Active | NCT03217747 | I/II | No | Adverse Events, Markers of CD8 response |
| ENGAGE-1[1] | GSK3174998 +/− Pembrolizumab | Completed | NCT02528357 | I | No | Serious and Non-serious Adverse Events |
| TACTI-002[1] | Eftilagimod alpha + Pembrolizumab | Completed | NCT03625323 | II | Depends on trial arm | Objective Response Rate |

Trial data obtained from clinicaltrials.gov

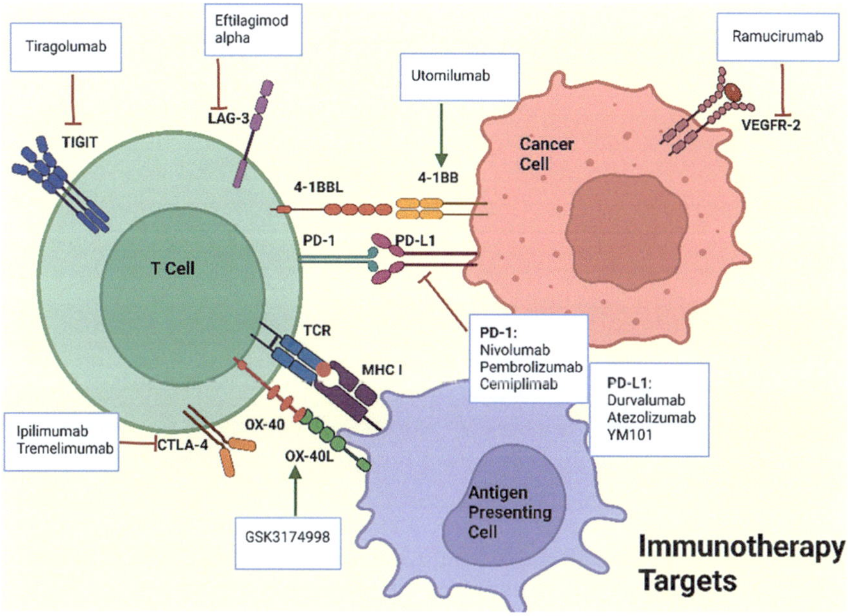


**Fig. 8.1** Immunotherapy pathways and targets

## 8.4 Antibody Drug Conjugates

An alternative approach to combination immune modulators is the addition of bispecific antibodies and antibody-drug conjugates (ADCs) to immunotherapy, mostly ICIs. As many of the ADCs were initially utilized in hematologic malignancies, most of the initial research involved hematologic agents. Pre-clinical studies found that ADCs with microtubule inhibitors improved immune-mediated treatment response by both increasing tumor-presenting antigens and enhancing the maturation of dendritic cells; similar outcomes were seen with pyrrolobenzodiazepine dimer or tubulysin ADCs [56–58]. Bispecific agents have also shown promise with antitumor activity when used in combination with the immune checkpoint blockade in early studies, such as YM101, a bispecific antibody against PD-L1 and TGF-B (transforming growth factor-beta) [59].

Given the success in pre-clinical studies, many of these novel combinations have advanced to phase 1/2 trials. Sacituzumab govitecan, which had initial success in metastatic breast cancer, is currently being investigated in lung cancer in combination with ICIs; including with atezolizumab (MORPHEUS) and with pembrolizumab with or without chemotherapy (EVOKE-02) [60–62]. Another TROP-2 ADC, datopotamab deruxtecan, is under evaluation in combination with durvaluamb and carboplatin in the first line in the ADVANZAR trial [63]. TROPION-Lung02, phase Ib trial, found the combination of datopotamab deruxtecan with pembrolizumab and with/without chemotherapy (cisplatin 75 mg/m$^2$ or carboplatin

AUC 5) safe and tolerable with 61% patients reported grade 3 adverse events and ORR of the triplet regimen of 60% (95% CI, 36–81%) [64]. Another ongoing phase Ib trial is analyzing the combination of pembrolizumab and trastuzumab deruxtecan in metastatic NSCLC as well as metastatic breast cancer [65]. The clinical benefit weighted against the added toxicity of these novel agents will ultimately determine the utility of this approach in NSCLC and the results of these ongoing clinical trials will be enlightening.

## 8.5 Adoptive Cellular Therapies

In recent years, chimeric antigen receptor cells (CAR-T), tumor-infiltrating lymphocytes (TILs), and T-cell receptor-engineered T cells (TCT-T) collectively called "adoptive cell therapies" (ACT) have entered the forefront of cancer treatment [66–68]. Success with TILs in solid tumors has been modest despite their discovery in 1988, when T cells were isolated from tumor cells and reinfused, but there has been some advancement with TILs in melanoma [69, 70]. Recently, there has been some progress with lifileucel in NSCLC patients who were resistant to ICIs, with ORR of 21.4% and responses seen in 6 of the 28 patients including patients who were PD-L1 negative, had low TMB or STK11 mutations [71]. In addition to the logistical challenges of TILs, both intrinsic and extrinsic resistance has been observed, such as TIL quiescent genes among others [70].

To overcome this seemingly early resistance, investigators have utilized the combination of ICIs with TILs in NSCLC, notably in a phase I study of nivolumab with TILs, where 6 out of 13 evaluable patients had a response, and some patients had durable responses [72]. Another TIL, LN-145, evaluated with durvalumab was withdrawn due to toxicities [73]. Currently recruiting trials include a trial of L-TIL and tislelizumab in ICI resistance NSCLC and TBio-4101 with pembrolizumab (STARLING trial) [NCT05576077] [NCT05878028].

CAR-T cells have also had a slower adoption in solid tumors with lung cancer being no exception. However, initial *in vitro* and animal studies did demonstrate clinical benefit notably when combined with PD-L1 blockade [74]. One of the major limitations to CAR-T implementation in lung cancer is identifying a target antigen that is consistently expressed on tumor cells [75]. There are several ongoing trials evaluating several different antigens including carcinoembryonic antigen (CEA), human epidermal growth factor receptor 2 (HER2), PD-1, EGFR, and Mesothelin, among others [75]. A phase 1 trial of mesothelin CAR-T in combination with pembrolizumab in patients with pleural disease had promising results with median OS of 23.9 months since CAR-T infusion and 2 patients had a complete metabolic response on PET scan [76]. A study in China evaluated an EGFR-directed CAR-T, and 7 out of the 11 patients had a clinical response [77]. Not all targets have been successful, for example, a CAR-T targeting VEGFR2 had no objective responses in solid metastatic tumors [NCT01218867]. Toxicity also remains a concern, with pulmonary edema reported previously [78].

TCT-T cells while similar to CAR-T differ in their ability to recognize antigens on cellular membranes and intracellular proteins which improves their versatility [79]. Several phase I trials have proven the safety and efficacy of TCT-T in solid tumors including NSCLC [80–82]. TCT-T cells have even been investigated in combination with PD-L1 blockade in melanoma [83]. Further trials with TCT-T and immune modulators are warranted to determine the efficacy and safety of this novel treatment modality.

## 8.6 Vaccines

Recognition of specific tumor-associated antigens is a critical component of the immune-mediated response against malignant cells. These tumor-specific antigens or "neoantigens" are unique to tumor cells and are typically generated by the frequent genetic mutations in the DNA of tumor cells [84–86]. Given the tumor-specific nature of neoantigens, they are excellent targets for tumor-specific vaccines as they allow tumor-specific immune-mediated response [87, 88]. Increased expression of these tumor neoantigens is associated with increased tumor mutation burden (TMB), a known positive prognostic factor in ICI treatment response [89, 90].

This prompted a phase I investigation into a personalized neoantigen-vaccine NEO-PV-01 used in combination with pembrolizumab and carboplatin/pemetrexed in non-squamous NSCLC in the first line; initial results reported no serious adverse events and evidence of increased CD4+ cells in the tumor in the biopsy obtained after treatment [91]. Other ongoing early-phase clinical trials of neoantigen vaccine include PANDA-VAC evaluated in combination with pembrolizumab in squamous NSCLC and PNeoVCA in combination with pembrolizumab in advanced solid tumors [NCT04266730] [92].

An alternative type of vaccine-mediated treatment includes the use of oncolytic viruses in combination with cancer vaccines [93, 94]. Promising results in preclinical studies prompted a phase 1 trial evaluating the combination of an oncolytic virus and MAGE-A3 adenovirus vaccine (AdMA3), which demonstrated the overall safety of this regimen [95, 96]. It should be noted that as a result of their cancer specificity, these vaccines typically do not elicit an autoimmune response and therefore the typical immune-mediated adverse events of ICIs are not seen with this vaccine-mediated treatment modality which improves the toxicity profile of combination treatments [97].

## 8.7 Immunotherapy and Radiation

The first connection between radiation and the immune response was inadvertently made with the discovery of the "abscopal effect" when response to treatment was observed outside the radiation field [98]. Further, this abscopal event appears to require functional immune systems as it was relatively absent in immune deficit settings [99]. This concept was later demonstrated with the observation that tumor cells release tumor-associated antigens and increase the expression of MHC class I, after being exposed to radiation, resulting in increased antigen-presenting dendritic cells thereby increasing the immune-mediated response [100–102]. Additionally, radiation has been shown to alter the tumor microenvironment favorably and increase levels of oxidative phosphorylation (OXPHOS), facilitating and improving the immune-mediated tumor response [103–107]. All of these factors likely explain the clinical response seen with radiation and ICI despite low PD-L1 and TMB status [108].

This synergy between radiation and the immune-mediated response was explored in the metastatic and locally advanced settings in NSCLC. In the PEMBRO-RT trial, patients were enrolled regardless of PD-L1 status and prior treatment and received either pembrolizumab alone or after 3 doses of 8 Gy to a single tumor site [109]. This method improved median OS median to 15.9 months (95% CI, 7.1 months to not reached) vs 7.6 months (95% CI, 6.0–13.9 months) in the control arm without radiation (hazard ratio, 0.66; 95% CI 0.37–1.18; $P = .16$). MD Anderson Cancer Center (MDACC) trial evaluated a similar population, but these patients were required to have lung or liver lesions that would be treatable with RT and one additional noncontiguous lesion. In the trial, the lung or liver lesion was treated with pembrolizumab with or with concurrent radiation with SBRT 50 Gy in 4 fractions or if not feasible, fractionated RT with 45 Gy in 15 fractions [110]. Responses were similar with median PFS of 9.1 months (95% CI 3.6–18.4 months) ($p = 0.52$) vs 5.1 months (95% CI 3.4–12.7 months) in the pembrolizumab alone group [110]. Given the smaller size of these studies, there was limited statistical power, but in a combined analysis median OS was 19.2 months (95% CI 14.6–23.8) (HR 0.67, 0.54–0.84) ($p = 0{\cdot}0004$) in radiation with pembrolizumab group vs 8.7 months (95% CI 6.4–11.0) with pembrolizumab alone [111].

In locally advanced, nonresectable NSCLC, combination chemotherapy with radiation followed by durvalumab has become the standard of care after the PACIFIC trial [112]. In the trial, patients either received durvalumab or placebo every 2 weeks for up to 12 months, 1–42 days after completing chemo-radiation, improved median PFS of 16.8 months (95% CI 13.0–18.1) was observed with durvalumab vs 5.6 months (95% CI 4.6–7.8) with placebo (HR 0.52, 95% CI 0.42–0.65) ($P < 0.001$) [112]. Given the intensity of this regimen, toxicity and tolerability can be limiting in certain patient population. Designed to have decreased toxicity compared to the stand CRT regimen, the DOLPHIN trial evaluated the combination of durvalumab and concurrent radiation with an ORR of 90.9% (95% CI 75.7–98.1) [113]. The combination of radiation and ICIs in oligometastatic NSCLC has also been successful, with improved survival of median PFS 19.7 months (95% CI 7.6–31.7) with the administration of pembrolizumab after radiation of an oligometastatic site compared to an historical median PFS of 6.6 months [114, 115].

## 8.8 Conclusions

While ICIs and immune-mediated treatments have revolutionized the treatment of lung cancer in the last decade, resistance remains a challenge. Combination treatments and novel agents seek to overcome this resistance with success across several modalities including radiation, ADCs, TILs, CAR-T, TCT-T, TILs, vaccines, and oncolytic viruses, among others. The advancement of next-generation sequencing and the development of "Precision Medicine" has allowed many of these personalized novel therapeutics to come to the forefront of NSCLC treatment [116]. Despite these advancements, there are some limitations to widespread adoption of these strategies. While a lesser concern, the cost of these novel therapeutics compared to traditional chemotherapy counterparts is substantial and could limit implementation. Additionally, the requirement for hospital admission or close observation after administration could also be a limiting factor in certain settings, namely community practice.

Each of these novel therapeutics is associated with its own toxicity profiles, some more significant than others. The layering or sequencing of therapies can create a compounding effect on toxicity as has previously been observed with EGFR tyrosine kinase inhibitors and ICIs with the potential life-threatening complication of pneumonitis [117]. Some of these agents, namely ADCs, have toxicities that can be new to oncologists and can require the assistance of specialists including ophthalmology, neurology, and dermatology, many of whom may not able available in all practice settings [118]. The IL-2/inflammatory response (CRS) seen with many adoptive cellular therapies can also limit the widespread implementation as lower functional status and certain co-morbidities would be inhibitory. Additionally, there is limited response to our current immunotherapy agents, namely ICIs, in certain driver mutated lung cancer, such as anaplastic lymphoma kinase [ALK] and epidermal growth factor receptor [EGFR] with increased risk of toxicity [119]. It remains to be seen if these novel agents will be effective in the diverse driver mutated population.

Despite the fact that PDL1 status is routinely used as a marker of response to ICI, current data demonstrates a lack of prognostic accuracy due to tumor heterogeneity, insufficient tumor sampling, and variations among assays [120–122]. The definition of positivity >1% vs >50% has also been debated which can further complicate the matter [123]. Better prognostic and predictive biomarkers are needed for both ICI and immunotherapy in general. Given these potential challenges and complications, the optimal sequencing of the various treatments is essential. This also pertains to the peri-operative and curative intent setting as more and more of these agents are moving to the first line. The results of current trials and future trials will likely dictate treatment protocols in NSCLC in the future and these novel therapeutics could lead to durable responses and even increased cure rates.

## References

1. Mattiuzzi C, Lippi G. Current cancer epidemiology. J Epidemiol Glob Health. 2019;9(4):217–22.
2. Thai AA, Solomon BJ, Sequist LV, Gainor JF, Heist RS. Lung cancer. Lancet. 2021;398(10299):535–54.
3. Kris MG, Johnson BE, Berry LD, Kwiatkowski DJ, Iafrate AJ, Wistuba II, et al. Using multiplexed assays of oncogenic drivers in lung cancers to select targeted drugs. JAMA. 2014;311(19):1998–2006.

4. Couzin-Frankel J. Cancer immunotherapy. Science. 2013;342(6165):1432–3.
5. Shiravand Y, Khodadadi F, Kashani SMA, Hosseini-Fard SR, Hosseini S, Sadeghirad H, et al. Immune checkpoint inhibitors in cancer therapy. Curr Oncol Tor Ont. 2022;29(5):3044–60.
6. Mazieres J, Drilon A, Lusque A, Mhanna L, Cortot AB, Mezquita L, et al. Immune checkpoint inhibitors for patients with advanced lung cancer and oncogenic driver alterations: results from the IMMUNOTARGET registry. Ann Oncol. 2019;30(8):1321–8.
7. Reck M, Rodríguez-Abreu D, Robinson AG, Hui R, Csőszi T, Fülöp A, et al. Pembrolizumab versus chemotherapy for PD-L1–positive non–small-cell lung cancer. N Engl J Med. 2016;375(19):1823–33.
8. Herbst RS, Giaccone G, de Marinis F, Reinmuth N, Vergnenegre A, Barrios CH, et al. Atezolizumab for first-line treatment of PD-L1–selected patients with NSCLC. N Engl J Med. 2020;383(14):1328–39.
9. Sezer A, Kilickap S, Gümüş M, Bondarenko I, Özgüroğlu M, Gogishvili M, et al. Cemiplimab monotherapy for first-line treatment of advanced non-small-cell lung cancer with PD-L1 of at least 50%: a multicentre, open-label, global, phase 3, randomised, controlled trial. Lancet. 2021;397(10274):592–604.
10. Hellmann MD, Paz-Ares L, Bernabe Caro R, Zurawski B, Kim SW, Carcereny Costa E, et al. Nivolumab plus Ipilimumab in advanced non–small-cell lung cancer. N Engl J Med. 2019;381(21):2020–31.
11. Johnson ML, Cho BC, Luft A, Alatorre-Alexander J, Geater SL, Laktionov K, et al. Durvalumab with or without tremelimumab in combination with chemotherapy as first-line therapy for metastatic non–small-cell lung cancer: the phase III POSEIDON study. J Clin Oncol. 2023;41(6):1213–27.
12. Gandhi L, Rodríguez-Abreu D, Gadgeel S, Esteban E, Felip E, De Angelis F, et al. Pembrolizumab plus chemotherapy in metastatic non–small-cell lung cancer. N Engl J Med. 2018;378(22):2078–92.
13. West H, McCleod M, Hussein M, Morabito A, Rittmeyer A, Conter HJ, et al. Atezolizumab in combination with carboplatin plus nab-paclitaxel chemotherapy compared with chemotherapy alone as first-line treatment for metastatic non-squamous non-small-cell lung cancer (IMpower130): a multicentre, randomised, open-label, phase 3 trial. Lancet Oncol. 2019;20(7):924–37.
14. Gogishvili M, Melkadze T, Makharadze T, Giorgadze D, Dvorkin M, Penkov K, et al. Cemiplimab plus chemotherapy versus chemotherapy alone in non-small cell lung cancer: a randomized, controlled, double-blind phase 3 trial. Nat Med. 2022;28(11):2374–80.
15. Paz-Ares L, Ciuleanu TE, Cobo M, Schenker M, Zurawski B, Menezes J, et al. First-line nivolumab plus ipilimumab combined with two cycles of chemotherapy in patients with non-small-cell lung cancer (CheckMate 9LA): an international, randomised, open-label, phase 3 trial. Lancet Oncol. 2021;22(2):198–211.
16. Wakelee H, Liberman M, Kato T, Tsuboi M, Lee SH, Gao S, et al. Perioperative pembrolizumab for early-stage non–small-cell lung cancer. N Engl J Med. 2023;389(6):491–503.
17. Forde PM, Spicer J, Lu S, Provencio M, Mitsudomi T, Awad MM, et al. Neoadjuvant nivolumab plus chemotherapy in resectable lung cancer. N Engl J Med. 2022;386(21):1973–85.
18. Provencio M, Nadal E, González-Larriba JL, Martínez-Martí A, Bernabé R, Bosch-Barrera J, et al. Perioperative nivolumab and chemotherapy in stage III non–small-cell lung cancer. N Engl J Med. 2023;389(6):504–13.
19. Heymach JV, Harpole D, Mitsudomi T, Taube JM, Galffy G, Hochmair M, et al. Perioperative durvalumab for resectable non–small-cell lung cancer. N Engl J Med. 2023;389(18):1672–84.
20. Felip E, Altorki N, Zhou C, Csőszi T, Vynnychenko I, Goloborodko O, et al. Adjuvant atezolizumab after adjuvant chemotherapy in resected stage IB–IIIA non-small-cell lung cancer (IMpower010): a randomised, multicentre, open-label, phase 3 trial. Lancet. 2021;398(10308):1344–57.
21. Shu CA, Gainor JF, Awad MM, Chiuzan C, Grigg CM, Pabani A, et al. Neoadjuvant atezolizumab and chemotherapy in patients with resectable non-small-cell lung cancer: an open-label, multicentre, single-arm, phase 2 trial. Lancet Oncol. 2020;21(6):786–95.

22. O'Brien M, Paz-Ares L, Marreaud S, Dafni U, Oselin K, Havel L, et al. Pembrolizumab versus placebo as adjuvant therapy for completely resected stage IB–IIIA non-small-cell lung cancer (PEARLS/KEYNOTE-091): an interim analysis of a randomised, triple-blind, phase 3 trial. Lancet Oncol. 2022;23(10):1274–86.
23. Kluger HM, Tawbi HA, Ascierto ML, Bowden M, Callahan MK, Cha E, et al. Defining tumor resistance to PD-1 pathway blockade: recommendations from the first meeting of the SITC Immunotherapy Resistance Taskforce. J Immunother Cancer. 2020;8(1):e000398.
24. Kalbasi A, Ribas A. Tumour-intrinsic resistance to immune checkpoint blockade. Nat Rev Immunol. 2020;20(1):25–39.
25. McGranahan N, Furness AJS, Rosenthal R, Ramskov S, Lyngaa R, Saini SK, et al. Clonal neoantigens elicit T cell immunoreactivity and sensitivity to immune checkpoint blockade. Science. 2016;351(6280):1463–9.
26. Gao J, Shi LZ, Zhao H, Chen J, Xiong L, He Q, et al. Loss of IFN-γ pathway genes in tumor cells as a mechanism of resistance to anti-CTLA-4 therapy. Cell. 2016;167(2):397–404.e9.
27. Riaz N, Morris L, Havel JJ, Makarov V, Desrichard A, Chan TA. The role of neoantigens in response to immune checkpoint blockade. Int Immunol. 2016;28(8):411–9.
28. Hugo W, Zaretsky JM, Sun L, Song C, Moreno BH, Hu-Lieskovan S, et al. Genomic and transcriptomic features of response to anti-PD-1 therapy in metastatic melanoma. Cell. 2016;165(1):35–44.
29. Zingg D, Arenas-Ramirez N, Sahin D, Rosalia RA, Antunes AT, Haeusel J, et al. The histone methyltransferase Ezh2 controls mechanisms of adaptive resistance to tumor immunotherapy. Cell Rep. 2017;20(4):854–67.
30. Pereira C, Gimenez-Xavier P, Pros E, Pajares MJ, Moro M, Gomez A, et al. Genomic profiling of patient-derived xenografts for lung cancer identifies *B2M* inactivation impairing immunorecognition. Clin Cancer Res. 2017;23(12):3203–13.
31. Gettinger S, Choi J, Hastings K, Truini A, Datar I, Sowell R, et al. Impaired HLA class I antigen processing and presentation as a mechanism of acquired resistance to immune checkpoint inhibitors in lung cancer. Cancer Discov. 2017;7(12):1420–35.
32. Galon J, Bruni D. Approaches to treat immune hot, altered and cold tumours with combination immunotherapies. Nat Rev Drug Discov. 2019;18(3):197–218.
33. Thommen DS, Schreiner J, Müller P, Herzig P, Roller A, Belousov A, et al. Progression of lung cancer is associated with increased dysfunction of T cells defined by coexpression of multiple inhibitory receptors. Cancer Immunol Res. 2015;3(12):1344–55.
34. Joyce JA, Fearon DT. T cell exclusion, immune privilege, and the tumor microenvironment. Science. 2015;348(6230):74–80.
35. Chaput N, Lepage P, Coutzac C, Soularue E, Le Roux K, Monot C, et al. Baseline gut microbiota predicts clinical response and colitis in metastatic melanoma patients treated with ipilimumab. Ann Oncol. 2019;30(12):2012.
36. Derosa L, Hellmann MD, Spaziano M, Halpenny D, Fidelle M, Rizvi H, et al. Negative association of antibiotics on clinical activity of immune checkpoint inhibitors in patients with advanced renal cell and non-small-cell lung cancer. Ann Oncol. 2018;29(6):1437–44.
37. Chen X, Su C, Ren S, Zhou C, Jiang T. Pan-cancer analysis of KEAP1 mutations as biomarkers for immunotherapy outcomes. Ann Transl Med. 2020;8(4):141.
38. Skoulidis F, Goldberg ME, Greenawalt DM, Hellmann MD, Awad MM, Gainor JF, et al. *STK11/LKB1* mutations and PD-1 inhibitor resistance in *KRAS*-mutant lung adenocarcinoma. Cancer Discov. 2018;8(7):822–35.
39. Socinski MA, Jotte RM, Cappuzzo F, Orlandi F, Stroyakovskiy D, Nogami N, et al. Atezolizumab for first-line treatment of metastatic nonsquamous NSCLC. N Engl J Med. 2018;378(24):2288–301.
40. Reckamp KL, Redman MW, Dragnev KH, Minichiello K, Villaruz LC, Faller B, et al. Phase II randomized study of ramucirumab and pembrolizumab versus standard of care in advanced non-small-cell lung cancer previously treated with immunotherapy-lung-MAP S1800A. J Clin Oncol. 2022;40(21):2295–306.

41. Reckamp KL, Redman MW, Dragnev KH, Iams WT, Henick BS, Miao J, et al. SWOG S2302, PRAGMATICA-LUNG: a prospective randomized study of ramucirumab plus pembrolizumab (PR) versus standard of care (SOC) for participants previously treated with immunotherapy for stage IV or recurrent non-small cell lung cancer. J Clin Oncol. 2024;42(16_suppl):TPS8657.
42. Cho BC, Abreu DR, Hussein M, Cobo M, Patel AJ, Secen N, et al. Tiragolumab plus atezolizumab versus placebo plus atezolizumab as a first-line treatment for PD-L1-selected non-small-cell lung cancer (CITYSCAPE): primary and follow-up analyses of a randomised, double-blind, phase 2 study. Lancet Oncol. 2022;23(6):781–92.
43. Roche. Roche provides update on phase III Skyscraper-01 study in PD-L1-high metastatic non-small cell lung cancer [Internet]. 2024 [cited 2025 Mar 3]. Available from: www.roche.com/media/releases/med-cor-2024-11-26
44. Genentech. Genentech provides update of phase 2/3 Skyscraper-06 study in metastatic nonsquamous non–small cell lung cancer [Internet]. [cited 2025 Mar 3]. Available from: https://www.gene.com/media/press-releases/15029/2024-07-03/genentech-provides-update-on-phase
45. Workman CJ, Cauley LS, Kim IJ, Blackman MA, Woodland DL, Vignali DAA. Lymphocyte activation gene-3 (CD223) regulates the size of the expanding T cell population following antigen activation in vivo1. J Immunol. 2004;172(9):5450–5.
46. Huang CT, Workman CJ, Flies D, Pan X, Marson AL, Zhou G, et al. Role of LAG-3 in regulatory T cells. Immunity. 2004;21(4):503–13.
47. Kisielow M, Kisielow J, Capoferri-Sollami G, Karjalainen K. Expression of lymphocyte activation gene 3 (LAG-3) on B cells is induced by T cells. Eur J Immunol. 2005;35(7):2081–8.
48. Felip E, Majem M, Doger B, Clay TD, Carcereny E, Bondarenko I, et al. A phase II study (TACTI-002) in first-line metastatic non–small cell lung carcinoma investigating eftilagimod alpha (soluble LAG-3 protein) and pembrolizumab: updated results from a PD-L1 unselected population. J Clin Oncol. 2022;40(16_suppl):9003.
49. Krebs MG, Forster M, Majem M, Peguero J, Iams W, Clay T, et al. Eftilagimod alpha (a soluble LAG-3 protein) combined with pembrolizumab in second-line metastatic NSCLC refractory to anti–programmed cell death protein 1/programmed death-ligand 1-based therapy: final results from a phase 2 study. JTO Clin Res Rep. 2024;5(11):100725.
50. Fisher TS, Kamperschroer C, Oliphant T, Love VA, Lira PD, Doyonnas R, et al. Targeting of 4-1BB by monoclonal antibody PF-05082566 enhances T-cell function and promotes anti-tumor activity. Cancer Immunol Immunother. 2012;61(10):1721–33.
51. Tolcher AW, Sznol M, Hu-Lieskovan S, Papadopoulos KP, Patnaik A, Rasco DW, et al. Phase Ib study of utomilumab (PF-05082566), a 4-1BB/CD137 agonist, in combination with pembrolizumab (MK-3475) in patients with advanced solid tumors. Clin Cancer Res. 2017;23(18):5349–57.
52. Sapski S, Beha N, Kontermann R, Müller D. Tumor-targeted costimulation with antibody-fusion proteins improves bispecific antibody-mediated immune response in presence of immunosuppressive factors. Onco Targets Ther. 2017;6(12):e1361594.
53. Thapa B, Kato S, Nishizaki D, Miyashita H, Lee S, Nesline MK, et al. OX40/OX40 ligand and its role in precision immune oncology. Cancer Metastasis Rev. 2024;43(3):1001–13.
54. Massarelli E, Lam VK, Parra ER, Rodriguez-Canales J, Behrens C, Diao L, et al. High OX-40 expression in the tumor immune infiltrate is a favorable prognostic factor of overall survival in non-small cell lung cancer. J Immunother Cancer. 2019;7(1):351.
55. Postel-Vinay S, Lam VK, Ros W, Bauer TM, Hansen AR, Cho DC, et al. First-in-human phase I study of the OX40 agonist GSK3174998 with or without pembrolizumab in patients with selected advanced solid tumors (ENGAGE-1). J Immunother Cancer. 2023;11(3):e005301.
56. Müller P, Martin K, Theurich S, Schreiner J, Savic S, Terszowski G, et al. Microtubule-depolymerizing agents used in antibody–drug conjugates induce antitumor immunity by stimulation of dendritic cells. Cancer Immunol Res. 2014;2(8):741–55.

57. Rios-Doria J, Harper J, Rothstein R, Wetzel L, Chesebrough J, Marrero A, et al. Antibody–drug conjugates bearing pyrrolobenzodiazepine or tubulysin payloads are immunomodulatory and synergize with multiple immunotherapies. Cancer Res. 2017;77(10):2686–98.
58. Boshuizen J, Pencheva N, Krijgsman O, Altimari DD, Castro PG, De Bruijn B, et al. Cooperative targeting of immunotherapy-resistant melanoma and lung cancer by an AXL-targeting antibody–drug conjugate and immune checkpoint blockade. Cancer Res. 2021;81(7):1775–87.
59. Yi M, Zhang J, Li A, Niu M, Yan Y, Jiao Y, et al. The construction, expression, and enhanced anti-tumor activity of YM101: a bispecific antibody simultaneously targeting TGF-β and PD-L1. J Hematol Oncol. 2021;14(1):27.
60. Aditya B, Hurvitz SA, Tolaney SM, Delphine L, Kevin P, Mafalda O, et al. Sacituzumab govitecan in metastatic triple-negative breast cancer. N Engl J Med. 2021;384(16):1529–41.
61. Johnson ML, Solomon BJ, Awad MM, Cho BC, Gainor JF, Goldberg SB, et al. MORPHEUS: a phase Ib/II multi-trial platform evaluating the safety and efficacy of cancer immunotherapy (CIT)-based combinations in patients (pts) with non-small cell lung cancer (NSCLC). J Clin Oncol. 2018;36(15_suppl):TPS9105.
62. Garon EB, Liu SV, Owen SP, Reck M, Neal JW, Vicente D, et al. EVOKE-02: a phase 2 study of sacituzumab govitecan (SG) plus pembrolizumab (pembro) with or without platinum chemotherapy in first-line metastatic non–small cell lung cancer (NSCLC). J Clin Oncol. 2022;40(16_suppl):TPS9146.
63. Aggarwal C, Cheema P, Arrieta O, Bonanno L, Borghaei H, Hu Y, et al. P2.04-02 AVANZAR: phase III study of datopotamab deruxtecan (dato-DXd) + durvalumab + carboplatin as 1L treatment of advanced/mNSCLC. J Thorac Oncol. 2023;18(11):S305–6.
64. Goto Y, Su WC, Levy BP, Rixe O, Yang TY, Tolcher AW, et al. TROPION-Lung02: datopotamab deruxtecan (Dato-DXd) plus pembrolizumab (pembro) with or without platinum chemotherapy (Pt-CT) in advanced non-small cell lung cancer (aNSCLC). J Clin Oncol. 2023;41(16_suppl):9004.
65. Borghaei H, Besse B, Bardia A, Mazieres J, Popat S, Augustine B, et al. Trastuzumab deruxtecan (T-DXd; DS-8201) in combination with pembrolizumab in patients with advanced/metastatic breast or non-small cell lung cancer (NSCLC): a phase Ib, multicenter, study. J Clin Oncol. 2020;38(15_suppl):TPS1100.
66. Dougé A, El Ghazzi N, Lemal R, Rouzaire P. Adoptive T cell therapy in solid tumors: state-of-the art, current challenges, and upcoming improvements. Mol Cancer Ther. 2024;23(3):272–84.
67. Li Y, Sharma A, Schmidt-Wolf IGH. Evolving insights into the improvement of adoptive T-cell immunotherapy through PD-1/PD-L1 blockade in the clinical spectrum of lung cancer. Mol Cancer. 2024;23(1):80.
68. Xu MY, Zeng N, Liu CQ, Sun JX, An Y, Zhang SH, et al. Enhanced cellular therapy: revolutionizing adoptive cellular therapy. Exp Hematol Oncol. 2024;13(1):47.
69. Rosenberg SA, Restifo NP. Adoptive cell transfer as personalized immunotherapy for human cancer. Science. 2015;348(6230):62–8.
70. Li B. Why do tumor-infiltrating lymphocytes have variable efficacy in the treatment of solid tumors? Front Immunol. 2022;13:973881.
71. Schoenfeld AJ, Lee SM, Doger de Spéville B, Gettinger SN, Häfliger S, Sukari A, et al. Lifileucel, an autologous tumor-infiltrating lymphocyte monotherapy, in patients with advanced non–small cell lung cancer resistant to immune checkpoint inhibitors. Cancer Discov. 2024;14(8):1389–402.
72. Creelan BC, Wang C, Teer JK, Toloza EM, Yao J, Kim S, et al. Tumor-infiltrating lymphocyte treatment for anti-PD-1-resistant metastatic lung cancer: a phase 1 trial. Nat Med. 2021;27(8):1410–8.
73. Lee SM, Haigentz M, Villaruz LC, Gorbatchevsky I, Suzuki S, Tanamly S, et al. A phase 2 study to assess the efficacy and safety of autologous tumor-infiltrating lymphocytes (TIL, LN-145) alone and in combination with anti-PD-L1 inhibitor durvalumab in patients with locally advanced or metastatic NSCLC. J Clin Oncol. 2018;36(15_suppl):TPS3107.

74. Gulati P, Rühl J, Kannan A, Pircher M, Schuberth P, Nytko KJ, et al. Aberrant Lck signal via CD28 costimulation augments antigen-specific functionality and tumor control by redirected T cells with PD-1 blockade in humanized mice. Clin Cancer Res. 2018;24(16):3981–93.
75. Zeltsman M, Dozier J, McGee E, Ngai D, Adusumilli PS. CAR T-cell therapy for lung cancer and malignant pleural mesothelioma. Depth Rev Chimeric Antigen Recept T Cell-Based Ther. 2017;187:1–10.
76. Adusumilli PS, Zauderer MG, Rivière I, Solomon SB, Rusch VW, O'Cearbhaill RE, et al. A phase I trial of regional mesothelin-targeted CAR T-cell therapy in patients with malignant pleural disease, in combination with the anti–PD-1 agent pembrolizumab. Cancer Discov. 2021;11(11):2748–63.
77. Feng K, Guo Y, Dai H, Wang Y, Li X, Jia H, et al. Chimeric antigen receptor-modified T cells for the immunotherapy of patients with EGFR-expressing advanced relapsed/refractory non-small cell lung cancer. Sci China Life Sci. 2016;59(5):468–79.
78. Morgan RA, Yang JC, Kitano M, Dudley ME, Laurencot CM, Rosenberg SA. Case report of a serious adverse event following the administration of T cells transduced with a chimeric antigen receptor recognizing ERBB2. Mol Ther. 2010;18(4):843–51.
79. Baulu E, Gardet C, Chuvin N, Depil S. TCR-engineered T cell therapy in solid tumors: state of the art and perspectives. Sci Adv. 2023;9(7):eadf3700.
80. Lu YC, Parker LL, Lu T, Zheng Z, Toomey MA, White DE, et al. Treatment of patients with metastatic cancer using a major histocompatibility complex class II–restricted T-cell receptor targeting the cancer germline antigen MAGE-A3. J Clin Oncol. 2017;35(29):3322–9.
81. Foy SP, Jacoby K, Bota DA, Hunter T, Pan Z, Stawiski E, et al. Non-viral precision T cell receptor replacement for personalized cell therapy. Nature. 2023;615(7953):687–96.
82. Blumenschein GR, Devarakonda S, Johnson M, Moreno V, Gainor J, Edelman MJ, et al. Phase I clinical trial evaluating the safety and efficacy of ADP-A2M10 SPEAR T cells in patients with MAGE-A10$^{+}$ advanced non-small cell lung cancer. J Immunother Cancer. 2022;10(1):e003581.
83. Veatch J, Paulson K, Asano Y, Martin L, Lee B, Hall ET, et al. Merkel polyoma virus specific T-cell receptor transgenic T-cell therapy in PD-1 inhibitor refractory Merkel cell carcinoma. J Clin Oncol. 2022; https://doi.org/10.1200/JCO.2022.40.16_suppl.954.
84. Liu Z, Lv J, Dang Q, Liu L, Weng S, Wang L, et al. Engineering neoantigen vaccines to improve cancer personalized immunotherapy. Int J Biol Sci. 2022;18(15):5607–23.
85. Biswas N, Chakrabarti S, Padul V, Jones LD, Ashili S. Designing neoantigen cancer vaccines, trials, and outcomes. Front Immunol. 2023;14:1105420.
86. Ho SY, Chang CM, Liao HN, Chou WH, Guo CL, Yen Y, et al. Current trends in neoantigen-based cancer vaccines. Pharm Basel (Switz). 2023;16(3):392.
87. Xie N, Shen G, Gao W, Huang Z, Huang C, Fu L. Neoantigens: promising targets for cancer therapy. Signal Transduct Target Ther. 2023;8(1):9.
88. Ye L, Creaney J, Redwood A, Robinson B. The current lung cancer neoantigen landscape and implications for therapy. J Thorac Oncol. 2021;16(6):922–32.
89. Rizvi NA, Hellmann MD, Snyder A, Kvistborg P, Makarov V, Havel JJ, et al. Mutational landscape determines sensitivity to PD-1 blockade in non–small cell lung cancer. Science. 2015;348(6230):124–8.
90. Hellmann MD, Nathanson T, Rizvi H, Creelan BC, Sanchez-Vega F, Ahuja A, et al. Genomic features of response to combination immunotherapy in patients with advanced non-small-cell lung cancer. Cancer Cell. 2018;33(5):843–852.e4.
91. Awad MM, Govindan R, Balogh KN, Spigel DR, Garon EB, Bushway ME, et al. Personalized neoantigen vaccine NEO-PV-01 with chemotherapy and anti-PD-1 as first-line treatment for non-squamous non-small cell lung cancer. Cancer Cell. 2022;40(9):1010–1026.e11.
92. Lou Y. A phase I pilot study of personalized neoantigen peptide-based vaccine in combination with pembrolizumab in advanced solid tumors (PNeoVCA). J Clin Oncol. 2024; https://doi.org/10.1200/JCO.2022.40.16_suppl.954.
93. Bridle BW, Stephenson KB, Boudreau JE, Koshy S, Kazdhan N, Pullenayegum E, et al. Potentiating cancer immunotherapy using an oncolytic virus. Mol Ther. 2010;18(8):1430–9.

94. Pol JG, Zhang L, Bridle BW, Stephenson KB, Rességuier J, Hanson S, et al. Maraba virus as a potent oncolytic vaccine vector. Mol Ther. 2014;22(2):420–9.
95. Pol JG, Acuna SA, Yadollahi B, Tang N, Stephenson KB, Atherton MJ, et al. Preclinical evaluation of a MAGE-A3 vaccination utilizing the oncolytic Maraba virus currently in first-in-human trials. Onco Targets Ther. 2019;8(1):e1512329.
96. Jonker DJ, Hotte SJ, Abdul Razak AR, Renouf DJ, Lichty B, Bell JC, et al. Phase I study of oncolytic virus (OV) MG1 maraba/MAGE-A3 (MG1MA3), with and without transgenic MAGE-A3 adenovirus vaccine (AdMA3) in incurable advanced/metastatic MAGE-A3-expressing solid tumours: CCTG IND.214. J Clin Oncol. 2017;35(15_suppl):e14637.
97. Kumari K, Singh A, Chaudhary A, Singh RK, Shanker A, Kumar V, et al. Neoantigen identification and dendritic cell-based vaccines for lung cancer immunotherapy. Vaccine. 2024;12(5):498.
98. Mole RH. Whole body irradiation; radiobiology or medicine? Br J Radiol. 1953;26(305):234–41.
99. Park B, Yee C, Lee KM. The effect of radiation on the immune response to cancers. Int J Mol Sci. 2014;15(1):927–43.
100. Twyman-Saint Victor C, Rech AJ, Maity A, Rengan R, Pauken KE, Stelekati E, et al. Radiation and dual checkpoint blockade activate non-redundant immune mechanisms in cancer. Nature. 2015;520(7547):373–7.
101. Sharabi AB, Lim M, DeWeese TL, Drake CG. Radiation and checkpoint blockade immunotherapy: radiosensitisation and potential mechanisms of synergy. Lancet Oncol. 2015;16(13):e498–509.
102. Sharabi AB, Nirschl CJ, Kochel CM, Nirschl TR, Francica BJ, Velarde E, et al. Stereotactic radiation therapy augments antigen-specific PD-1–mediated antitumor immune responses via cross-presentation of tumor antigen. Cancer Immunol Res. 2015;3(4):345–55.
103. Shang S, Liu J, Verma V, Wu M, Welsh J, Yu J, et al. Combined treatment of non-small cell lung cancer using radiotherapy and immunotherapy: challenges and updates. Cancer Commun. 2021;41(11):1086–99.
104. Chamoto K, Chowdhury PS, Kumar A, Sonomura K, Matsuda F, Fagarasan S, et al. Mitochondrial activation chemicals synergize with surface receptor PD-1 blockade for T cell-dependent antitumor activity. Proc Natl Acad Sci [Internet]. 2017 [cited 2024 Jun 23];114(5). Available from: https://pnas.org/doi/full/10.1073/pnas.1620433114
105. Demaria S, Golden EB, Formenti SC. Role of local radiation therapy in cancer immunotherapy. JAMA Oncol. 2015;1(9):1325–32.
106. Ashton TM, McKenna WG, Kunz-Schughart LA, Higgins GS. Oxidative phosphorylation as an emerging target in cancer therapy. Clin Cancer Res. 2018;24(11):2482–90.
107. Le M, McNeill FE, Seymour CB, Rusin A, Diamond K, Rainbow AJ, et al. Modulation of oxidative phosphorylation (OXPHOS) by radiation- induced biophotons. Environ Res. 2018;163:80–7.
108. Kordbacheh T, Honeychurch J, Blackhall F, Faivre-Finn C, Illidge T. Radiotherapy and anti-PD-1/PD-L1 combinations in lung cancer: building better translational research platforms. Ann Oncol. 2018;29(2):301–10.
109. Theelen WSME, Peulen HMU, Lalezari F, van der Noort V, de Vries JF, Aerts JGJV, et al. Effect of pembrolizumab after stereotactic body radiotherapy vs pembrolizumab alone on tumor response in patients with advanced non-small cell lung cancer: results of the PEMBRO-RT phase 2 randomized clinical trial. JAMA Oncol. 2019;5(9):1276–82.
110. Welsh J, Menon H, Chen D, Verma V, Tang C, Altan M, et al. Pembrolizumab with or without radiation therapy for metastatic non-small cell lung cancer: a randomized phase I/II trial. J Immunother Cancer. 2020;8(2):e001001.
111. Theelen WSME, Chen D, Verma V, Hobbs BP, Peulen HMU, Aerts JGJV, et al. Pembrolizumab with or without radiotherapy for metastatic non-small-cell lung cancer: a pooled analysis of two randomised trials. Lancet Respir Med. 2021;9(5):467–75.

112. Antonia SJ, Villegas A, Daniel D, Vicente D, Murakami S, Hui R, et al. Durvalumab after chemoradiotherapy in stage III non–small-cell lung cancer. N Engl J Med. 2017;377(20):1919–29.
113. Tachihara M, Tsujino K, Ishihara T, Hayashi H, Sato Y, Kurata T, et al. Durvalumab plus concurrent radiotherapy for treatment of locally advanced non–small cell lung cancer: the DOLPHIN phase 2 nonrandomized controlled trial. JAMA Oncol. 2023;9(11):1505.
114. Bauml JM, Mick R, Ciunci C, Aggarwal C, Davis C, Evans T, et al. Pembrolizumab after completion of locally ablative therapy for oligometastatic non–small cell lung cancer: a phase 2 trial. JAMA Oncol. 2019;5(9):1283.
115. Cantor DJ, Davis C, Ciunci C, Aggarwal C, Evans T, Cohen RB, et al. Brief report: long-term follow-up of adjuvant pembrolizumab after locally ablative therapy for oligometastatic NSCLC. JTO Clin Res Rep. 2024;5(6):100667.
116. Lancaster EM, Jablons D, Kratz JR. Applications of next-generation sequencing in neoantigen prediction and cancer vaccine development. Genet Test Mol Biomark. 2020;24(2):59–66.
117. Chan DWK, Choi HCW, Lee VHF. Treatment-related adverse events of combination EGFR tyrosine kinase inhibitor and immune checkpoint inhibitor in EGFR-mutant advanced non-small cell lung cancer: a systematic review and meta-analysis. Cancer. 2022;14(9):2157.
118. Wei Q, Li P, Yang T, Zhu J, Sun L, Zhang Z, et al. The promise and challenges of combination therapies with antibody-drug conjugates in solid tumors. J Hematol Oncol. 2024;17(1):1.
119. Addeo A, Passaro A, Malapelle U, Banna GL, Subbiah V, Friedlaender A. Immunotherapy in non-small cell lung cancer harbouring driver mutations. Cancer Treat Rev. 2021;96:102179.
120. McLaughlin J, Han G, Schalper KA, Carvajal-Hausdorf D, Pelekanou V, Rehman J, et al. Quantitative assessment of the heterogeneity of PD-L1 expression in non–small-cell lung cancer. JAMA Oncol. 2016;2(1):46–54.
121. Sundar R, Soong R, Cho BC, Brahmer JR, Soo RA. Immunotherapy in the treatment of non-small cell lung cancer. Lung Cancer. 2014;85(2):101–9.
122. Zang X, Allison JP. The B7 family and cancer therapy: costimulation and coinhibition. Clin Cancer Res. 2007;13(18):5271–9.
123. Meng X, Huang Z, Teng F, Xing L, Yu J. Predictive biomarkers in PD-1/PD-L1 checkpoint blockade immunotherapy. Cancer Treat Rev. 2015;41(10):868–76.

# Immunotherapy in Melanoma

# 9

Yan Xing, Helena T. Wu, Swapnil Rajurkar, Tingting Tan, and Vanessa Hsu

## 9.1 Introduction

Melanoma, a malignancy originating from melanocytes, has historically been associated with high mortality rates, particularly in its advanced stages [1]. Before the advent of effective immunotherapy, treatment options for advanced melanoma were limited and often yielded poor outcomes [2]. The emergence of immunotherapy has marked a significant breakthrough in cancer treatment, especially for melanoma, offering durable responses and improved long-term survival. The evaluation of novel immunotherapeutic agents and combinations relies heavily on rigorous clinical trials conducted in phases, from initial safety assessments in Phase I to efficacy evaluations in Phase II and pivotal studies in Phase III. These trials are crucial in determining whether new therapies are safe and effective, ultimately leading to regulatory approvals by health authorities and subsequent changes in clinical practice guidelines [3].

The field of melanoma treatment has undergone a remarkable transformation in the past decade, shifting from a disease with historically poor prognosis to one where immunotherapy has ushered in an era of improved survival rates [4]. This paradigm shift is largely attributable to the development and implementation of

Y. Xing (✉) · V. Hsu
City of Hope Comprehensive Cancer Center, Duarte, CA, USA
e-mail: yxing@coh.org

H. T. Wu
Data Science Institute, The University of Chicago, Chicago, IL, USA

S. Rajurkar
City of Hope National Medical Center, Upland, CA, USA

T. Tan
Department of Medical Oncology, City of Hope National Medical Center,
Newport Beach, CA, USA



R. Salgia, P. Kulkarni (eds.), *Immunotherapies in Solid Tumors*, Cancer Treatment and Research 129, https://doi.org/10.1007/978-3-031-97242-3_9

various immunotherapeutic strategies, including immune checkpoint inhibitors (ICIs) targeting molecules such as PD-1, CTLA-4, and LAG-3, as well as cell-based therapies like tumor-infiltrating lymphocytes (TIL) and innovative combination approaches [5]. Recent clinical trials have highlighted the significant potential of neoadjuvant immunotherapy, suggesting it may become a new standard of care for patients with resectable melanoma [3]. While these advancements are significant, challenges remain, particularly concerning resistance to immunotherapy and the need for more personalized treatment strategies. Furthermore, specific melanoma subtypes like mucosal and uveal melanoma present unique challenges and opportunities for the development of targeted immunotherapeutic interventions [6, 7].

## 9.2 Neoadjuvant Immunotherapy in Melanoma

### 9.2.1 Overview and Rationale

Neoadjuvant immunotherapy, administered prior to surgical resection, represents an increasingly utilized strategy in melanoma treatment [8]. This approach is predicated on several potential advantages. By initiating systemic treatment early, it addresses the risk of micrometastatic disease, which is often present even in seemingly localized melanoma. Furthermore, delivering immunotherapy while the tumor and its microenvironment are intact can elicit a more robust and systemic anti-tumor immune response compared to adjuvant therapy administered after surgery [9]. The presence of the entire tumor mass allows for a broader presentation of tumor-specific antigens, potentially leading to a more diverse and effective activation of the immune system. Additionally, neoadjuvant therapy provides a unique opportunity to assess the pathological response to treatment in the resected tumor specimen, which has emerged as a valuable biomarker for predicting long-term clinical outcomes.

### 9.2.2 Key Clinical Trials and Findings

The phase III NADINA trial has provided compelling evidence for the benefit of neoadjuvant immunotherapy in resectable Stage III melanoma [3]. This study demonstrated that two cycles of neoadjuvant treatment with the combination of ipilimumab and nivolumab followed by surgery and response-driven adjuvant nivolumab significantly improved event-free survival (EFS) compared to adjuvant nivolumab alone. The estimated 12-month EFS rate was substantially higher in the neoadjuvant group, indicating a significant reduction in the risk of disease progression, recurrence, or death. Notably, the NADINA trial incorporated a de-escalation strategy based on the pathological response to neoadjuvant therapy, where patients with a major pathological response (MPR) received observation post-surgery, potentially reducing the need for further adjuvant treatment in this subgroup. These findings suggest that neoadjuvant ipilimumab plus nivolumab could become the new standard of care for resectable Stage III melanoma due to the significant improvement in EFS.

The SWOG S1801 trial also supports the use of neoadjuvant immunotherapy in melanoma, demonstrating improved outcomes for patients who received at least one dose (up to three doses) of neoadjuvant pembrolizumab and after surgery compared to adjuvant pembrolizumab alone [10]. The consistency of positive results across these phase II and III trials reinforces the benefit of administering immunotherapy in the neoadjuvant setting.

The OpACIN and PRADO studies have explored different dosing regimens of neoadjuvant ipilimumab and nivolumab to optimize treatment activity and safety [11, 12]. These studies reported high major pathological response (MPR) rates with combination neoadjuvant immunotherapy. However, it is important to note that these regimens were also associated with significant toxicities. This suggests a need for careful consideration of the balance between efficacy and tolerability when selecting neoadjuvant immunotherapy regimens, as well as the exploration of less toxic but still effective options like the combination of nivolumab and relatlimab, which has shown promising MPR rates with a more favorable toxicity profile [11, 12].

### 9.2.3 Long-Term Outcomes and Prognostic Markers

Long-term follow-up data from neoadjuvant immunotherapy trials (Table 9.1) are demonstrating sustained benefits in recurrence-free survival (RFS) and overall survival (OS) [13]. The extent of pathological response achieved after neoadjuvant therapy, particularly the achievement of a major pathological response (≤10% viable tumor) or a complete pathological response (no viable tumor), has emerged as a strong prognostic marker for these long-term outcomes [14]. Patients who achieve a pCR or MPR after neoadjuvant treatment tend to have significantly improved long-term survival and a lower risk of recurrence compared to those with a lesser response. Furthermore, recurrences in patients with a pCR may occur later and are potentially more salvageable. This underscores the importance of pathological response as a key endpoint in neoadjuvant immunotherapy trials and as a guide for predicting individual patient outcomes. The neoadjuvant approach also opens the door for personalized treatment strategies, where the intensity and duration of adjuvant therapy can be tailored based on an individual's response to the initial neoadjuvant immunotherapy [14].

**Table 9.1** Summary of key neoadjuvant immunotherapy trials in melanoma [3, 11, 12]

| Trial name | Treatment arms | Sample size | Pathological response rate (MPR/pCR) | Median EFS | Median OS | Follow-up time | Key findings |
|---|---|---|---|---|---|---|---|
| NADINA | Ipib (80 mg) + Nivo (240 mg) (neoadjuvant) vs. Nivo (adjuvant) | 423 R (1:1) | MPR: 56.6–59%, pCR: 45.8–47.2% | 12-month EFS: 83.7% (neo); 57.2% (adj) | Not yet mature | Median 9.9 months | Neoadjuvant ipi + nivo significantly improved EFS compared to adjuvant Nivo |
| SWOG S1801 | Pembro (neoadjuvant-adjuvant) vs. Pembro (adjuvant) | 313 R (1:1) | MPR: 42% (neo-adj); 24% (adj) | 2-year EFS: 72% (neo-adj); 49% (adj) | Not reported | Median 14.7 months | Neoadjuvant-adjuvant pembrolizumab improved EFS |
| OpACIN | Ipi (3 mg/kg) + Nivo (1 mg/kg) neoadjuvant | 20 R (1:1) | MPR: 67% | 5-year EFS: 70% (neo); 60% (adj) | 5-year OS: 90% (neo); 70% (adj) | 69 months | High MPR rate but significant toxicity |
| OpACIN-neo | Arm A: Ipi (3 mg/kg) + nivo (1 mg/kg) vs. Arm B: Ipi (1 mg/kg) + Nivop (3 mg/kg) vs. Arm C: Ipi (3 mg/kg) × 2 cycles followed by nivo (3 mg/kg) every 2 weeks × 2 cycles neoadjuvant | 86 R (1:1:1) | MPR: 60% | 3-year EFS: 87% (arm A); 77% (arm B); 81% (arm C) | 3-year OS: 90% (arm A); 93% (arm B); 92% (arm C) | 47 months | Tolerable dosing schedule (arm B) with reduced toxicity and high MPR rate |
| PRADO | Ipi (1 mg/kg) + Nivo (3 mg/kg) neoadjuvant single arm | 99 | MPR: 61% | 3-year EFS: 76% | 3-yeaer OS: 90% | 37.9 months | Confirmed high MPR rate with ipilimumab (1 mg/kg) + nivolumab (3 mg/kg) neoadjuvant regimen |

Abbreviations: *R (1:1)* Randomized 1:1 assignment, *ipi* ipilimumab, *nivo* nivolumab, *pembro* pembrolizumab

## 9.3 Adjuvant Immunotherapy in Melanoma

### 9.3.1 Current Recommendations

Current guidelines recommend adjuvant immunotherapy for patients with resected Stage IIB, IIC, III, and resected Stage IV melanoma to reduce the risk of recurrence [15]. Adjuvant treatment with anti-PD-1 antibodies such as pembrolizumab and nivolumab has become a standard of care in these settings. For patients with resected Stage IV melanoma, adjuvant nivolumab in combination with Ipilimumab is also considered a potential option [16]. The selection of adjuvant therapy is often individualized based on factors such as the stage of melanoma, sentinel node tumor burden, *BRAF* mutation status, and the patient's overall health and risk of immune-related toxicities.

### 9.3.2 Comparison with Neoadjuvant Therapy

Recent clinical trial data, particularly from the NADINA trial, suggest that neoadjuvant immunotherapy may offer superior outcomes compared to adjuvant therapy alone in certain stages of melanoma, specifically stage III [3]. The NADINA trial demonstrated a significant improvement in event-free survival with neoadjuvant ipilimumab plus nivolumab followed by adjuvant therapy only in patients without a major pathological response, compared to the standard approach of adjuvant nivolumab alone. This emerging evidence challenges the traditional adjuvant-only paradigm for resectable Stage III melanoma and supports the consideration of neoadjuvant immunotherapy as a potentially more effective strategy.

### 9.3.3 Strategies to Improve Adjuvant Therapy

Efforts are underway to further enhance the effectiveness of adjuvant therapies in melanoma (Table 9.2). One promising avenue of research involves combining adjuvant immune checkpoint inhibitors with other immunomodulatory agents, such as neoantigen vaccines [17]. The rationale behind this approach is to potentially broaden and strengthen the anti-tumor immune response, leading to improved long-term outcomes and a reduced risk of relapse. Early studies investigating these combination strategies have shown encouraging trends, warranting further investigation in larger clinical trials.

**Table 9.2** Summary of key recent adjuvant immunotherapy trials in melanoma [18–23]

| Trial name | Treatment arms | Sample size | Median PFS | Median OS | Follow-up time | Key findings |
|---|---|---|---|---|---|---|
| CheckMate 76K | Adjuvant nivo vs. placebo | 790 R (2:1) | 12-month RFS: 89% nivo; 79.4% placebo | 12-month DMFS: 92.3% nivolumab; 86.7% placebo | Ongoing | Adjuvant nivolumab significantly improved RFS in resected stage IIB/C melanoma |
| KEYNOTE-716 | Adjuvant pembrolizumab vs. placebo | 976 R (1:1) | 36-month RFS: 76.2% pembro; 63.4% placebo<br>Median RFS not reached | 36-month DMFS: 84.4% pembrolizumab; 74.7% placebo<br>Median DMFS not reached | 39.4 months | Adjuvant pembrolizumab significantly improved RFS in resected stage IIB or IIC melanoma |
| CheckMate 238 | Adjuvant nivo vs. adjuvant ipi | 906 R (1:1) | Median RFS: 61 months nivolumab; 24.1 months ipilimumab | 5-year DMFS: 58% nivo; 51% ipi<br>Median DMFS not reached<br>5-year OS: 76% nivo; 72% ipi | 61.5 months | Adjuvant nivolumab is suitable for resected stage III/IV melanoma at high risk of recurrence with a more tolerable safety profile than ipilimumab |
| CheckMate 915 | Adjuvant nivo + ipi vs. adjuvant nivo | 1844 R (1:1) | 24-month RFS: 64.6% combination; 63.2% nivolumab<br>Median RFS not reached | 2-year DMFS: 75.4% combination; 77.4% nivo<br>2 year OS: 89.8% combination; 91.8% nivo | 28 months | Adjuvant nivo and ip did not improve RFS against adjuvant nivo in resected stage IIIB-D or stage IV melanoma |
| Multipeptide vaccines | 12MP + tet vs. 12MP + 6MHP | 167 R (1:1) | Median RFS: 2.7 years 12MP + tet; 13.3 years 12MP + 6MHP | 10-year OS: 56% 12MP + tet; 68% 12MP + 6MHP | 12.2 years | There is value in adding cognate T cell help to cancer vaccine |
| KEYNOTE-942 | Adjuvant mRNA-4157 + pembrolizumab vs. adjuvant pembrolizumab | 157 R (2:1) | 18-month RFS: 79% mRNA-4157 + pembro; 62% pembro alone | 18-month DMFS: 92% mRNA-4157 + pembro; 77% pembro<br>OS not specified | 23 months | Adjuvant mRNA-4157 plus pembro prolonged RFS in resected high-risk melanoma with a manageable safety profile |

Abbreviations: *RFS* recurrence-free survival, *DMFS* distant metastasis-free survival, *12MP* 12 class I peptides, *tet* tetanus peptide, *6MHP* 6 melanoma helper peptide, *ipi* ipilimumab, *nivo* nivolumab, *pembro* pembrolizumab

## 9.4 Stage IV

### 9.4.1 First-Line Immunotherapy

For patients with unresectable or metastatic melanoma, first-line immunotherapy has become the cornerstone of treatment (Table 9.3) [5]. Recommended options include single-agent anti-PD-1 therapy with nivolumab or pembrolizumab, as well as combination immunotherapy regimens. The combination of ipilimumab (anti-CTLA-4) and nivolumab (anti-PD-1) has demonstrated significant clinical benefit, particularly in patients with poor prognostic features such as liver or brain metastases, *BRAF* mutations, or high LDH levels [15]. Another effective first-line combination is nivolumab plus relatlimab, an inhibitor of LAG-3, another immune checkpoint protein. This combination has shown improved progression-free survival and overall response rates compared to nivolumab monotherapy in treatment-naive metastatic melanoma, regardless of *BRAF* mutation status [5].

The combination of PD-1 and LAG-3 blockade with nivolumab and relatlimab has emerged as another valuable first-line immunotherapy option for metastatic melanoma [5]. The RELATIVITY-047 study demonstrated the superiority of this combination over nivolumab alone in terms of progression-free survival and overall response rates in treatment-naive patients [5].

### 9.4.2 Second-Line Treatment Options

Recent years have witnessed the approval and investigation of several novel immunotherapy agents and combinations for metastatic melanoma. Lifileucel (Amtagvi), a TIL therapy, received FDA accelerated approval in February 2024 for the treatment of adult patients with unresectable or metastatic melanoma who have previously been treated with a PD 1 blocking antibody, and if their melanoma is *BRAF V600* positive, a *BRAF* inhibitor with or without a *MEK* inhibitor [1]. This cellular therapy involves extracting a patient's own T cells from their tumor, expanding them in the laboratory, and then infusing them back into the patient to target and destroy cancer cells. Clinical trial data supporting this approval showed that approximately 30% of patients experienced tumor shrinkage, and about half of the responders had remissions lasting at least 12 months after a single TIL treatment [24].

### 9.4.3 Novel Immunotherapy Agents and Combinations

Ongoing research continues to explore new immunotherapy combinations and modalities to further improve outcomes for metastatic melanoma patients [25]. This includes investigating combinations of checkpoint inhibitors with targeted therapies like tyrosine-kinase inhibitors (TKIs), as well as other novel immunotherapeutic agents and strategies. For instance, studies are evaluating the combination of lifileucel with pembrolizumab in treatment-naive patients [26].

**Table 9.3** Summary of key phase 3 trials in stage IV melanoma [5, 6, 26–32]

| Trial name | Treatment arms | Sample size | Median PFS | Median OS | Follow-up time | Key findings |
|---|---|---|---|---|---|---|
| CheckMate-067 | Ipi (3 mg/kg) + Nivo (1 mg/kg) vs. Nivo 3 mg/kg vs. Ipi 3 mg/kg | 945 R (1:1:1) | Ipi + Nivo: 11.5 months; Nivo: 6.9 months; Ipi: 2.9 months | Ipi + Nivo: 71.9 months; Nivo: 36.9 months; Ipi: 19.9 months | 10 years | Combination therapy significantly improved PFS and OS |
| REALITIVITY-047 | Opdualag vs. Nivo monotherapy | 714 R (1:1) | 10.1 months (nivob-rela); 4.6 months (nivo) | 51 months (nivob-rela); 34.1 months (nivo) | 33.8 months | For small disease burden; combination significantly improved PFS and OS |
| DREAMseq | Nivo + Ipi followed by dabrafenib + trametinib vs. reverse sequential combination | 265 R (1:1) | 11.8 months (started on ipi/nivo); 8.5 months (started on dabrafenib/trametinib) | 2-year OS: 71.8% (started on ipi/nivo); 51.5% (started on dabrafenib/trametinib) | 27.7 months | For *BRAF* positive melanoma; combination nivolumab/ipilimumab followed by *BRAF* and *MEK* inhibitor treatment sequence significantly improved OS |
| EBIN | Ipi + Nivo and then Nivo; Encorafenib (*BRAF* inhibitor) + Binimetinib (*MEK* inhibitor) and then Nivo + Ipi and Nivo | 262 R (1:1) | 7.2 months; 9 months | 2 year OS: 68% encorafenib/binimetinib induction; 74% ipi/nivo | 21 months | For *BRAF V600E/K* metastatic melanoma; encorafenib/binimetinib induction did not significantly improve PFS; Immunotherapy should remain the first-line treatment. Patients with elevated LDH or liver metastasis may benefit from encorafenib/binimetinib induction |

| | | | | | | |
|---|---|---|---|---|---|---|
| Pembrolizumab + T-VEC vs. pembrolizumab + placebo | Pembro + T-VEC; Pembro + placebo | 692 R (1:1) | 14.3 months (Pembro-T-VEC); 8.5 months (pembro-placebo) | Not reached (combination); 49.2 months (placebo) | Not specified | Combination did not significantly improve PFS or OS |
| MDX010–20 | Ipi + gp100 vs. Ipi vs. gp100 | 676 R (3:1:1) | 2.76 months (ipi + gp100); 2.86 months (ipi); 2.76 months (gp100) | 10.0 months (ipi + gp100); 10.1 months (ipi); 6.4 months (gp100) | 55 months | Ipilimumab with or without gp100 vaccine showed improved OS compared to gp100 alone |

Abbreviations: *ipi* ipilimumab, *nivo* nivolumab, *pembro* pembrolizumab

## 9.5 Addressing Resistance to Immunotherapy

Despite the remarkable success of immunotherapy in melanoma, a significant challenge remains in overcoming resistance, which can be either primary (tumors that do not initially respond) or secondary (tumors that initially respond but later progress). Resistance to anti-PD-1 immunotherapy is a complex phenomenon involving various factors intrinsic to the tumor and extrinsic factors within the tumor microenvironment and the host.

Several mechanisms contribute to immunotherapy resistance. Dysregulation of the IFN-γ signaling pathway, often due to loss of *PTEN* expression or mutations in *JAK1/2* genes, can impair the anti-tumor immune response [27]. Insufficient antigen presentation by tumor cells, which can result from HLA downregulation or a low tumor mutation burden leading to a lack of neoantigens, can also hinder T-cell recognition. An immunosuppressive tumor microenvironment, characterized by the presence of regulatory T cells (Tregs), myeloid-derived suppressor cells (MDSCs), and elevated levels of IDO, can suppress the activity of anti-tumor T cells [27]. Alterations in intrinsic oncogenic pathways, such as mutations in the WNT/β-catenin pathway, can create an immunologically "cold" tumor microenvironment that is less responsive to immunotherapy [27]. Finally, T-cell exhaustion, a state of T-cell dysfunction resulting from chronic antigen stimulation, can limit the effectiveness of immunotherapy.

Strategies to overcome immunotherapy resistance are actively being explored. These include combinations of different immunotherapy agents (e.g., ipilimumab and nivolumab), therapies targeting the tumor microenvironment to reverse immunosuppression, personalized vaccines designed to elicit immune responses against tumor-specific neoantigens, and adoptive cell therapies like TIL that can overcome some resistance mechanisms.

## 9.6 Advancements in Immunotherapy for Specific Melanoma Subtypes

### 9.6.1 Mucosal Melanoma

Mucosal melanoma is a rare and aggressive subtype of melanoma that arises from melanocytes in mucosal surfaces. Treating mucosal melanoma presents unique challenges due to its rarity, distinct genetic characteristics (often lacking *BRAF* mutations), and generally poorer response to conventional immunotherapy compared to cutaneous melanoma [15]. However, recent advancements in immunotherapy offer hope for improving outcomes in this challenging disease. Combination checkpoint inhibition with ipilimumab and nivolumab has shown some efficacy [6]. Adoptive cell therapy using TIL has also demonstrated clinically meaningful and durable efficacy in advanced mucosal melanoma [6]. Furthermore, research is ongoing to investigate novel combinations of immunotherapy with TKIs and anti-angiogenic agents, particularly in acral and mucosal melanoma which often lack targetable *BRAF* mutations [6].

### 9.6.2 Uveal Melanoma

Uveal melanoma is a rare cancer that originates in the eye. It has a distinct genetic profile, with mutations in *GNAQ* or *GNA11* being common drivers, unlike cutaneous melanoma where *BRAF* mutations are more frequent [15]. Historically, uveal melanoma has shown limited response to the immune checkpoint inhibitors that have been effective in cutaneous melanoma [7]. However, recent advancements have brought new treatment options. Tebentafusp, a bispecific fusion protein that targets both glycoprotein 100 (gp100) on melanoma cells and CD3 on T cells, received FDA approval for metastatic uveal melanoma and has shown sustained benefit in a small proportion of patients [1]. Adoptive cell transfer therapies and other novel molecules are also being investigated as potential immunotherapeutic approaches for uveal melanoma [7].

### 9.6.3 Emerging Trends and Future Directions in Melanoma Immunotherapy

The field of melanoma immunotherapy is rapidly evolving, with several promising trends and future directions. There is an increasing focus on personalized immunotherapy approaches, utilizing biomarkers to predict which patients are most likely to respond to specific treatments. Biomarkers such as tumor mutation burden (TMB), PD-L1 expression levels, and gene expression signatures are being investigated for their ability to guide treatment decisions and optimize patient selection for different immunotherapeutic strategies.

The development of personalized neoantigen vaccines represents another exciting avenue for enhancing anti-tumor immune responses [33]. These vaccines are designed to target the unique mutations present in an individual patient's tumor, potentially eliciting a highly specific and effective anti-cancer immune response, particularly when combined with checkpoint inhibitors [33].

Research in adoptive cell therapies is expanding beyond TIL to include engineered T-cell receptors (TCRs) and other novel cellular immunotherapies that may offer improved targeting and efficacy in melanoma [5]. Understanding and modulating the gut microbiome is also emerging as a critical area of investigation, as the composition of the gut microbiota has been shown to influence responses to immunotherapy. Strategies aimed at optimizing the gut microbiome may enhance the efficacy of immunotherapeutic interventions. Finally, liquid biopsies, such as the analysis of circulating tumor DNA (ctDNA), are showing promise for monitoring treatment response, detecting early signs of recurrence, and guiding treatment adjustments in a non-invasive manner [34].

## 9.7 Conclusion

Melanoma immunotherapy has achieved remarkable progress, transforming the treatment landscape and significantly improving outcomes for patients with this once largely fatal disease. Recent clinical trials, particularly those evaluating neoadjuvant approaches, hold the promise of establishing new standards of care for resectable melanoma. While significant advancements have been made, challenges such as resistance to therapy and the need for more effective treatments for specific melanoma subtypes persist. Continued research into novel immunotherapeutic agents, combination strategies, personalized approaches guided by biomarkers, and innovative cellular therapies is crucial to further enhance the efficacy and durability of responses in patients with melanoma. The future of melanoma immunotherapy holds great potential for further improving the lives of individuals affected by this disease.

## References

1. Fateeva A, Eddy K, Chen S. Current state of melanoma therapy and next steps: battling therapeutic resistance. Cancer. 2024;16(8):1571.
2. Sorino C, Iezzi S, Ciuffreda L, Falcone I. Immunotherapy in melanoma: advances, pitfalls, and future perspectives. Front Mol Biosci [Internet]. 2024 [cited 2025 Apr 12];11. Available from: https://www.frontiersin.orghttps://www.frontiersin.org/journals/molecular-biosciences/articles/10.3389/fmolb.2024.1403021/full.
3. Blank CU, Lucas MW, Scolyer RA, Wiel BA van de, Menzies AM, Lopez-Yurda M, et al. Neoadjuvant nivolumab and ipilimumab in resectable stage III melanoma. N Engl J Med. 2024;391(18):1696–708.
4. Gorantla VC, Kirkwood JM. State of melanoma: an historic overview of a field in transition. Hematol Oncol Clin North Am. 2014;28(3):415–35.
5. Mooradian MJ, Sullivan RJ. Immunotherapy in melanoma: recent advancements and future directions. Cancer. 2023;15(16):4176.
6. Jung S, Johnson DB. Management of acral and mucosal melanoma: medical oncology perspective. Oncologist. 2022;27(8):703–10.
7. Uveal melanoma: recent advances in immunotherapy [Internet]. [cited 2025 Apr 6]. Available from: https://www.wjgnet.com/2218-4333/full/v15/i1/23.htm.
8. Neoadjuvant anti-PD-1-based immunotherapy: evolving a new standard of care. J ImmunoTher Cancer [Internet]. [cited 2025 Apr 6]. Available from: https://jitc.bmj.com/content/13/1/e010833.
9. Hong WX, Haebe S, Lee AS, Westphalen CB, Norton JA, Jiang W, et al. Intratumoral immunotherapy for early-stage solid tumors. Clin Cancer Res. 2020;26(13):3091–9.
10. Patel SP, Othus M, Chen Y, Wright GP, Yost KJ, Hyngstrom JR, et al. Neoadjuvant–adjuvant or adjuvant-only pembrolizumab in advanced melanoma. N Engl J Med. 2023;388(9):813–23.
11. Versluis JM, Menzies AM, Sikorska K, Rozeman EA, Saw RPM, van Houdt WJ, et al. Survival update of neoadjuvant ipilimumab plus nivolumab in macroscopic stage III melanoma in the OpACIN and OpACIN-neo trials. Ann Oncol. 2023;34(4):420–30.
12. Reijers ILM, Menzies AM, Lopez-Yurda M, Versluis JM, Rozeman EA, Saw RPM, et al. Impact of personalized response-directed surgery and adjuvant therapy on survival after neoadjuvant immunotherapy in stage III melanoma: comparison of 3-year data from PRADO and OpACIN-neo. Eur J Cancer. 2025;214:115141.
13. Sharon CE, Tortorello GN, Ma KL, Huang AC, Xu X, Giles LR, et al. Long-term outcomes to neoadjuvant pembrolizumab based on pathological response for patients with resectable stage III/IV cutaneous melanoma☆. Ann Oncol. 2023;34(9):806–12.
14. Junior DS do RL, Cidale BMA, Pereira AZL, de Menezes JN, Bertolli E, Belfort FA, et al. Emerging indications for neoadjuvant systemic therapies in cutaneous malignancies. Med Sci. 2024;12(3):35.
15. Pavlick AC, Ariyan CE, Buchbinder EI, Davar D, Gibney GT, Hamid O, et al. Society for Immunotherapy of Cancer (SITC) clinical practice guideline on immunotherapy for the treatment of melanoma, version 3.0. J Immunother Cancer. 2023;11(10):e006947.

16. Sondak VK, Atkins MB, Messersmith H, Provenzano A, Seth R, Agarwala SS. Systemic therapy for melanoma: ASCO guideline update Q and A. JCO Oncol Pract. 2024;20(2):173–7.
17. Collins JM, Redman JM, Gulley JL. Combining vaccines and immune checkpoint inhibitors to prime, expand, and facilitate effective tumor immunotherapy. Expert Rev Vaccines. 2018;17(8):697–705.
18. Kirkwood JM, Del Vecchio M, Weber J, Hoeller C, Grob JJ, Mohr P, et al. Adjuvant nivolumab in resected stage IIB/C melanoma: primary results from the randomized, phase 3 CheckMate 76K trial. Nat Med. 2023;29(11):2835–43.
19. Luke JJ, Ascierto PA, Khattak MA, de la Cruz Merino L, Del Vecchio M, Rutkowski P, et al. Pembrolizumab versus placebo as adjuvant therapy in resected stage IIB or IIC melanoma: final analysis of distant metastasis-free survival in the phase III KEYNOTE-716 study. J Clin Oncol. 2024;42(14):1619–24.
20. Adjuvant nivolumab versus ipilimumab in resected stage III/IV melanoma: 5-year efficacy and biomarker results from CheckMate 238—PMC [Internet]. [cited 2025 Apr 12]. Available from: https://pmc.ncbi.nlm.nih.gov/articles/PMC10472092/.
21. Weber JS, Schadendorf D, Del Vecchio M, Larkin J, Atkinson V, Schenker M, et al. Adjuvant therapy of nivolumab combined with ipilimumab versus nivolumab alone in patients with resected stage IIIB-D or stage IV melanoma (CheckMate 915). J Clin Oncol. 2023;41(3):517–27.
22. Multipeptide vaccines for melanoma in the adjuvant setting: long-term survival outcomes and post-hoc analysis of a randomized phase II trial. Nat Commun [Internet]. [cited 2025 Apr 12]. Available from: https://www.nature.com/articles/s41467-024-46877-6.
23. Weber JS, Carlino MS, Khattak A, Meniawy T, Ansstas G, Taylor MH, et al. Individualised neoantigen therapy mRNA-4157 (V940) plus pembrolizumab versus pembrolizumab monotherapy in resected melanoma (KEYNOTE-942): a randomised, phase 2b study. Lancet. 2024;403(10427):632–44.
24. Kwong MLM, Yang JC. Lifileucel: FDA-approved T-cell therapy for melanoma. Oncologist. 2024;29(8):648–50.
25. Qin Z, Zheng M. Advances in targeted therapy and immunotherapy for melanoma (review). Exp Ther Med. 2023;26(3):416.
26. Thomas SS, Gogas H, Hong YK, In GK, de Spéville D, Uribe B, Furness AJS, et al. Efficacy and safety of lifileucel, an autologous tumor-infiltrating lymphocyte cell therapy, and pembrolizumab in patients with immune checkpoint inhibitor-naive unresectable or metastatic melanoma: updated results from IOV-COM-202 cohort 1A. J Clin Oncol. 2024;42(16_suppl):9505.
27. Zielińska MK, Ciążyńska M, Sulejczak D, Rutkowski P, Czarnecka AM. Mechanisms of resistance to anti-PD-1 immunotherapy in melanoma and strategies to overcome it. Biomol Ther. 2025;15(2):269.
28. Improved survival with ipilimumab in patients with metastatic melanoma. N Engl J Med [Internet]. [cited 2025 Apr 12]. Available from: https://www.nejm.org/doi/full/10.1056/NEJMoa1003466.
29. Randomized, double-blind, placebo-controlled, global phase III trial of talimogene laherparepvec combined with pembrolizumab for advanced melanoma. J Clin Oncol [Internet]. [cited 2025 Apr 12]. Available from: https://ascopubs.org/doi/full/10.1200/JCO.22.00343.
30. Atkins MB, Lee SJ, Chmielowski B, Tarhini AA, Cohen GI, Truong TG, et al. Combination dabrafenib and trametinib versus combination nivolumab and ipilimumab for patients with advanced BRAF-mutant melanoma: the DREAMseq trial—ECOG-ACRIN EA6134. J Clin Oncol. 2023;41(2):186–97.
31. Three-year overall survival with nivolumab plus relatlimab in advanced melanoma from RELATIVITY-047. J Clin Oncol [Internet]. [cited 2025 Apr 12]. Available from: https://ascopubs.org/doi/10.1200/JCO.24.01124.
32. Final, 10-year outcomes with nivolumab plus ipilimumab in advanced melanoma. N Engl J Med [Internet]. [cited 2025 Apr 12]. Available from: https://www.nejm.org/doi/full/10.1056/NEJMoa2407417.

33. Aurisicchio L, Pallocca M, Ciliberto G, Palombo F. The perfect personalized cancer therapy: cancer vaccines against neoantigens. J Exp Clin Cancer Res. 2018;37(1):86.
34. Bartolomucci A, Nobrega M, Ferrier T, Dickinson K, Kaorey N, Nadeau A, et al. Circulating tumor DNA to monitor treatment response in solid tumors and advance precision oncology. Npj Precis Oncol. 2025;9(1):1–19.

# Role of Immunotherapy in Ovarian Cancer: Advances, Challenges, and Future Perspectives

**10**

Pankaj Garg, Gargi Singhal, Siddhika Pareek, Ajaz Khan, TingTing Tan, Deric Wheeler, and Sharad S. Singhal

## Abbreviations

| | |
|---|---|
| ACT | Adoptive Cell Therapy |
| AI | Artificial Intelligence |
| APC | Antigen-Presenting Cell |
| BRCA | Breast Cancer Gene |
| CAR-T | Chimeric Antigen Receptor T-Cell |
| CAMs | Complementary and Alternative Medicines |
| CRISPR | Clustered Regularly Interspaced Short Palindromic Repeats |

P. Garg
Department of Chemistry, GLA University, Mathura, Uttar Pradesh, India

G. Singhal
Undergraduate Medical Sciences, S.N. Medical College Agra, Agra, Uttar Pradesh, India

S. Pareek
Department of Medical Oncology & Therapeutics Research, City of Hope National Medical Center, Duarte, CA, USA

A. Khan
Department of Medical Oncology, Zion, IL, USA

T. Tan
Department of Medical Oncology, City of Hope National Medical Center, Newport Beach, CA, USA

D. Wheeler
Department of Human Oncology, School of Medicine and Public Health, University of Wisconsin, Madison, WI, USA

Carbone Cancer Center, University of Wisconsin, Madison, WI, USA

S. S. Singhal (✉)
Department of Medical Oncology & Therapeutics Research, Beckman Research Institute, City of Hope, Comprehensive Cancer Center and National Medical Center, Duarte, CA, USA
e-mail: ssinghal@coh.org



R. Salgia, P. Kulkarni (eds.), *Immunotherapies in Solid Tumors*, Cancer Treatment and Research 129, https://doi.org/10.1007/978-3-031-97242-3_10

| | |
|---|---|
| CTLA-4 | Cytotoxic T-Lymphocyte Associated Protein-4 |
| DCs | Dendritic Cells |
| HLA | Human Leukocyte Antigen |
| ICI | Immune Checkpoint Inhibitors |
| ML | Machine Learning |
| MHC | Major Histocompatibility Complex |
| MSI | Microsatellite Instability |
| OV | Oncolytic Virus |
| PARP | Poly (ADP-Ribose) Polymerase |
| PD-1 | Programmed Cell Death Protein 1 |
| PD-L1 | Programmed Cell Death Ligand 1 |
| PFS | Progression-Free Survival |
| TCR | T-Cell Receptor |
| TILs | Tumor-Infiltrating Lymphocytes |
| TMB | Tumor Mutational Burden |
| VEGF | Vascular Endothelial Growth Factor |

## 10.1 Introduction

Ovarian cancer (OC) has emerged as one of the leading gynecologic malignancies, with high global infection and mortality rates [1]. OC is exceptional in the sense that it is primarily diagnosed at an advanced stage because there is no early detection test, and the symptoms are not manifested until the growth is in the advanced stage [2]. Thus, it is still considered as the most lethal cancer of the female reproductive tract. Treatment of advanced stages of OC is very limited, largely contributing to the mortality rate of OC. The silent progression of this malignancy emphasizes an urgent need for improving the understanding of OC risk factors, getting diagnosed in the initial stages, and employing innovative therapeutic management plans [3]. OC incidence rates differ from region to region and with age, but developed countries tend to have a higher incidence rate. There are numerous other risk factors associated with this cancer type; one such genetic risk includes susceptible BRCA1/BRCA2 gene mutations, which significantly increase the lifespan risk of OC. Other risk factors include age, postmenopausal status, and parity factors whereby nulliparous women have marginally elevated risk [4]. In addition to definite risk factors, many preceding investigations have established genetic predisposition, where a family history of OC greatly enhances susceptibility. These risk factors support the extended understanding of the occurrence of OC and emphasize the need to focus on high-risk populations [5].

OC remains a difficult disease to predict, and the five-year survival rate for the disease has not risen above 50% across most populations. This poor five-year survival rate is to a greater extent understandable because OC is often diagnosed in an advanced stage when the tumor has already spread to different organs. OC in its initial stages offers a much better prognosis; however, as the symptoms are nonspecific, diagnosis at an early stage is rare. These disparities in survival based on the stage of diagnosis reinforce the call for better screening techniques and diagnostic instruments to improve the five-year survival rate for OC patients [6].

### 10.1.1 Current Treatment Modalities and Limitations

The existing first-line management strategies for OC are surgery, chemotherapy, and targeted therapy, each having its own goal and disadvantage. Initial management of OC frequently involves surgery, the main objective of which is to eliminate the main primary tumor mass as much as possible [7]. This procedure of debulking is important, as the quantity of tumor left behind influences patient outcome whereby shrinking the tumor mass improves survival. If debulking surgery is performed optimally, it helps in multiplying the efficiency of successive treatments and boosts the probability for long-term remission of the patient [8].

Chemotherapy comes in the second line of OC treatment after surgery, especially platinum-based drugs like cisplatin or carboplatin accompanied by paclitaxel. Given as a postoperative treatment, the primary purpose of chemotherapy is to get rid of any residual cancer cells and/or to prevent a relapse [9]. Chemotherapy may also be administered before surgery when the surgeon is unable to perform debulking surgery initially, owing to the massive infiltration of the tumor or the poor health of the patient; this is known as neoadjuvant therapy. Many OC patients show primary chemosensitivity to platinum-containing drugs; however, most patients inevitably become resistant to such therapy and develop recurrence, which necessitates additional treatment strategies [10].

Over the recent past, targeted treatments have offered other approaches to deal with OC, especially to patients with certain gene abnormalities. For instance, PARP inhibitors have benefitted individuals with BRCA1 or BRCA2 mutations, which tries to fix DNA damage in cancer cells causing cell death. Moreover, angiogenic molecules such as bevacizumab target the formation of new blood vessels within the tumor, hence starving the growing cancer cells of oxygen and other nutrients [10, 11] While some of these targeted therapies are effective and offer a progression-free survival (PFS), they are not considered curative. These drawbacks support the concept of exploring other unique therapeutic approaches that could help overcome the resistance and increase the survival rate in women with advanced or relapsed OC [12].

### 10.1.2 Limitations and Resistance

One of the key problems of OC treatment is the chemo-resistance that significantly reduces the lifespan of standard chemotherapy [13]. A number of OC patients get good initial responses to platinum-based chemotherapy regimens; however, many patients develop resistance, leading to the recurrence of the tumor mass. Several mechanisms play a crucial part in this resistance. One such related effect is the development of genetic mutations within cancer cells that can cause changes in drug targets, causing chemotherapy agents to lose effectiveness [14]. Additionally, enhanced efflux pump activity in resistant cancer cells pumps out chemotherapeutic agents from the cellular environment and decreases concentrates of the drug within the cell, lowering its lethality rate. Aberrations in these pathways, and particularly

DNA repair, are also involved. Alterations in DNA repair pathways, especially in cancers with BRCA mutations, also play a key role. BRCA mutations initially make tumors more sensitive to DNA-damaging agents, but later, countering pathways restore repair function and allow DNA repair. These resistance mechanisms are the underlying factors that impair attainment of a durable remission, thus pointing toward the need for alternative treatment strategies that can evade or counteract these pathways [15].

Another problem related to the treatment of OC is that patients may not achieve a long-term cure. Despite initial treatments, OC may reoccur and has higher levels of resistance to first-line treatments. This recurrence is particularly concerning for patients on platinum-based regimes because there are few remaining options for second-line treatments. In these patients, the chance of gaining a sustained response worsens, as with each time there is a relapse, the treatment planning spindles toward managing symptoms and maintaining the patient's quality of life [16]. The very high recurrence rate and lack of a definitive remedy emphasize the need for exploring new agents that would be effective in preventing or significantly delaying recurrence, perhaps by integrating existing agents or using immunotherapy.

The toxicity of chemotherapy regimens and targeted therapy agents affects the quality of life of patients, which makes the management of OC even more challenging. For example, for platinum-based chemotherapy adverse effects are nausea, fatigue, neuropathy, and hematologic toxicity that, in turn, restrict the doses of chemotherapy agents [17]. Targeted therapy with molecular drugs also has side effects; for example, anti-angiogenic bevacizumab raises rates of hypertension, bleeding, and gastrointestinal perforation. These side effects may require dose modification or temporary discontinuation of the therapy that weakens the treatment's efficacy. Furthermore, issues of cumulative toxicity often deprive the patient of further lines of therapy in the future as the disease advances. These and other limitations/resistance factors exemplify the great need for effective therapies with reduced toxicities to enable patients to gain a better quality of life [17, 18].

### 10.1.3 Unmet Needs in OC Treatment

There are several key gaps in OC treatment that interactively conspire to contribute to suboptimal patient outcomes. The first main concern of the current endometrial cancer diagnosis is the inefficiency of early detection strategies. Epithelial OC (EOC) frequently presents no symptoms in the initial stages, and the current diagnostic markers, viz., CA-125 and transvaginal ultrasound have inadequate sensitivity and specificity to enable early diagnosis. Unfortunately, just over half of all EOC cases are diagnosed at or before stage III, and as is the case with stage III, survival rates are lower, and treatments can be even more difficult when the cancer is diagnosed at stage IV [19].

One of the other major problems is that the rate of OC recurrence is rather high, even after necessary primary therapy. While the majority of patients have a satisfactory treatment outcome to first-line treatment, which includes surgery and platinum-based chemotherapy, more than 70% have recurrence and failure within 2–3 years in the majority of instances [20]. Recurrent OC is generally known as cancer that returns after treatment and which is usually treated with fewer effective treatment options. This stresses the need for therapies that could provide long-lasting results because recurrence rates remain high. Also, the heterogeneous nature of OC necessitates tailored treatment strategies [21]. High-grade serous ovarian and BRCA-associated endometriosis, and clear cell carcinoma are the most nuanced molecular subtypes and exhibit different sensitivities to treatment. However, treatment remains predominantly non-sophisticated and molecular analysis profiles and even targeted therapies are poor and rarely specific to the tumor type [22].

The side effects of current therapies are another unmet need, as both anticancer agents and molecular-targeted drugs are toxic to the body. These side effects are not only those that affect the quality of life of patients after diagnosis but also those that affect doses and treatment duration. Moreover, most of the molecular targeted agents like PARP inhibitors and anti-angiogenic agents are helpful only in a subset of patients, leaving the majority of patients with advanced disease with limited therapeutic options [23]. Innovation in immunotherapy for OC should therefore be pursued further. Immunotherapy has transformed treatment in some cancers including melanoma and lung cancer, but it has not produced the same impact in OC because the tumor environment inhibits immune activity. To address this issue, new approaches to increase the immune response and maintain anti-tumor immunity in OC patients need to be developed. Many of these needs remain unmet and will require enhanced detection, newer and less toxic remedies, mollification of treatment methods, and immunotherapeutic methodologies [24]. Both cooperative research and higher rates of clinical trial participation are therefore necessary in order to advance the treatment of OC.

## 10.2 Immunotherapy: The Future for OC

Immunotherapy continued as a revolutionary treatment in cancer management because the approach helps the immune system identify and destroy cancerous cells. Immunotherapy works differently from other therapies like chemotherapy and radiation therapy as it directly affects cancer cells [25]. The immune system can detect an abnormal cell primarily through molecular markers: tumor-associated antigens (TAAs) and tumor-specific antigens (TSAs). However, tumors on the other hand generate ways through which the immune system cannot detect cancer cells; for example, immune checkpoint pathways (PD-1/PD-L1 and CTLA-4), cytokines such as TGF-β, or the ability to create an immunosuppressive microenvironment around the tumor [26].

Immunotherapy aims to overcome these barriers through several strategies:

(i) ***Immune checkpoint inhibitors (ICIs):*** Inhibit antibodies such as PD-1 and CTLA-4 to protect T cells from suppression and to reactivate the immune surveillance.

(ii) ***Adoptive cell therapy (ACT):*** Includes *ex vivo* engineering or *in vivo* enlargement of cells that have immunity to cancer, for example, tumor-infiltrating lymphocytes (TILs) or CAR T cells.
(iii) ***Cancer vaccines:*** Meant to stimulate an immune response after injecting tumor antigens back into the body.
(iv) ***Oncolytic viruses:*** Genetically manipulated viruses, create selective targeted cancer cell killing and stimulation of immune system.
(v) ***Cytokine therapy:*** Uses other agonist factors, such as interleukins or interferons, to increase the immune response.

Concerning OC, immunotherapy seems to be relatively helpful because this approach focuses on abnormalities of the immunologic system of the cancer patients. Nevertheless, challenges still exist that consist of the dissimilarities of the OC microenvironment as well as the inefficiency of current immunotherapeutic approaches as a single treatment modality. Thus, further research for exploring new immunotherapy approaches, combined with chemotherapy, targeted therapy, or other immune modulators is being actively pursued (Fig. 10.1) [27].

### 10.2.1 Development of Immunotherapy in Cancer Management: An Overview

It is important to mention that cancer immunotherapy is relatively an old approach for the treatment of cancer. The idea of immunotherapies dated back to early nineteenth century where William Coley experimented with bacterial toxins to boost the immune system of cancer patients. Coley did not follow a standard approach toward the therapy he implemented, and also generated the concept that immune activation could bring stamina and regression of tumors [28].

The early of the mid-twentieth century underlined cytokine-based therapies, by the use of interferons and interleukin-2(IL-2) as an adjuvant form of therapy for treating diseases like melanoma and renal cell carcinoma through immune activation. However, these therapies were associated with severe toxicities and variable efficacy patterns that required a more specific treatment regimen [29]. Since the early twenty-first century, ICIs have changed the cancer immunotherapy scenario; antibodies such as ipilimumab (CTLA-4) and pembrolizumab (PD-1) have been demonstrated globally, with success in treating medical maladies like melanoma, non-small cell lung cancer (NSCLC), and renal cell carcinoma. These therapies were revolutionary because they revealed the fact that manipulating immune checkpoints favors effective and sustainable results, even for metastasized cancers [30].

An immunotherapy-based approach in OC was initiated by the time it was realized as an immunogenic cancer type that exhibits TILs in tumor biopsies. Initial strategies were aimed toward OC vaccines that exploited antigens such as

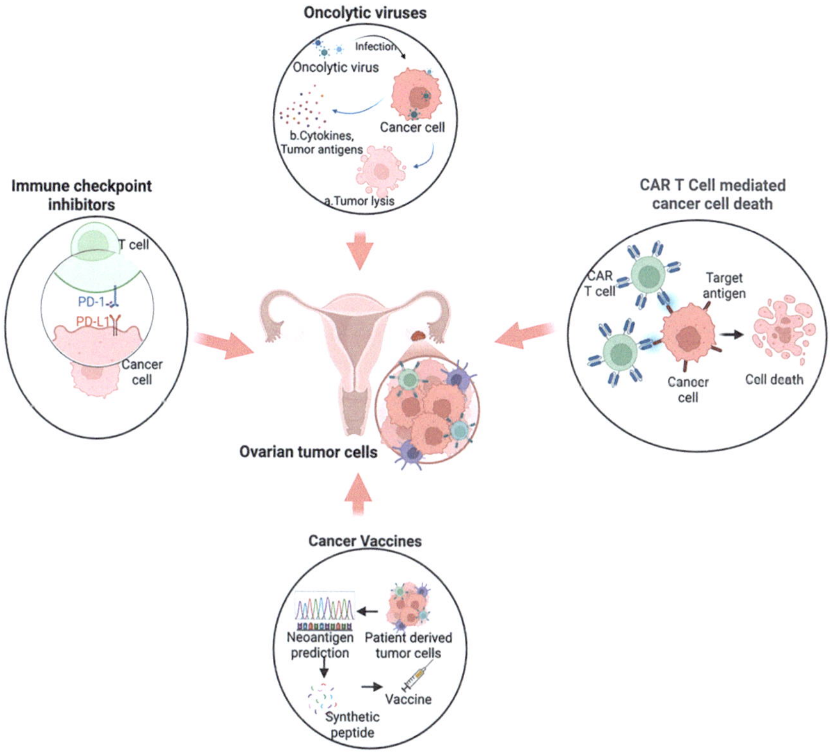


**Fig. 10.1** **Immunotherapeutic landscape in ovarian cancer.** Schematic representation of major immunotherapeutic strategies for ovarian cancer tumor cells including immune checkpoint inhibitors, CAR-T cells mediated cancer cell death, cancer vaccines, and oncolytic viruses. The figure highlights the mechanisms of action and interplay within the tumor microenvironment

MUC1, CA 125, and NY-ESO 1; however, the outcomes of these strategies were not very encouraging. The incorporation of ICIs in OC trials provided an insight into the benefits of immunotherapy; however, the immunotherapy monotone response has been reported as minimal mainly due to TME-induced immunosuppression [31]. New developments such as combination therapy and utilization of CAR T-cell therapy with targets of ovarian-specific antigens (mesothelin and MUC16) have extended the immunotherapy horizon. It remains as an active area of research with ongoing clinical trials for developing new anticancer agents, approaches to their usage, and biomarker identification to select patients who can benefit from therapy. Thus, immunotherapy has now moved from a promising idea to a standard of care in current-day clinical oncology, providing better insight to women diagnosed with OC. All the same, the fact that it continues to evolve means that it has the potential to revolutionize the current therapeutic scenario, with much better disease prognoses and treatment outcomes [32].

## 10.3 Immune Evasion in OC

### 10.3.1 Tumor Microenvironment and Strategies of Immune Evasion

The OC tumor microenvironment (TME) takes an active part in immune escape and tumor development. It is a dynamic system involving cancer cells, stroma, immune cells, and the components from the TME. Tumor-associated macrophages, myeloid-derived suppressor cells, and T cells are targeted in the development of OC cells within a TME. For instance, secreted remodeling cancer-associated fibroblasts (CAFs) and mesenchymal stromal cells release cytokines TGF-β and VEGF, which impede attraction and activation of immune cells [33]. Tumor hypoxia in the TME has a several-fold effect on promoting immunosuppression through regulating the expression of immune checkpoint molecules and proliferating regulatory T cells (Tregs) and myeloid-derived suppressor cells (MDSCs). Collectively, these patterns of regulation prevent strong and efficient antitumor immune reactions and enable OC cells to escape immune detection [34].

### 10.3.2 Role of Immune Checkpoint Molecules (e.g., PD-1, PD-L1, CTLA-4)

The immune checkpoint molecules are the proteins that have a major contribution in the TME such as PD-1, PD-L1, and CTLA-4. These are special proteins that help to maintain immune tolerance; OC is adept at escaping immune-mediated killing. It has a receptor on T cells known as programmed death-1 (PD-1), and a ligand, programmed death ligand-1 (PD-L1), which is overexpressed in a number of cancers, including OC, which limits the T-cell-mediated immune response [35]. In sync, PD-1 binds with PD-L1 and disables T cells, thus inhibiting the immune system's ability to target cancer cells. CTLA-4, a potent inhibitory receptor on T cells, antagonizes CD28 for B7 molecules on antigen-presenting cells. This interaction inhibits T-cell activation and the lack of any physiological response that facilitates full immune evasion [36]. These immune checkpoint pathways have been exploited in other cancers with ICIs, but when applied to OC, the efficacy is diminished because of the suppressive nature of the TME, highlighting the need for combination strategies for improved treatment efficacy (Fig. 10.2).

### 10.3.3 Tumor Immune Cell Infiltration and Its Role in OC Prognosis

The relative distribution and density of infiltrating immune cells in ovarian tumors are associated with the prognosis of affected patients. The infiltration of TILs and especially CD8+ cytotoxic T cells are related to better survival outcomes. On the other hand, immunosuppressive cells including Tregs and myeloid-derived

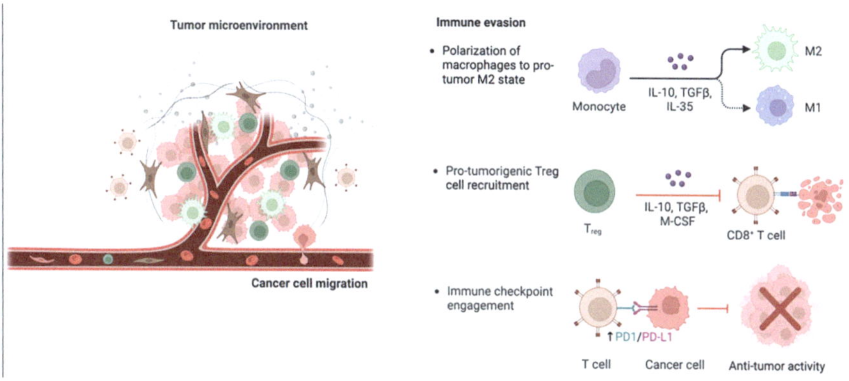


**Fig. 10.2 Mechanisms of immune evasion in ovarian cancer.** Schematic representation of immune evasion strategies in the ovarian cancer tumor microenvironment. Key mechanisms include polarization of macrophages toward the immunosuppressive M2 phenotype via IL-10, TGFβ, and IL-35 signaling; recruitment of pro-tumorigenic regulatory T cells (Tregs) that suppress $CD8^+$ T-cell activity through IL-10, TGFβ, and M-CSF; and immune checkpoint engagement via PD-1/PD-L1 interactions, leading to suppression of anti-tumor immunity

suppressor cells (MDSCs) are negative predictors of survival because they sharply suppress the function of effector T cells and promote tumor progression, respectively [37]. Furthermore, changes in macrophages at the TME play a crucial role in disease progression because they become more polarized. Tumor-associated macrophages (TAMs) in the TME are M2-polarized cells that secrete anti-inflammatory cytokines that support angiogenesis and promote tissue remodeling, while M1 macrophages possess antitumor activity [38]. However, in the OC TME, TAMs are mainly M2-like, which in turn further reduces antitumor immunity.

In conclusion, OC is secluded from immune identification and its destruction can be mediated by consecutive strategies, the TME's immunosuppressive element, activation of the immune checkpoint path, and infiltration of immune-suppressive cells. Knowledge of these mechanisms is therefore essential in developing successful immunotherapeutic approaches for combating immune tolerance in OC [39].

## 10.4 Checkpoint Inhibitors for OC

### 10.4.1 Check Points and Classification of Checkpoint Inhibitors

Checkpoint inhibitors are a class of immunotherapeutic agents that target pathways in an immuno-suppressive system to enhance the ability of T-cell receptors to identify cancerous cells. PD-1/PD-L1 and T-cell immune checkpoint receptor CTLA-4 are two key players in immune checkpoint pathways addressed in cancer treatment. PD-1 is presented on T cells and PD-L1 is presented on tumor cells; the interaction between these two results in T-cell exhaustion and immune diminution [40]. Engagement of these receptors with their ligands inhibits T-cell function, while blocking this interaction with monoclonal antibodies, like pembrolizumab (anti-PD-1) or atezolizumab (anti-PD-L1), restores this activity. Likewise, CTLA-4 interferes with CD28 relating to the clash for B7 molecules on antigen-presenting cells to delimit T-cell activation. Ipilimumab, an anti-CTLA-4 antibody, enhances immune activation by disrupting this pathway [41]. In OC, ICIs target the immunosuppressive TME; however, their efficacy remains limited as a sole therapy agent, thereby prompting interest in combination with chemotherapy, targeted therapy, or other immunotherapies [42].

### 10.4.2 Pharmacotherapy of PD-1/PD-L1 and CTLA-4 Inhibitors: Clinical Trials and Outcomes

Several clinical trials have used ICIs in OC, with most being the members of the PD-1/PD-L1 and CTLA-4. Phase II trials have tested both pembrolizumab and nivolumab (PD-1 inhibitors) in recurrent OC and demonstrated modest but evidence-based activity [43]. For instance, the KEYNOTE-100 trial examined pembrolizumab treatment in heavily pretreated OC patients and detected an overall response rate (ORR) of approximately 8%, with a better response in the patients with high PD-L1 biomarker expression. Nivolumab also elicited a 15% ORR in a phase II trial of patients with recurrent OC [44]. Similarly, other PD-L1 inhibitors like atezolizumab and durvalumab have been investigated and reported to have moderate efficacy. For instance, atezolizumab's combination with bevacizumab was reported to show a significant improvement in progression-free survival in some clinical trials but failed to show similar interactions in different patient categories [45]. Single-agent trials using ipilimumab (anti-CTLA-4) have demonstrated low response rates, but grouping it with nivolumab has shown synergistic effects, attaining an ORR of 31%. These studies exhibit the future of ICIs in treating OC, especially when incorporated with other therapy regimens [46].

### 10.4.3 Complications Concerning to Response Rates and Resistance Mechanisms

Immunotherapy with ICIs has shown an average clinical effectiveness in OC due to low response rates and resistance. One such reported issue is the immunosuppressive properties of the OC TME, impairing the infiltration and actions of effector T cells. Tregs, MDSCs, and M2-polarization-expressing macrophages compromise anti-tumor immunity and decrease checkpoint blockades [47]. Also, a lot of ovarian tumors with low mutational burden are often accompanied by reduced TILs, which means that the tumor is not recognized by the immune system. Further mechanisms of resistance are linked to the change in the markers of immune activation on the cancer cell surface, overexpression of TIM-3, and LAG-3 immune checkpoints when necessary [48]. Other possible alterations include the JAK/STAT and PI3K/AKT pathways. Additionally, adaptive resistance can happen by altering antigens for presentation, which involves downregulation of major histocompatibility complex (MHC) molecules [49]. To address these issues, combination strategies are being investigated in forthcoming studies; ICIs with other immunotherapies or chemotherapy, or agents targeting the TME to enhance response rates and overcome resistance mechanisms in OC [50].

## 10.5 Adoptive Cell Therapy (ACT) for OC

### 10.5.1 Types of ACT: TILs, CAR-T Cells, and TCR-Engineered T Cells

ACT is a novel immunotherapeutic strategy wherein healthy immune cells isolated from a patient can be cultured *in vitro* or genetically modified before being administered back into the same patient with the intent of triggering a highly effective anti-tumor response [51]. In OC, ACT strategies have primarily focused on three types of immune cells:

- ***Tumor-infiltrating lymphocytes (TILs):*** TIL-based ACT comprises of harvesting lymphocytes from the TME, culturing the harvested lymphocytes, then reintroducing the cultured lymphocytes back into the patient. TILs act upon tumor-specific antigens and hence are exclusive toward the tumor cells. Single TILs are precisely cytotoxic and are sensitive to tumor cells. However, the immunosuppressive TME in OC often reduces the effectiveness of this approach because it suppresses immune activity [52].
- ***Chimeric antigen receptor T (CAR-T) cells:*** CAR-T cells are designed to express synthetic receptors that identify tumor-associated antigens such as mesothelin or MUC16 to OC. CAR-T therapy has had great outcomes in hematological neoplasia, but challenges arise when applied to solid tumors, such as OC, due to diverse antigens and the hostile TME [53].
- ***T-cell receptor (TCR)-engineered T cells:*** The TCR plotted T cells are genetically retargeted here to express receptors for specific intracellular tumor antigens presented by MHC molecules. It can target a wider range of antigens/peptides, but the problem of specific and optimal antigen presentation and MHC compatibility is a challenge in OC [54].

### 10.5.2 Survivors' Stories and Challenges to Curing OC

ACT has been tried with some success in OC, especially in recurrent or refractory disease. For instance, CAR-T cells targeting mesothelin showed significant safety and antitumor activity in patients who had relapsed/multiple mesotheliomas. Similarly, TIL therapy has also been reported as effective to treat some OC patients, with research showing evidence of long-term remission of the diseases [55]. Nevertheless, there are still concerns to the usefulness of ACT in OC. As mentioned earlier, the OC TME is immunosuppressive as it contains Tregs, MDSCs, and cytokines that inhibit the activity of the transferred cells. In addition, ovarian tumor cells are antigenically distinct and thus the ACT strategies delimit the targeting of tumor cells [39]. Consequently, toxicities including cytokine release syndrome (CRS) and neurotoxicity due to CAR-T therapy restrict its applicability in many clinical cases. Additionally, there are some technical problems associated with the manufacturing and delivery of specialized and personified cell therapies that affect their clinical implementation [56].

### 10.5.3 Prospective and Novel Approaches to Applying ACT in OC

The present constraints have instigated researchers to develop new approaches to improve the effectiveness and safety of ACT in OC. For CAR-T therapy, escalating efforts are made for reaching dual-targeting CAR-T cells that would target multiple antigens to address the heterogeneity in tumors [57]. Furthermore, modifying CAR-T cells to secrete cytokines or making them resistant to immunosuppressive factors present in the TME is still under exploration [58]. Adding TILs with ICIs or cytokines, such as IL-2, has enhanced their effectiveness and duration *in-vivo*. Additionally, TCR-engineered T cells are being optimized to recognize tumor antigens without affecting other targets through the use of high-affinity receptors [59].

Another line of future research is the application of allogeneic ACT platforms, including "off-the-shelf" CAR-T cells from healthy donors, to minimize the development of personal approaches. The improvement of "gene editing technology" such as CRISPR/Cas9 to raise the specificity and function of ACT products also seems highly promising [60]. Finally, ongoing investigations related to biomarker findings are proving useful in identifying patients who will respond best to ACT, resulting in improved treatment outcomes. Despite several fierce challenges in OC treatment and care, ACT continues to develop through newer innovative combination strategies and may become a groundbreaking therapy modality for the treatment of OC [61].

## 10.6 Cancer Vaccines in OC

### 10.6.1 Types of Cancer Vaccines: Peptide-Based, DNA/RNA-Based, Dendritic Cell Vaccines

Cancer vaccines progressed with an aim of advancing immunological awareness toward malignant cells, differentiating the tumor from composing cells while presenting tumor-specific antigens. In OC, three main types of vaccines are under investigation [62]:

- ***Peptide-based vaccines:*** These vaccines employ short peptides derived from tumor-associated antigens that include NY-ESO-1, WT1, and HER 2, to stimulate a T-cell-mediated immune response [63]. Peptide-based vaccines are comparatively cheaper and simple to produce and have shown safety and immunogenicity in phase I/II trials. However, their effectiveness may be reduced by low antigen presentation and low immunogenicity, which has been reported in some patients [64].

- ***DNA/RNA-based vaccines:*** These vaccines introduce nucleic acids encoding tumor antigens and produce antigens within the host cells in the event of disease. In OC, DNA vaccines have been recommended based on antigens such as survivin and VEGF. There are other types of vaccines based on RNA, but the aforementioned types are more popular due to factors such as high efficiency of the antigen's expression and multiple antigen targets [65].
- ***Dendritic cell (DC) vaccines:*** DC vaccines consist of pulsing dendritic cells, the most effective antigen-presenting cells in the body, with tumor antigens, in an aim to stimulate T cells [66]. For example, autoantigen-based DC vaccines containing peptides derived from mesothelin or MUC1 have been examined in ovarian carcinoma. DC vaccines are very selective as they prove to be extremely difficult in terms of production and synthesis, thus making them less available [67].

### 10.6.2 The Treatment and Therapeutic Efficacy: Clinical Trails

Studies on cancer vaccines for OC have shown inspiring results but are still far from clinical practice. For example, the IMA901 vaccine, containing different peptides of tumor-associated antigens as components, revealed immunogenicity and extended survival in a subset of patients [68]. Similarly, the OVA-301 trial aimed at recording the immune response of patients who received a DC vaccine loaded with tumor lysates in recurrent OC and showed improved immune responses in some of the patients. Other related trials of VGX-3100, a DNA vaccine that targets HPV-related antigens, have proven safe and potentially active against gynecologic cancers, including OC [69]. Despite this progress, the therapeutic outcomes in OC are still rather limited, as vaccines are typically employed to augment the effects of other treatments, including ICIs or chemotherapy.

### 10.6.3 Obstacles to Vaccine Effectiveness and Immunocompetent OC Patients

Several factors act as barriers to achieving success with cancer vaccines in OC. One such barrier is a highly immunosuppressive TME, which hinders proper antigen loading of dendritic cells and T-cell stimulation. Patients with high-frequency derived Tregs, MDSCs, and inhibitory cytokines, including TGF-β and IL-10, impaired vaccine-induced immunity [70]. Another limitation is that OC antigens are rarely immunogenic; the tumors have a low mutation rate and therefore a low expression of neoantigens that stimulate vaccination. Also, the antigen variability of ovarian tumors may cause the escape of undesignated tumor cells, with reduced effectiveness of the vaccine [71]. Further, the absence of predictive biomarkers that could indicate which patients may benefit from vaccine therapy only makes the matters worse. Last but not least, practicalities like hindered vaccine storage and transportation and required individual vaccine preparation (as with DC vaccines) contribute to the overall cost of creating and administrating vaccine-based therapies, limiting their extensive use.

In conclusion, cancer vaccines demonstrate potential value for OC treatment, especially if used as an adjunct to or in combination with other immunomodulatory or targeted therapies. By overcoming issues with immune suppression, selection of the antigen, and patient classification, their full potential as therapeutic agents will be realized [72].

## 10.7 Oncolytic Viruses and OC

### 10.7.1 Oncolytic Viruses (OVs) as a Type of Antitumor Agent

OVs are live viruses that are designed to replicate within tumor cells and have no reproducibility in normal cells. Their therapeutic effects rely on two primary mechanisms: exerting direct toxic effects via the lysis of tumor cells and stimulating immune effector mechanisms [73]. When OVs enter cancer cells they replicate inside them, causing cell lysis and releasing tumor-associated antigens (TAAs). This antigen initiates an immune response and turns the tumor into an immune surveillance active site [74]. Furthermore, OVs also regulate the TME through the suppression of immunosuppressive biomarkers, thus opening up the space for infiltration of effector immune cells including CTLs. Some OVs are designed to express therapeutic transgenes such as immune adjuvants like granulocyte-macrophage colony-stimulating factor (GM-CSF) to enhance OV immunogenicity. These specific characteristics make OVs an attractive strategy for combating an immunosuppressive TME in OC, which poses a significant challenge to the overall management of the disease [75].

### 10.7.2 New OV Specific to OC Under Research

Several OVs are being explored for their potential use in OC treatment, including:

- ***Herpes simplex virus (HSV):*** Engineered strains such as T-VEC (Talimogene laherparepvec) exhibit potential against OC. T-VEC is transduced to express GM-CSF, which is capable of overcoming tumor immune tolerance and stimulating dendritic cells to initiate a T-cell response [76].
- ***Adenoviruses:*** ONYX-015 belongs to the class of adenoviruses that are adenoviral vectors, selectively replicating in the p53-deficient cancer cells that are characteristic of OC [77].
- ***Reoviruses***: Reolysin (pelareorep), a naturally occurring reovirus, is selective for cancer cells with an activated Ras pathway, which is often dysregulated in OC [78].

- ***Vaccinia virus:*** Second-generation MVs like JX-594, also known as pexastimogene devacirepvec, are engineered by incorporating the T7-TK gene to selectively kill tumor cells, downregulate the expression of immune-suppressive cytokines, and upregulate immune-stimulatory cytokines and chemokines [79].
- ***Measles virus:*** The measles virus has been attenuated so that the resulting vaccine targets cancer cells that express CD46, which is an overexpressed antigen in OC cells [80].

### 10.7.3 Preclinical and Clinical Effects

Investigations on OVs have shown promising outcomes in cell culture and tumor-bearing rodent models of ovarian malignancy. For instance, therapies founded on herpes simplex virus (HSV) have proven to induce destruction of OC cells and elicit good immune reactions in animal models [81]. Similarly, reoviruses exhibit potent cytopathic impacts in OC cells with mutated Ras. In OC, there have been positive clinical trial reports related to the use of OVs [82]. T-VEC has been proven to be safe and effective in patients with advanced solid tumors such as OC, but it is seemingly more effective when used in conjunction with ICIs [83]. Likewise, pelareorep has demonstrated its capacity to create tumor-specific immune responses and to increase survival simultaneously with chemotherapy in early-stage clinical trials [84].

Although these results indicate a more favorable scenario, the clinical use of OVs for OC remains constrained [85]. Some challenges that remain include the delivery of nanoparticles to the tumor site, overcoming the immunogenic reaction against viral carriers as well as the sentinel nature of OCs. Synergistic combinations with other agents, including ICIs or chemotherapy, are being investigated. Consequently, OVs are considered to be a promising and developing approach for OC treatment, taking advantage of the immune-stimulating properties and the direct cytotoxic effect of the virus on tumor cells. Further studies are ongoing to enhance the effectiveness of OVs and to better define their potential to eliminate the drawbacks of existing therapies [86].

## 10.8 Combined Regimens in Immunotherapy of OC

### 10.8.1 Understanding the Logic of Conjugating Immunotherapy to Chemotherapy, Radiotherapy, or Targeted Therapy

The idea for combining immunotherapy with other therapeutic modalities in OC lies in the potential to overcome the limitations of single-agent treatments. The systemic use of cytotoxic agents such as chemotherapy and radiotherapy effectively bring down tumor mass and metabolic load, but these effects are associated with immune impairing consequences and resistance. These therapies can evoke immunogenic cell death (ICD), liberating tumor-associated antigens (TAAs) along with shifting the TME from anti-inflammatory to pro-inflammatory, which augments immunotherapy [87]. PARP inhibitors and other agents including anti-angiogenic agents like bevacizumab have related benefits in ovarian carcinoma because they restore key pathways required for tumor growth. These agents, when used concurrently to immunotherapy, can have an even more profound impact on antitumor immunity. This is because of their conjoint effects on the TME, improved vasculature for immune cell infiltration, and enhanced immune stimulation due to shared pathways [88, 89].

### 10.8.2 Synergistic Effects and Recent Clinical Trial Outcomes

Combined treatment regimens aim to maximize interactions between various forms of therapy. For instance:

- ***Checkpoint inhibitors and chemotherapy:*** Trials such as IMagyn050 compared atezolizumab (anti-PD-L1) with platinum-based chemotherapy and bevacizumab in OC. Although the overall outcomes were not decent, some categories of patients receiving these treatments developed significant positive effects, thus highlighting the issue of patient segmentation [90].
- ***PARP inhibitors and immunotherapy:*** The synergetic effect of niraparib with pembrolizumab for patients with HER2-negative OC was evidenced by positive activity in the TOPACIO/KEYNOTE-162 phase II trial. This synergism originates from the fact that PARP inhibitors enhance DNA damage and neoantigen presentation, priming the immune system for checkpoint blockade [91].
- ***Radiotherapy and checkpoint inhibitors:*** Researchers from Yonsei University demonstrated the fact that radiotherapy increases PD-L1 levels and enhances the ability of cancer cell antigen presentation, making tumors more responsive to ICIs. The early Phase II trials assessing this combination in OC have also validated this immune activation, but with lesser evidence, which emphasizes the need for further evaluation [92].

### 10.8.3 Selective Research Combination Strategies and Their Successful Implementation

One related trial reported the combination of pembrolizumab and bevacizumab for patients with platinum-resistant OC, along with the maintenance of cyclophosphamide. This combinatorial regimen produced a durable response that was well attributed by immune checkpoint inhibition, angiogenesis inhibition, and immunogenic cell death induced by cyclophosphamide [93]. Another example is a case series from the MEDIOLA trial, olaparib, a PARP inhibitor, with durvalumab, a 4D-L1 antibody in BRCA-mutated OC. Remarkable exhibition of tumor regression as well as improved PFS highlights the potential of targeted immunity and immune-based combinations [94, 95].

However, there are some hurdles, such as the recognition of biomarkers that would help to predict which combination is more likely to produce a better response, how toxicities are shared between the ICIs, and to understand the interpretation of mechanisms that make the tumors resistant to treatment. The future work holds for fine-tuning combination strategies based on molecular profiling and immunogenic investigations [96]. Finally, the use of additional agents can enhance the efficacy of immunotherapy, making combination therapies a breakthrough direction in the treatment of OC. Considering its operation on various aspects of tumor-related characteristics, these strategies have high potential to enhance efficacy and to meet the needs of this challenging disease.

## 10.9 Biomarkers Associated with Immunotherapy Outcome of OC

### 10.9.1 Immunotherapy Efficacy in Biomarker Prediction

Recognition of successful biomarkers is crucial to raise the specificity and efficacy of immunotherapy in ovarian carcinoma. Biomarkers assist in identifying which patient is likely to improve after receiving a particular treatment solution so as to personalize the therapy. Commonly explored biomarkers include:

- ***PD-L1 expression:*** Tumor expression of PD-L1 and its presence in immune cells within the TME predict responses to ICIs targeting PD-1/PD-L1 [97].
- ***Tumor-infiltrating lymphocytes (TILs):*** TIL density and especially the presence of CD8+ cytotoxic T cells are related to better survival and significantly better immunotherapy outcomes in OC [98].
- ***Immune gene signatures:*** Transcriptomic assessments of immune signatures, including interferon-gamma signaling, can be used as a predictive biomarker for the identification of prospective responders to immunotherapy [99].

### 10.9.2 Tumor Mutational Burden (TMB), Microsatellite Instability (MSI), and Other Emerging Biomarkers

- ***Tumor mutational burden (TMB):*** A high TMB means a higher number of tumor neoantigens, which makes tumors more responsive to an immune checkpoint blockade. As discussed earlier, TMB is often lower in OC compared to other cancer types; however, specific subtypes are still potentially benefited by this biomarker [100].
- ***Microsatellite instability (MSI):*** In a nutshell, high MSI status identifies defects in the DNA mismatch repair (MMR) system that in turn will promote formation of neoantigens. High MSI OCs are not common, but they are sensitive to PD-1 inhibitors in clinical trials [101].

- ***BRCA mutations and homologous recombination deficiency (HRD):*** Although initially associated with PARP inhibitors only, BRCA mutations and HRD may modulate immune responses via promoting genomic instability and, therefore, neoantigen burden [102].
- ***Emerging biomarkers:*** Other possible biomarkers include circulating or tumor-infiltrating MDSCs, Tregs, and cytokine profiles in the TME. To a greater extent, these biomarkers epitomize the state of immunosuppression in the OC TME and give information on emergent resistance determinants [103].

### 10.9.3 Impact of Liquid Biopsy and Immune Profiling

- ***Liquid biopsy:*** Liquid biopsy techniques, which include the analysis of circulating tumor DNA (ctDNA), circulating tumor cells (CTCs), and exosomes, offer non-invasive methods to monitor biomarkers in real-time [104]. ctDNA provides data on TMB mutations and genomic alterations that can help determine immunotherapy response. Consequently, the content of exosomes, RNA, and protein can indicate changes in the TME and immune activity [105].
- ***Immune profiling:*** Among immune-related methods, flow cytometry, multiplex IHC, and scRNA-seq enable the assessment of the immune repertoire from the peripheral blood and TME, including its functional activity. These methods allow for the determination of the immune phenotypes that are potential predictors of immunotherapy responses or resistance [106]. Despite the scarcity of biomarker types that can predict immunotherapy efficacy in advanced OC, this field is rapidly evolving. Tumor genomics and characteristics and circulating tumor cell profiling and applications are developing to orient immunotherapy targeting. Further investigations will seek to optimize these biomarkers and incorporate them into treatment plans, so as to gain the most out of OC immunotherapy [107].

## 10.10 Emerging Approaches and Novel Immunotherapy Targets

### 10.10.1 Second-Generation Immune Checkpoint Receptors After PD-1/PD-L1

While PD-1/PD-L1 and CTLA-4 have been significant in immunotherapy, their poor outcome in OC has led to a search for other targets of immune checkpoints [108]. These novel targets include:

- ***LAG-3 (Lymphocyte activation gene-3):*** LAG-3 is a co-inhibitory receptor present on the exhausted T-cell population. The suppression of LAG-3 ameliorates T-cell function and exhibits strong combinatorial effects with PD-1 blockade in preclinical and first-line clinical trials [109].

- ***TIM-3 (T-cell immunoglobulin and mucin-domain containing-3):*** TIM-3 binds to T cells to inhibit their function; resulting in T-cell exhaustion. TIM-3 is on clinical trials for OC as well as for combination with other checkpoint blockades. This inhibition of TIM-3 is under investigation in OC clinical trials, particularly in combination with other ICIs [110].
- ***VISTA (V-domain Ig suppressor of T-cell activation):*** Another novel immune checkpoint is VISTA, which plays a crucial role as a suppressor of T cells and regulates immune response to cancer cells with a low inflammatory reaction [111].
- ***B7-H3 and B7-H4:*** These molecules are overexpressed in OC and could be potential candidates for immunotherapy developments [112].

### 10.10.2 Epigenetic and Metabolic Reprogramming in Enhancing Immunotherapy Outlook

Specific changes in the TME involving epigenetics and metabolic alterations are responsible for immune escape and resistance to immunotherapeutic intervention [113].

- ***Epigenetic reprogramming:*** Changes like DNA methylation and histone acetylation can suppress neoantigens or immune-related genes, dropping tumor immunogenicity [114]. Some understudied epigenetic drugs include the use of HDAC inhibitors in altering the TME to improve immune checkpoint function [115].
- ***Metabolic reprogramming:*** Tumors affect the metabolic environment of immune cells by taking up or releasing glucose to form lactate, and by reducing available amino acids such as tryptophan [116]. These approaches are based on blocking tumor metabolism: for example, inhibitors of the enzyme indole amine dioxygenase (IDO) targeting tryptophan metabolism or lactate dehydrogenase reverse this suppressive effect and activate T cells [117].
- ***Combination approaches:*** Combination of epigenetic or metabolic modulators with immunotherapies may improve the results of therapy in "cold" ovarian tumors with low immune infiltration [118].

### 10.10.3 Artificial Intelligence (AI) and Machine Learning (ML) Approaches in Immunotherapy Personalization

AI and ML are revolutionizing immunotherapy by facilitating the design of personalized treatment strategies:

- ***Predictive biomarker discovery:*** Advanced ML methods are applied to large and multi-level datasets encompassing genomics, transcriptomics, and proteomics to identify response of biomarkers to immunotherapy [119]. For example, AI can be employed for stratifying OC patients based on immune response characteristics at molecular and cellular levels [120].

- ***Drug response modeling:*** Cancer immunotherapy assessment utilizes ML-based tumor-immune interactions and the performance of specified immunotherapy regimens [121]. It helps clinicians to try multiple combinations *in silico* before use in real practice [122].
- ***Neoantigen prediction:*** AI technologies define tumor-specific neoantigens that are applicable to cancer-personalized vaccines or T-cell therapies, thus increasing their accuracy and effectiveness [123].
- ***Real-time monitoring:*** AI allows for the assessment of liquid biopsies and imaging to track tumor progression and response to therapy in a timely manner, allowing for the prompt identification of an alternative [124].

Altogether the current and emerging immunotherapies for OC indicate that next-generation checkpoint targets, epigenetic and metabolic reprogramming, and AI-directed personalization to immunotherapies will remain the frontier in OC treatment. These strategies are being developed to address existing shortcomings that will enhance the existing tool kit with targeted therapies and to identify molecular markers to support the ability to effectively treat patients with different cancer drugs and ultimately lead to better patient survival [125].

## 10.11 Challenges and Future Directions in Immunotherapy for OC

### 10.11.1 Major Obstacles in Advancing Immunotherapy for OC

Despite significant progress in immunotherapy, its application in OC remains limited by several challenges:

- ***Low tumor immunogenicity:*** OC has been described as a "cold" tumor with low infiltration density by immune cells and a low number of neoantigens. These immune suppressive characteristics trademark the maladaptive term of "cold" and limit the efficacy of ICIs and other immunotherapeutic strategies [42].
- ***Heterogeneity:*** The molecular and immunological nature of OC is another challenge because different types of tumors can have different genetic/immune backgrounds in response to treatment [126].
- ***Limited success in clinical trials:*** Interestingly, OC has not been proven to exhibit a significant clinical benefit in a few ICIs, as observed in some other tumor types that pose more challenges in devising new patient-specific subtypes and combination therapies [127].
- ***Access to immunotherapy:*** High costs, limited availability, and infrastructure requirements for advanced immunotherapies pose significant barriers, particularly in low- and middle-income countries [128].

### 10.11.2 Managing Resistance Patterns and Immune-Related Adverse Events

- ***Resistance mechanisms:*** To enhance immunotherapy performance, it is crucial to manage both primary and acquired resistance simultaneously [129].
- ***Immune escape:*** One of the major factors that have been reported to cause resistance include downregulation of MHC molecules, upregulation of inhibitory cytokines, and immunosuppressive cell infiltration such as myeloid-derived suppressor cells. Such approaches, as seen by using ICIs with agents targeting these pathways, are being explored [130].
- ***Checkpoint blockade resistance:*** The failure of PD-1/PD-L1 inhibitors can be managed by novel ICIs alone or in combination with epigenetic modulators/methylation or metabolic reprogramming agents [131].
- ***Immune-related adverse events (irAEs):*** Immunotherapies can cause a syndrome of autoimmune activation, including syndromes of systemic or organ-specific autoimmune manifestations like colitis, pneumonitis, or endocrinopathy [132].
- ***Management strategies:*** Biomarkers for early diagnosis, differentiating severity of irAEs, and effective management are paramount to protect patients' longevity and maintain high compliance with therapies [133].

### 10.11.3 Perspectives on Future Research and Clinical Applications

- ***Biomarker-driven therapies:*** The integration of predictive biomarkers such as tumor mutational burden (TMB), PD-L1 expression, and immune gene signatures is the key to transforming immunotherapy for OC patients. Improvement in mechanisms involving liquid biopsy and immune profiling enhances the capability of monitoring in a real-time manner as well as the ability to predict treatment response [134].
- ***Combination approaches:*** Combining immunotherapy with chemotherapy, radiotherapy, or targeted therapies (e.g., PARP inhibitors) holds promise for overcoming resistance and boosting efficacy [135]. Novel combinations, such as ICIs with OVs or epigenetic drugs, are being tested in preclinical and clinical studies [136].
- ***Personalized immunotherapy:*** AI and ML should be used in immunotherapy by weighing large data sets to create unique treatment plans as well as estimating an individual's prognosis [137].
- ***Innovative immunotherapies:*** CAR-T cell therapy, OV therapy, and cancer vaccines extend the list of treatment options. For instance, engineered CAR-T cells for specific OC antigens are being fine-tuned to deal with the limiting immunosuppressive environment [138].
- ***Prevention and early intervention:*** Other opportunities for immunotherapy include prophylactic applications with regard to implications in high-risk BRCA mutation carriers [139] (Tables 10.1 and 10.2).

**Table 10.1** Overview of immunotherapy approaches in ovarian cancer: mechanisms, clinical applications, and challenges

| Immunotherapy approach | Mechanism of action | Clinical trials/ examples | Challenges | References |
|---|---|---|---|---|
| Checkpoint inhibitors | Block immune checkpoint molecules (e.g., PD-1, PD-L1, CTLA-4) to restore T-cell activity. | Trials like JAVELIN Ovarian 200 with avelumab (anti-PD-L1). | Limited response rates, resistance mechanisms, immune-related adverse events. | [22, 23, 42, 43] |
| Adoptive cell therapy (ACT) | Infusion of modified immune cells such as CAR-T cells or TILs to directly attack cancer cells. | TILs in advanced ovarian cancer (NCT02482090); CAR-T cells targeting mesothelin. | Tumor microenvironment suppresses ACT, potential for severe toxicity. | [51, 52] |
| Cancer vaccines | Stimulate the immune system using tumor-specific antigens. | OCDC (a dendritic cell vaccine) in ovarian cancer trials. | Limited immune response, difficulty in breaking tumor tolerance. | [63, 66, 70] |
| Oncolytic viruses | Engineered viruses selectively infect and kill cancer cells while boosting immune response. | Preclinical studies with HSV-1 and reovirus. | Delivery challenges, immune suppression by tumors. | [73, 74, 81, 86] |
| Combination therapies | Combine immunotherapy with chemo, radio, or targeted therapies for synergistic effects. | Pembrolizumab with bevacizumab and chemotherapy (NCT02657889). | Managing increased toxicity and optimizing sequence of treatments. | [90, 91, 93, 94] |
| Epigenetic modulators | Reprogram the tumor microenvironment to enhance immune recognition and response. | Trials with DNA methyl transferase inhibitors (e.g., azacytidine). | Potential off-target effects, requires patient-specific optimization. | [50, 131, 136] |

Altogether, to overcome immunotherapy limitations in OC, efforts must be focused on the development of the new generation of immune-modulating biomaterials, including nanomaterials, a better understanding of immune system interactions with OC cells, and the application of an individualized approach to cancer treatment [140]. Through the eradication of treatment resistance, reduction of treatment-related risks, and increase of treatment efficiency, immunotherapy for OC is likely to exhibit a desirable effect in improving patients' survival rate and quality of life.

**Table 10.2** Comprehensive overview of immunotherapy strategies in ovarian cancer: mechanisms of action, clinical efficacy, and limitations

| Resistance mechanism | Description | Specific cancer types | Associated genes/ pathways | Limitations | References |
|---|---|---|---|---|---|
| Efflux pump activity | Overexpression of drug efflux pumps like P-glycoprotein (ABCB1) removes chemotherapy agents from cancer cells, reducing drug accumulation. | Ovarian cancer, colorectal cancer, lung cancer | P-glycoprotein (ABCB1), multidrug resistance-associated proteins (MRP1) | Can lead to cross-resistance to multiple drugs; limits effectiveness of various chemotherapies. | [12–15] |
| Alterations in DNA repair mechanisms | Enhanced DNA repair pathways, such as homologous recombination, restore damaged DNA, preventing the efficacy of DNA-damaging chemotherapies. | Ovarian cancer, breast cancer, prostate cancer | BRCA1/2, RAD51, Fanconi Anemia Pathway | Tumor cells may repair chemotherapy-induced DNA damage, rendering therapy ineffective. | [14–16] |
| Cell cycle arrest and apoptosis resistance | Tumor cells activate survival pathways that delay or prevent apoptosis, leading to resistance against chemotherapies inducing cell death. | Ovarian cancer, non-small cell lung cancer, glioblastoma | TP53, BCL-2 family proteins | Resistance to apoptosis can be hard to overcome, leading to continued tumor growth despite chemotherapy. | [17, 18] |
| TME alterations | The TME, including hypoxia and stromal components, can confer resistance by limiting drug penetration and activating anti-apoptotic signals. | Ovarian cancer, breast cancer, pancreatic cancer | Hypoxia-inducible factor (HIF-1), VEGF | Hypoxia in tumors limits drug penetration, and stromal cells can actively secrete growth factors that promote resistance. | [33, 34, 97, 98] |

(continued)

**Table 10.2** (continued)

| Resistance mechanism | Description | Specific cancer types | Associated genes/ pathways | Limitations | References |
|---|---|---|---|---|---|
| Epithelial-mesenchymal transition (EMT) | EMT results in the acquisition of stem-like properties and resistance to chemotherapy through enhanced survival mechanisms. | Ovarian cancer, breast cancer, melanoma | TWIST1, Snail, ZEB1 | EMT contributes to metastasis and immune evasion, complicating treatment options and patient outcomes. | [19, 20] |
| Autophagy activation | Chemoresistant ovarian cancer cells activate autophagy to survive in nutrient-poor conditions and in the presence of chemotherapy. | Ovarian cancer, pancreatic cancer, hepatocellular carcinoma | Beclin-1, LC3, mTOR | Autophagy can be both pro-survival and cytotoxic depending on the context, making it a complex mechanism to target. | [21–23] |
| Immune evasion mechanisms | Tumor cells evade immune detection through the activation of immune checkpoint molecules or by inducing immune cell dysfunction. | Ovarian cancer, melanoma, non-small cell lung cancer | PD-L1, CTLA-4, IDO1 | Resistance through immune checkpoint inhibition can be challenging to overcome, as tumor cells continue to exploit immune escape mechanisms. | [34–36] |

## 10.12 Clinical Significance

This chapter focuses on the prospects of immunotherapy in the treatment of OC and the possibility of surpassing conventional methods with immunological approaches including the use of ICIs, adoptive cell therapies, and cancer vaccines. Sophisticated strategies as well as biomarkers play a progressive role in organizing conventional treatments and immunotherapies for overcoming troubles such as resistance mechanisms and immune-related adverse events, thus, leading to the enhancement of patients' outcomes.

## 10.13 Conclusions and Future Directions

Immunotherapy has emerged as a revolutionary model offering hope in escaping the confines of conventional treatments in OC. Despite the progress in employing more effective treatments, like ICIs, adoptive cell therapies, cancer vaccines, and OVs, challenges have begun to emerge in the form of immune evasion, resistance mechanisms, and variations in patient responses. The complexity of the TME and chemoresistance necessitate further exploration and better approaches to intervention [141].

New developments, such as epigenetic therapy, metabolic reprogramming, application of AI in immunotherapy, and the identification of new biomarkers that may predict the result of immunotherapy will further help to individualize and improve the application of immunotherapy for OC. Additionally, the results of the strategies mentioned above exhibited combined effects, thereby emphasizing that combination treatment is more efficient. Nevertheless, immune-related adverse event management and the optimization of target selection remain essential [142].

In the future, more interdisciplinary cooperation of basic science, clinical investigation, and technological development will help to reach the immunotherapy maximum potential. Combined with the knowledge of these gaps in OC treatment, there is a possibility of the future looking stronger with lasting responses and fewer recurrent cases. In this chapter, we review how much more work should be done to further advance the field, fill the remaining gaps in OC, and to bring immunotherapy to further heights as the cornerstone in the treatment of this disease [143].

**Acknowledgments** The National Cancer Institute of the National Institutes of Health (P30CA33572) and the United States Department of Defense (W81XWH-22-1-0331, HT9425-25-1-0500) both provided funding for this project. Also appreciated is financial support from City of Hope's Beckman Research Institute. The figures were made using https://biorender.com.

**Declaration of Competing Interest** The authors have no conflicts of interest to disclose.

## References

1. Momenimovahed Z, Tiznobaik A, Taheri S, Salehiniya H. Ovarian cancer in the world: epidemiology and risk factors. Int J Women's Health. 2019;11:287–99.
2. Elias KM, Guo J, Bast RC Jr. Early detection of ovarian cancer. Hematol Oncol Clin North Am. 2018;32(6):903–14. Marth C, Abreu MH, Andersen KK, et al. Real-life data on treatment and outcomes in advanced ovarian cancer: an observational, multinational cohort study (RESPONSE trial). Cancer. 2022;128(16):3080–89. https://doi.org/10.1002/cncr.34350.
3. Ho WK, Hassan NT, Yoon SY, et al. Age-specific breast, and ovarian cancer risks associated with germline *BRCA1* or *BRCA2* pathogenic variants—an Asian study of 572 families. Lancet Reg Health West Pac. 2024;44:101017. Published 2024 Feb 5. https://doi.org/10.1016/j.lanwpc.2024.101017.

4. Zheng G, Baandrup L, Wang J, Hertzum-Larsen R, Hannibal CG, Faber MT, Sundström K, Kjær SK. Ovarian cancer risk factors in relation to family history. J Natl Cancer Inst. 2024;116(11):1767–74. https://doi.org/10.1093/jnci/djae164.
5. Chandra A, Pius C, Nabeel M, Nair M, Vishwanatha JK, Ahmad S, Basha R. Ovarian cancer: current status and strategies for improving therapeutic outcomes. Cancer Med. 2019;8(16):7018–31. https://doi.org/10.1002/cam4.2560.
6. Quesada S, Thomas QD, Colombo PE, Fiteni F. Optimal first-line medico-surgical strategy in ovarian cancers: are we there yet? Cancer. 2023;15(14):3556. https://doi.org/10.3390/cancers15143556.
7. Pinelli C, Guerrisi R, Brusadelli C, Artuso V, Majd HS, Bogani G, Ghezzi F, Casarin J. Interval debulking surgery for advanced ovarian cancer: when how and why? Gynecol Pelvic Med. 2021;4 https://doi.org/10.21037/gpm-20-61.
8. Rose PG, Fusco N, Fluellen L, Rodriguez M. Second-line therapy with paclitaxel and carboplatin for recurrent disease following first-line therapy with paclitaxel and platinum in ovarian or peritoneal carcinoma. J Clin Oncol. 1998;16(4):1494–7. https://doi.org/10.1200/JCO.1998.16.4.1494.
9. Coleridge SL, Bryant A, Kehoe S, Morrison J. Neoadjuvant chemotherapy before surgery versus surgery followed by chemotherapy for initial treatment in advanced ovarian epithelial cancer. Cochrane Database Syst Rev. 2021;7(7):CD005343. https://doi.org/10.1002/14651858.CD005343.pub6.
10. Xie Y, Xiao D, Li D, Peng M, Peng W, Duan H, Yang X. Combined strategies with PARP inhibitors for the treatment of BRCA wide type cancer. Front Oncol. 2024;14:1441222. https://doi.org/10.3389/fonc.2024.1441222.
11. Choi HY, Chang JE. Targeted therapy for cancers: from ongoing clinical trials to FDA-approved drugs. Int J Mol Sci. 2023;24(17):13618. https://doi.org/10.3390/ijms241713618.
12. Pokhriyal R, Hariprasad R, Kumar L, Hariprasad G. Chemotherapy resistance in advanced ovarian cancer patients. Biomarkers Cancer. 2019;11:1179299X19860815. https://doi.org/10.1177/1179299X19860815.
13. Havasi A, Cainap SS, Havasi AT, Cainap C. Ovarian cancer—insights into platinum resistance and overcoming it. Medicina. 2023;59:544. https://doi.org/10.3390/medicina59030544.
14. Damia G, Broggini M. Platinum resistance in ovarian cancer: role of DNA repair. Cancer. 2019;11(1):119. https://doi.org/10.3390/cancers11010119.
15. Matsuo K, Lin YG, Roman LD, Sood AK. Overcoming platinum resistance in ovarian carcinoma. Expert Opin Investig Drugs. 2010;19(11):1339–54. https://doi.org/10.1517/13543784.2010.515585.
16. Anand U, Dey A, Chandel AKS, Sanyal R, Mishra A, Pandey DK, De Falco V, Upadhyay A, Kandimalla R, Chaudhary A, Dhanjal JK, Dewanjee S, Vallamkondu J, Pérez de la Lastra JM. Cancer chemotherapy and beyond: current status, drug candidates, associated risks, and progress in targeted therapeutics. Genes Dis. 2022;10(4):1367–401. https://doi.org/10.1016/j.gendis.2022.02.007.
17. Li M, Kroetz DL. Bevacizumab-induced hypertension: clinical presentation and molecular understanding. Pharmacol Ther. 2018;182:152–60. https://doi.org/10.1016/j.pharmthera.2017.08.012.
18. Doherty JA, Jensen A, Kelemen LE, Pearce CL, Poole E, Schildkraut JM, Terry KL, Tworoger SS, Webb PM, Wentzensen N. Current gaps in ovarian cancer epidemiology: the need for new population-based research. J Natl Cancer Inst. 2017;109(10):djx144. https://doi.org/10.1093/jnci/djx144.
19. Ushijima K. Treatment for recurrent ovarian cancer-at first relapse. J Oncol. 2010;2010:497429. https://doi.org/10.1155/2010/497429.
20. Kleinmanns K, Bjørge L. Enhancing precision oncology in high-grade serous carcinoma: the emerging role of antibody-based therapies. npj Womens Health. 2024;2:7. https://doi.org/10.1038/s44294-024-00010-6.
21. Winterhoff B, Hamidi H, Wang C, Kalli KR, Fridley BL, Dering J, Chen HW, Cliby WA, Wang HJ, Dowdy S, Gostout BS, Keeney GL, Goode EL, Konecny GE. Molecular

classification of high grade endometrioid and clear cell ovarian cancer using TCGA gene expression signatures. Gynecol Oncol. 2016;141(1):95–100. https://doi.org/10.1016/j.ygyno.2016.02.023.
22. Min HY, Lee HY. Molecular targeted therapy for anticancer treatment. Exp Mol Med. 2022;54(10):1670–94. https://doi.org/10.1038/s12276-022-00864-3.
23. Yoon H, Kim A, Jang H. Immunotherapeutic approaches in ovarian cancer. Curr Issues Mol Biol. 2023;45:1233–49. https://doi.org/10.3390/cimb45020081.
24. Liu B, Zhou H, Tan L, et al. Exploring treatment options in cancer: tumor treatment strategies. Sig Transduct Target Ther. 2024;9:175. https://doi.org/10.1038/s41392-024-01856-7.
25. Yang K, Lu R, Mei J, et al. The war between the immune system and the tumor—using immune biomarkers as tracers. Biomark Res. 2024;12:51. https://doi.org/10.1186/s40364-024-00599-5.
26. Zhu S, Zhang T, Zheng L, et al. Combination strategies to maximize the benefits of cancer immunotherapy. J Hematol Oncol. 2021;14:156. https://doi.org/10.1186/s13045-021-01164-5.
27. Dobosz P, Dzieciątkowski T. The intriguing history of cancer immunotherapy. Front Immunol. 2019;10:2965. https://doi.org/10.3389/fimmu.2019.02965.
28. Muhammad S, Fan T, Hai Y, et al. Reigniting hope in cancer treatment: the promise and pitfalls of IL-2 and IL-2R targeting strategies. Mol Cancer. 2023;22:121. https://doi.org/10.1186/s12943-023-01826-7.
29. Shiravand Y, Khodadadi F, Kashani SMA, Hosseini-Fard SR, Hosseini S, Sadeghirad H, Ladwa R, O'Byrne K, Kulasinghe A. Immune checkpoint inhibitors in cancer therapy. Curr Oncol (Toronto, Ont). 2022;29(5):3044–60. https://doi.org/10.3390/curroncol29050247.
30. Tassi E, Bergamini A, Wignall J, Sant'Angelo M, Brunetto E, Balestrieri C, Redegalli M, Potenza A, Abbati D, Manfredi F, Cangi MG, Magliacane G, Scalisi F, Ruggiero E, Maffia MC, Trippitelli F, Rabaiotti E, Cioffi R, Bocciolone L, Candotti G, Bonini C. Epithelial ovarian cancer is infiltrated by activated effector T cells co-expressing CD39, PD-1, TIM-3, CD137 and interacting with cancer cells and myeloid cells. Front Immunol. 2023;14:1212444. https://doi.org/10.3389/fimmu.2023.1212444.
31. Mun SS, Meyerberg J, Peraro L, Korontsvit T, Gardner T, Malviya M, Kyi C, O'Cearbhaill RE, Liu C, Dao T, Scheinberg DA. Dual targeting ovarian cancer by Muc16 CAR T cells secreting a bispecific T cell engager antibody for an intracellular tumor antigen WT1. Cancer Immunol Immunother. 2023;72(11):3773–86. https://doi.org/10.1007/s00262-023-03529-w.
32. Guo J, Zeng X, Zhu Y, Yang D, Zhao X. Mesothelin-based CAR-T cells exhibit potent antitumor activity against ovarian cancer. J Transl Med. 2024;22(1):367. https://doi.org/10.1186/s12967-024-05174-y.
33. Garg P, Pareek S, Kulkarni P, Horne D, Salgia R, Singhal SS. Exploring the potential of TGFβ as a diagnostic marker and therapeutic target against cancer. Biochem Pharmacol. 2025;231:116646. https://doi.org/10.1016/j.bcp.2024.116646.
34. Garg P, Ramisetty SK, Raghu Subbalakshmi A, Krishna BM, Pareek S, Mohanty A, Kulkarni P, Horne D, Salgia R, Singhal SS. Gynecological cancer tumor microenvironment: unveiling cellular complexity and therapeutic potential. Biochem Pharmacol. 2024;229:116498. https://doi.org/10.1016/j.bcp.2024.116498.
35. Bose CK. Immune checkpoint blockers and ovarian cancer. Indian J Med Paediatr Oncol. 2017;38(2):182–9. https://doi.org/10.4103/ijmpo.ijmpo_73_16.
36. Han Y, Liu D, Li L. PD-1/PD-L1 pathway: current research in cancer. Am J Cancer Res. 2020;10(3):727–42.
37. Fanale D, Dimino A, Pedone E, Brando C, Corsini LR, Filorizzo C, Fiorino A, Lisanti MC, Magrin L, Randazzo U, Bazan Russo TD, Russo A, Bazan V. Prognostic and predictive role of tumor-infiltrating lymphocytes (TILs) in ovarian cancer. Cancer. 2022;14(18):4344. https://doi.org/10.3390/cancers14184344.
38. Zhang W, Wang M, Ji C, Liu X, Gu B, Dong T. Macrophage polarization in the tumor microenvironment: emerging roles and therapeutic potentials. Biomed Pharmacother. 2024;177:116930. https://doi.org/10.1016/j.biopha.2024.116930.

39. Blanc-Durand F, Clemence Wei Xian L, Tan DSP. Targeting the immune microenvironment for ovarian cancer therapy. Front Immunol. 2023;14:1328651. https://doi.org/10.3389/fimmu.2023.1328651.
40. Wojtukiewicz MZ, Rek MM, Karpowicz K, Górska M, Polityńska B, Wojtukiewicz AM, Moniuszko M, Radziwon P, Tucker SC, Honn KV. Inhibitors of immune checkpoints-PD-1, PD-L1, CTLA-4-new opportunities for cancer patients and a new challenge for internists and general practitioners. Cancer Metastasis Rev. 2021;40(3):949–82. https://doi.org/10.1007/s10555-021-09976-0.
41. Córdova-Bahena L, Velasco-Velázquez MA. Anti-PD-1 and anti-PD-L1 antibodies as immunotherapy against cancer: a structural perspective. Rev Investig Clin. 2020;73(1):008–16. https://doi.org/10.24875/RIC.20000341.
42. Pawłowska A, Rekowska A, Kuryło W, Pańczyszyn A, Kotarski J, Wertel I. Current understanding on why ovarian cancer is resistant to immune checkpoint inhibitors. Int J Mol Sci. 2023;24(13):10859. https://doi.org/10.3390/ijms241310859.
43. Zhao L, Zhai Y, Niu G. Research progress of immune checkpoint inhibitors in ovarian cancer. Explor Immunol. 2024;4:853–70. https://doi.org/10.37349/ei.2024.00177.
44. Matulonis UA, Shapira-Frommer R, Santin AD, Lisyanskaya AS, Pignata S, Vergote I, Raspagliesi F, Sonke GS, Birrer M, Provencher DM, Sehouli J, Colombo N, González-Martín A, Oaknin A, Ottevanger PB, Rudaitis V, Katchar K, Wu H, Keefe S, Ruman J, et al. Antitumor activity and safety of pembrolizumab in patients with advanced recurrent ovarian cancer: results from the phase II KEYNOTE-100 study. Ann Oncol. 2019;30(7):1080–7. https://doi.org/10.1093/annonc/mdz135.
45. Velimirovici MD, Feier CVI, Vonica RC, Faur AM, Muntean C. Efficacy and safety of atezolizumab as a PD-L1 inhibitor in the treatment of cervical cancer: a systematic review. Biomedicine. 2024;12(6):1291. https://doi.org/10.3390/biomedicines12061291.
46. Khan B, Qahwaji RM, Alfaifi MS, Mobashir M. Nivolumab and ipilimumab acting as tormentors of advanced tumors by unleashing immune cells and associated collateral damage. Pharmaceutics. 2024;16(6):732. https://doi.org/10.3390/pharmaceutics16060732.
47. Yang C, Xia BR, Zhang ZC, Zhang YJ, Lou G, Jin WL. Immunotherapy for ovarian cancer: adjuvant, combination, and neoadjuvant. Front Immunol. 2020;11:577869. https://doi.org/10.3389/fimmu.2020.577869.
48. Hudry D, Le Guellec S, Meignan S, Bécourt S, Pasquesoone C, El Hajj H, Martínez-Gómez C, Leblanc É, Narducci F, Ladoire S. Tumor-infiltrating lymphocytes (TILs) in epithelial ovarian cancer: heterogeneity, prognostic impact, and relationship with immune checkpoints. Cancer. 2022;14(21):5332. https://doi.org/10.3390/cancers14215332.
49. Anderson AC, Joller N, Kuchroo VK. Lag-3, Tim-3, and TIGIT: co-inhibitory receptors with specialized functions in immune regulation. Immunity. 2016;44(5):989–1004. https://doi.org/10.1016/j.immuni.2016.05.001.
50. Varayathu H, Sarathy V, Thomas BE, Mufti SS, Naik R. Combination strategies to augment immune check point inhibitors efficacy—implications for translational research. Front Oncol. 2021;11:559161. https://doi.org/10.3389/fonc.2021.559161.
51. Rosenberg SA, Restifo NP, Yang JC, Morgan RA, Dudley ME. Adoptive cell transfers: a clinical path to effective cancer immunotherapy. Nat Rev Cancer. 2008;8(4):299–308. https://doi.org/10.1038/nrc2355.
52. Wang S, Sun J, Chen K, et al. Perspectives of tumor-infiltrating lymphocyte treatment in solid tumors. BMC Med. 2021;19:140. https://doi.org/10.1186/s12916-021-02006-4.
53. Morello A, Sadelain M, Adusumilli PS. Mesothelin-targeted CARs: driving T cells to solid tumors. Cancer Discov. 2016;6(2):133–46. https://doi.org/10.1158/2159-8290.CD-15-0583.
54. Greenbaum U, Dumbrava EI, Biter AB, Haymaker CL, Hong DS. Engineered T-cell receptor T cells for cancer immunotherapy. Cancer Immunol Res. 2021;9(11):1252–61. https://doi.org/10.1158/2326-6066.CIR-21-0269.
55. Chen J, Hu J, Gu L, Ji F, Zhang F, Zhang M, Li J, Chen Z, Jiang L, Zhang Y, Shi R, Ma L, Jia S, Zhang Y, Zhang Q, Liang J, Yao S, Hu Z, Guo Z. Anti-mesothelin CAR-T immunotherapy

in patients with ovarian cancer. Cancer Immunol Immunother. 2023;72(2):409–25. https://doi.org/10.1007/s00262-022-03238-w.
56. Morris EC, Neelapu SS, Giavridis T, Sadelain M. Cytokine release syndrome and associated neurotoxicity in cancer immunotherapy. Nat Rev Immunol. 2022;22(2):85–96. https://doi.org/10.1038/s41577-021-00547-6.
57. Choudhery MS, Arif T, Mahmood R, Harris DT. CAR-T-cell-based cancer immunotherapies: potentials, limitations, and future prospects. J Clin Med. 2024;13:3202. https://doi.org/10.3390/jcm13113202.
58. Tang L, Pan S, Wei X, Xu X, Wei Q. Arming CAR-T cells with cytokines and more: innovations in the fourth-generation CAR-T development. Mol Ther. 2023;31(11):3146–62. https://doi.org/10.1016/j.ymthe.2023.09.021.
59. Matsueda S, Chen L, Li H, et al. Recent clinical researches and technological development in TIL therapy. Cancer Immunol Immunother. 2024;73:232. https://doi.org/10.1007/s00262-024-03793-4.
60. Garg P, Singhal G, Pareek S, Kulkarni P, Horne D, Nath A, Salgia R, Singhal SS. Unveiling the potential of gene editing techniques in revolutionizing cancer treatment: a comprehensive overview. Biochim Biophys Acta Rev Cancer. 2025;1880(1):189233. https://doi.org/10.1016/j.bbcan.2024.189233.
61. Atallah GA, Abd Aziz NH, Teik CK, Shafiee MN, Kampan NC. New predictive biomarkers for ovarian cancer. Diagnostics. 2021;11(3):465. https://doi.org/10.3390/diagnostics11030465.
62. Chow S, Berek JS, Dorigo O. Development of therapeutic vaccines for ovarian cancer. Vaccine. 2020;8(4):657. https://doi.org/10.3390/vaccines8040657.
63. Zhou H, Ma Y, Liu F, Li B, Qiao D, Ren P, Wang M. Current advances in cancer vaccines targeting NY-ESO-1 for solid cancer treatment. Front Immunol. 2023;14:1255799. https://doi.org/10.3389/fimmu.2023.1255799.
64. Abd-Aziz N, Poh CL. Development of peptide-based vaccines for cancer. J Oncol. 2022;2022:9749363. https://doi.org/10.1155/2022/9749363.
65. Saha C, Bojdo J, Dunne NJ, Duary RK, Buckley N, McCarthy HO. Nucleic acid vaccination strategies for ovarian cancer. Front Bioeng Biotechnol. 2022;10:953887. https://doi.org/10.3389/fbioe.2022.953887.
66. Santos PM, Butterfield LH. Dendritic cell-based cancer vaccines. J Immunol. 2018;200(2):443–9. https://doi.org/10.4049/jimmunol.1701024.
67. Lee KW, Yam JWP, Mao X. Dendritic cell vaccines: a shift from conventional approach to new generations. Cells. 2023;12(17):2147. https://doi.org/10.3390/cells12172147.
68. Bedke J, Stenzl A. IMA901: a peptide vaccine in renal cell carcinoma. Expert Opin Investig Drugs. 2013;22(10):1329–36. https://doi.org/10.1517/13543784.2013.822066.
69. Trimble CL, Morrow MP, Kraynyak KA, Shen X, Dallas M, Yan J, Edwards L, Parker RL, Denny L, Giffear M, Brown AS, Marcozzi-Pierce K, Shah D, Slager AM, Sylvester AJ, Khan A, Broderick KE, Juba RJ, Herring TA, Boyer J, et al. Safety, efficacy, and immunogenicity of VGX-3100, a therapeutic synthetic DNA vaccine targeting human papillomavirus 16 and 18 E6 and E7 proteins for cervical intraepithelial neoplasia 2/3: a randomised, double-blind, placebo-controlled phase 2b trial. Lancet. 2015;386(10008):2078–88. https://doi.org/10.1016/S0140-6736(15)00239-1.
70. Fan T, Zhang M, Yang J, Zhu Z, Cao W, Dong C. Therapeutic cancer vaccines: advancements, challenges, and prospects. Signal Transduct Target Ther. 2023;8(1):450. https://doi.org/10.1038/s41392-023-01674-3.
71. Martin SD, Brown SD, Wick DA, Nielsen JS, Kroeger DR, Twumasi-Boateng K, Holt RA, Nelson BH. Low mutation burden in ovarian cancer may limit the utility of neoantigen-targeted vaccines. PLoS One. 2016;11(5):e0155189. https://doi.org/10.1371/journal.pone.0155189.
72. Van Tilbeurgh M, Lemdani K, Beignon AS, Chapon C, Tchitchek N, Cheraitia L, Marcos Lopez E, Pascal Q, Le Grand R, Maisonnasse P, Manet C. Predictive markers of immunogenicity and efficacy for human vaccines. Vaccine. 2021;9(6):579. https://doi.org/10.3390/vaccines9060579.

73. Chiocca EA, Rabkin SD. Oncolytic viruses and their application to cancer immunotherapy. Cancer Immunol Res. 2014;2(4):295–300. https://doi.org/10.1158/2326-6066.CIR-14-0015.
74. Davola ME, Mossman KL. Oncolytic viruses: how "lytic" must they be for therapeutic efficacy? Onco Targets Ther. 2019;8(6):e1581528. https://doi.org/10.1080/2162402X.2019.1596006.
75. Tian Y, Xie D, Yang L. Engineering strategies to enhance oncolytic viruses in cancer immunotherapy. Signal Transduct Target Ther. 2022;7(1):117. https://doi.org/10.1038/s41392-022-00951-x.
76. Harrington KJ, Puzanov I, Hecht JR, Hodi FS, Szabo Z, Murugappan S, Kaufman HL. Clinical development of talimogene laherparepvec (T-VEC): a modified herpes simplex virus type-1-derived oncolytic immunotherapy. Expert Rev Anticancer Ther. 2015;15(12):1389–403. https://doi.org/10.1586/14737140.2015.1115725.
77. Mantwill K, Klein FG, Wang D, Hindupur SV, Ehrenfeld M, Holm PS, Nawroth R. Concepts in oncolytic adenovirus therapy. Int J Mol Sci. 2021;22(19):10522. https://doi.org/10.3390/ijms221910522.
78. Müller L, Berkeley R, Barr T, Ilett E, Errington-Mais F. Past, present and future of oncolytic reovirus. Cancer. 2020;12(11):3219. https://doi.org/10.3390/cancers12113219.
79. Cousin S, Toulmonde M, Kind M, et al. Phase 2 trial of intravenous oncolytic virus JX-594 combined with low-dose cyclophosphamide in patients with advanced breast cancer. Exp Hematol Oncol. 2022;11:104. https://doi.org/10.1186/s40164-022-00338-2.
80. Engeland CE, Ungerechts G. Measles virus as an oncolytic immunotherapy. Cancer. 2021;13(3):544. https://doi.org/10.3390/cancers13030544.
81. Yin ZS, Wang Z. Strategies for engineering oncolytic viruses to enhance cancer immunotherapy. Front Pharmacol. 2024;15:1450203. https://doi.org/10.3389/fphar.2024.1450203.
82. Hirasawa K, Nishikawa SG, Norman KL, Alain T, Kossakowska A, Lee PW. Oncolytic reovirus against ovarian and colon cancer. Cancer Res. 2002;62(6):1696–701.
83. Ferrucci PF, Pala L, Conforti F, Cocorocchio E. Talimogene laherparepvec (T-VEC): an intralesional cancer immunotherapy for advanced melanoma. Cancer. 2021;13(6):1383. https://doi.org/10.3390/cancers13061383.
84. Mahalingam D, Chen S, Xie P, Loghmani H, Heineman T, Kalyan A, Kircher S, Helenowski IB, Mi X, Maurer V, Coffey M, Mulcahy M, Benson A, Zhang B. Combination of pembrolizumab and pelareorep promotes anti-tumour immunity in advanced pancreatic adenocarcinoma (PDAC). Br J Cancer. 2023;129(5):782–90. https://doi.org/10.1038/s41416-023-02344-5.
85. Garg P, Malhotra J, Kulkarni P, Horne D, Salgia R, Singhal SS. Emerging therapeutic strategies to overcome drug resistance in cancer cells. Cancer. 2024;16(13):2478. https://doi.org/10.3390/cancers16132478.
86. Kaufman HL, Kohlhapp FJ, Zloza A. Oncolytic viruses: a new class of immunotherapy drugs. Nature reviews. Drug Des Discov. 2015;14(9):642–62. https://doi.org/10.1038/nrd4663.
87. Nikolaidi A, Fountzilas E, Fostira F, Psyrri A, Gogas H, Papadimitriou C. Neoadjuvant treatment in ovarian cancer: new perspectives, new challenges. Front Oncol. 2022;12:820128. https://doi.org/10.3389/fonc.2022.820128.
88. Hockings H, Miller RE. The role of PARP inhibitor combination therapy in ovarian cancer. Ther Adv Med Oncol. 2023;15:17588359231173183. https://doi.org/10.1177/17588359231173183.
89. Alvarez Secord A, O'Malley DM, Sood AK, Westin SN, Liu JF. Rationale for combination PARP inhibitor and antiangiogenic treatment in advanced epithelial ovarian cancer: a review. Gynecol Oncol. 2021;162(2):482–95. https://doi.org/10.1016/j.ygyno.2021.05.018.
90. Kurtz JE, Lauraine EP, Oaknin A, Leither K, Cibula D, Denys H. Atezolizumab combined with bevacizumab and platinum-based therapy for platinum-sensitive ovarian cancer: placebo-controlled randomized phase III ATALANTE/ENGOT-ov29 trial. J Clin Oncol. 2023;41(30):1–17. https://doi.org/10.1200/JCO.23.00529.
91. Wu Z, Cui P, Tao H, Zhang S, Ma J, Liu Z, Wang J, Qian Y, Chen S, Huang Z, Zheng X, Huang D, Hu Y. The synergistic effect of PARP inhibitors and immune checkpoint inhibitors. Clin Med Insights Oncol. 2021;15:1179554921996288. https://doi.org/10.1177/1179554921996288.

92. Wen L, Tong F, Zhang R, Chen L, Huang Y, Dong X. The research progress of PD-1/PD-L1 inhibitors enhancing radiotherapy efficacy. Front Oncol. 2021;11:799957. https://doi.org/10.3389/fonc.2021.799957.
93. Andrikopoulou A, Liontos M, Skafida E, Koutsoukos K, Apostolidou K, Kaparelou M, Rouvalis A, Bletsa G, Dimopoulos MA, Zagouri F. Pembrolizumab in combination with bevacizumab and oral cyclophosphamide in heavily pre-treated platinum-resistant ovarian cancer. Int J Gynecol Cancer. 2023;33(4):571–6. https://doi.org/10.1136/ijgc-2022-003941.
94. Domchek SM, Postel-Vinay S, Im SA, Park YH, Delord JP, Italiano A, Alexandre J, You B, Bastian S, Krebs MG, Wang D, Waqar SN, Lanasa M, Rhee J, Gao H, Rocher-Ros V, Jones EV, Gulati S, Coenen-Stass A, Kozarewa I, et al. Olaparib and durvalumab in patients with germline BRCA-mutated metastatic breast cancer (MEDIOLA): an open-label, multicentre, phase 1/2, basket study. Lancet Oncol. 2020;21(9):1155–64. https://doi.org/10.1016/S1470-2045(20)30324-7.
95. Lampert EJ, Zimmer A, Padget M, Cimino-Mathews A, Nair JR, Liu Y, Swisher EM, Hodge JW, Nixon AB, Nichols E, Bagheri MH, Levy E, Radke MR, Lipkowitz S, Annunziata CM, Taube JM, Steinberg SM, Lee JM. Combination of PARP inhibitor Olaparib, and PD-L1 inhibitor durvalumab, in recurrent ovarian cancer: a proof-of-concept phase II study. Clin Cancer Res. 2020;26(16):4268–79. https://doi.org/10.1158/1078-0432.CCR-20-0056.
96. Lei Y, Li X, Huang Q, Zheng X, Liu M. Progress and challenges of predictive biomarkers for immune checkpoint blockade. Front Oncol. 2021;11:617335. https://doi.org/10.3389/fonc.2021.617335.
97. Jiang X, Wang J, Deng X, et al. Role of the tumor microenvironment in PD-L1/PD-1-mediated tumor immune escape. Mol Cancer. 2019;18:10. https://doi.org/10.1186/s12943-018-0928-4.
98. Cui J-W, Li Y, Yang Y, Yang H-K, Dong J-M, Xiao Z-H, et al. A tumor immunotherapy resistance: revealing the mechanism of PD-1/PD-L1-mediated tumor immune escape. Biomed Pharmacother. 2024;171:116203. https://doi.org/10.1016/j.biopha.2024.116203.
99. Hwang S, Kwon AY, Jeong JY, et al. Immune gene signatures for predicting durable clinical benefit of anti-PD-1 immunotherapy in patients with non-small cell lung cancer. Sci Rep. 2020;10:643. https://doi.org/10.1038/s41598-019-57218-9.
100. McGrail DJ, Pilié PG, Rashid NU, Voorwerk L, Slagter M, Kok M, Jonasch E, Khasraw M, Heimberger AB, Lim B, Ueno NT, Litton JK, Ferrarotto R, Chang JT, Moulder SL, Lin SY. High tumor mutation burden fails to predict immune checkpoint blockade response across all cancer types. Ann Oncol. 2021;32(5):661–72. https://doi.org/10.1016/j.annonc.2021.02.006.
101. Li K, Luo H, Huang L, et al. Microsatellite instability: a review of what the oncologist should know. Cancer Cell Int. 2020;20:16. https://doi.org/10.1186/s12935-019-1091-8.
102. Mangogna A, Munari G, Pepe F, Maffii E, Giampaolino P, Ricci G, Fassan M, Malapelle U, Biffi S. Homologous recombination deficiency in ovarian cancer: from the biological rationale to current diagnostic approaches. J Pers Med. 2023;13(2):284. https://doi.org/10.3390/jpm13020284.
103. Hao Z, Li R, Wang Y, et al. Landscape of myeloid-derived suppressor cell in tumor immunotherapy. Biomark Res. 2021;9:77. https://doi.org/10.1186/s40364-021-00333-5.
104. Wang H, Zhang Y, Zhang H, Cao H, Mao J, Chen X, Wang L, Zhang N, Luo P, Xue J, Qi X, Dong X, Liu G, Cheng Q. Liquid biopsy for human cancer: cancer screening, monitoring, and treatment. MedComm. 2024;5(6):e564. https://doi.org/10.1002/mco2.564.
105. Baev V, Koppers-Lalic D, Costa-Silva B. Liquid biopsy: current status and future perspectives. Cancer. 2023;15(12):3205. https://doi.org/10.3390/cancers15123205.
106. Nussbaum YI, Manjunath Y, Suvilesh KN, Warren WC, Shyu CR, Kaifi JT, Ciorba MA, Mitchem JB. Current and prospective methods for assessing anti-tumor immunity in colorectal cancer. Int J Mol Sci. 2021;22(9):4802. https://doi.org/10.3390/ijms22094802.
107. Garg P, Krishna M, Subbalakshmi AR, Ramisetty S, Mohanty A, Kulkarni P, Horne D, Salgia R, Singhal SS. Emerging biomarkers and molecular targets for precision medicine in cervical cancer. Biochim Biophys Acta Rev Cancer. 2024;1879(3):189106. https://doi.org/10.1016/j.bbcan.2024.189106.

108. Qin S, Xu L, Yi M, et al. Novel immune checkpoint targets: moving beyond PD-1 and CTLA-4. Mol Cancer. 2019;18:155. https://doi.org/10.1186/s12943-019-1091-2.
109. Ruffo E, Wu RC, Bruno TC, Workman CJ, Vignali DAA. Lymphocyte-activation gene 3 (LAG3): the next immune checkpoint receptor. Semin Immunol. 2019;42:101305. https://doi.org/10.1016/j.smim.2019.101305.
110. Sauer N, Janicka N, Szlasa W, Skinderowicz B, Kołodzińska K, Dwernicka W, Oślizło M, Kulbacka J, Novickij V, Karłowicz-Bodalska K. TIM-3 as a promising target for cancer immunotherapy in a wide range of tumors. Cancer Immunol Immunother. 2023;72(11):3405–25. https://doi.org/10.1007/s00262-023-03516-1.
111. Hosseinkhani N, Derakhshani A, Shadbad MA, Argentiero A, Racanelli V, Kazemi T, Mokhtarzadeh A, Brunetti O, Silvestris N, Baradaran B. The role of V-domain Ig suppressor of T cell activation (VISTA) in cancer therapy: lessons learned and the road ahead. Front Immunol. 2021;12:676181. https://doi.org/10.3389/fimmu.2021.676181.
112. Zhou L, Duan Y, Fu K, Zhang M, Li K, Yin R. The role of B7-H4 in ovarian cancer immunotherapy: current status, challenges, and perspectives. Front Immunol. 2024;15:1426050. https://doi.org/10.3389/fimmu.2024.1426050.
113. Cao J, Yan Q. Cancer epigenetics, tumor immunity, and immunotherapy. Trends Cancer. 2020;6(7):580–92. https://doi.org/10.1016/j.trecan.2020.02.003.
114. Liu Z, Ren Y, Weng S, Xu H, Li L, Han X. A new trend in cancer treatment: the combination of epigenetics and immunotherapy. Front Immunol. 2022;13:809761. https://doi.org/10.3389/fimmu.2022.809761.
115. Borcoman E, Kamal M, Marret G, Dupain C, Castel-Ajgal Z, Le Tourneau C. HDAC inhibition to prime immune checkpoint inhibitors. Cancer. 2022;14(1):66. https://doi.org/10.3390/cancers14010066.
116. Xia L, Oyang L, Lin J, Tan S, Han Y, Wu N, Yi P, Tang L, Pan Q, Rao S, Liang J, Tang Y, Su M, Luo X, Yang Y, Shi Y, Wang H, Zhou Y, Liao Q. The cancer metabolic reprogramming and immune response. Mol Cancer. 2021;20(1):28. https://doi.org/10.1186/s12943-021-01316-8.
117. Song X, Si Q, Qi R, Liu W, Li M, Guo M, Wei L, Yao Z. Indoleamine 2,3-dioxygenase 1: a promising therapeutic target in malignant tumor. Front Immunol. 2021;12:800630. https://doi.org/10.3389/fimmu.2021.800630.
118. Gomez S, Tabernacki T, Kobyra J, Roberts P, Chiappinelli KB. Combining epigenetic and immune therapy to overcome cancer resistance. Semin Cancer Biol. 2020;65:99–113. https://doi.org/10.1016/j.semcancer.2019.12.019.
119. Prelaj A, Miskovic V, Zanitti M, Trovo F, Genova C, Viscardi G, Rebuzzi SE, Mazzeo L, Provenzano L, Kosta S, Favali M, Spagnoletti A, Castelo-Branco L, Dolezal J, Pearson AT, Lo Russo G, Proto C, Ganzinelli M, Giani C, Ambrosini E, Pedrocchi ALG. Artificial intelligence for predictive biomarker discovery in immuno-oncology: a systematic review. Ann Oncol. 2024;35(1):29–65. https://doi.org/10.1016/j.annonc.2023.10.125.
120. Garg P, Mohanty A, Ramisetty S, Kulkarni P, Horne D, Pisick E, Salgia R, Singhal SS. Artificial intelligence and allied subsets in early detection and preclusion of gynecological cancers. Biochim Biophys Acta Rev Cancer. 2023;1878(6):189026. https://doi.org/10.1016/j.bbcan.2023.189026.
121. Butner JD, Dogra P, Chung C, Pasqualini R, Arap W, Lowengrub J, Cristini V, Wang Z. Mathematical modeling of cancer immunotherapy for personalized clinical translation. Nat Comput Sci. 2022;2(12):785–96. https://doi.org/10.1038/s43588-022-00377-z.
122. Garg P, Singhal G, Kulkarni P, Horne D, Salgia R, Singhal SS. Artificial intelligence-driven computational approaches in the development of anticancer drugs. Cancer. 2024;16(22):3884. https://doi.org/10.3390/cancers16223884.
123. Cai Y, Chen R, Gao S, Li W, Liu Y, Su G, Song M, Jiang M, Jiang C, Zhang X. Artificial intelligence applied in neoantigen identification facilitates personalized cancer immunotherapy. Front Oncol. 2023;12:1054231. https://doi.org/10.3389/fonc.2022.1054231.
124. Foser S, Maiese K, Digumarthy SR, Puig-Butille JA, Rebhan C. Looking to the future of early detection in cancer: liquid biopsies, imaging, and artificial intelligence. Clin Chem. 2024;70(1):27–32. https://doi.org/10.1093/clinchem/hvad196.

125. Demircan NC, Boussios S, Tasci T, Öztürk MA. Current and future immunotherapy approaches in ovarian cancer. Ann Transl Med. 2020;8(24):1714. https://doi.org/10.21037/atm-20-4499.
126. Wang T, Tian L, Wei B, et al. Effect of fibroblast heterogeneity on prognosis and drug resistance in high-grade serous ovarian cancer. Sci Rep. 2024;14:26617. https://doi.org/10.1038/s41598-024-77630-0.
127. Colombo I, Karakasis K, Suku S, Oza AM. Chasing immune checkpoint inhibitors in ovarian cancer: novel combinations and biomarker discovery. Cancer. 2023;15:3220. https://doi.org/10.3390/cancers15123220.
128. Shih YT, Pan IW, Teich N. Global challenges in access to and implementation of precision oncology: the health care manager and health economist perspective. Proc Am Soc Clin Oncol. 2022;42:429–37. https://doi.org/10.1200/EDBK_359650.
129. Sharma P, Hu-Lieskovan S, Wargo JA, Ribas A. Primary, adaptive, and acquired resistance to cancer immunotherapy. Cell. 2017;168(4):707–23. https://doi.org/10.1016/j.cell.2017.01.017.
130. Beatty GL, Gladney WL. Immune escape mechanisms as a guide for cancer immunotherapy. Clin Cancer Res. 2015;21(4):687–92. https://doi.org/10.1158/1078-0432.CCR-14-1860.
131. Dai M, Liu M, Yang H, et al. New insights into epigenetic regulation of resistance to PD-1/PD-L1 blockade cancer immunotherapy: mechanisms and therapeutic opportunities. Exp Hematol Oncol. 2022;11:101. https://doi.org/10.1186/s40164-022-00356-0.
132. Ibis B, Aliazis K, Cao C, Yenyuwadee S, Boussiotis VA. Immune-related adverse effects of checkpoint immunotherapy and implications for the treatment of patients with cancer and autoimmune diseases. Front Immunol. 2023;14:1197364. https://doi.org/10.3389/fimmu.2023.1197364.
133. Brahmer JR, Lacchetti C, Schneider BJ, Atkins MB, Brassil KJ, Caterino JM, Chau I, Ernstoff MS, Gardner JM, Ginex P, Hallmeyer S, National Comprehensive Cancer Network. Management of immune-related adverse events in patients treated with immune checkpoint inhibitor therapy: American Society of Clinical Oncology clinical practice guideline. J Clin Oncol. 2018;36(17):1714–68. https://doi.org/10.1200/JCO.2017.77.6385.
134. Yin X, Song Y, Deng W, Blake N, Luo X, Meng J. Potential predictive biomarkers in antitumor immunotherapy: navigating the future of antitumor treatment and immune checkpoint inhibitor efficacy. Front Oncol. 2024;14:1483454. https://doi.org/10.3389/fonc.2024.1483454.
135. Joshi S, Durden DL. Combinatorial approach to improve cancer immunotherapy: rational drug design strategy to simultaneously hit multiple targets to kill tumor cells and to activate the immune system. J Oncol. 2019;2019:5245034. https://doi.org/10.1155/2019/5245034.
136. Chianese A, Santella B, Ambrosino A, Stelitano D, Rinaldi L, Galdiero M, Zannella C, Franci G. Oncolytic viruses in combination therapeutic approaches with epigenetic modulators: past, present, and future perspectives. Cancer. 2021;13(11):2761. https://doi.org/10.3390/cancers13112761.
137. Liao J, Li X, Gan Y, Han S, Rong P, Wang W, Li W, Zhou L. Artificial intelligence assists precision medicine in cancer treatment. Front Oncol. 2023;12:998222. https://doi.org/10.3389/fonc.2022.998222.
138. Ponterio E, Haas TL, De Maria R. Oncolytic virus and CAR-T cell therapy in solid tumors. Front Immunol. 2024;15:1455163. https://doi.org/10.3389/fimmu.2024.1455163.
139. Liu T, Yu J, Gao Y, Ma X, Jiang S, Gu Y, Ming WK. Prophylactic interventions for hereditary breast and ovarian cancer risks and mortality in BRCA1/2 carriers. Cancer. 2023;16(1):103. https://doi.org/10.3390/cancers16010103.
140. Corradetti B, Pisano S, Conlan RS, Ferrari M. Nanotechnology and immunotherapy in ovarian cancer: tracing new landscapes. J Pharmacol Exp Ther. 2019;370(3):636–46. https://doi.org/10.1124/jpet.118.254979.
141. Satora M, Kułak K, Zaremba B, Grunwald A, Świechowska-Starek P, Tarkowski R. New hopes and promises in the treatment of ovarian cancer focusing on targeted treatment—a narrative review. Front Pharmacol. 2024;15:1416555. https://doi.org/10.3389/fphar.2024.1416555.

142. Ghemrawi R, Abuamer L, Kremesh S, Hussien G, Ahmed R, Mousa W, Khoder G, Khair M. Revolutionizing cancer treatment: recent advances in immunotherapy. Biomedicine. 2024;12(9):2158. https://doi.org/10.3390/biomedicines12092158.
143. Adhikary S, Pathak S, Palani V, Acar A, Banerjee A, Al-Dewik NI, Essa MM, Mohammed SGAA, Qoronfleh MW. Current technologies and future perspectives in immunotherapy towards a clinical oncology approach. Biomedicine. 2024;12(1):217. https://doi.org/10.3390/biomedicines12010217.

# Pancreatic Cancer Immunotherapy: A Team-Based Approach

# 11

Krushangi Patel, Percy Lee, Julius Weng, Laleh Melstrom, Mustafa Raoof, Aaron Lewis, and Vincent Chung

## 11.1 Introduction

Pancreatic cancer remains one of the most challenging cancers to treat. The estimated number of new pancreatic cancer cases in 2025 is 67,440 according to the American Cancer Society and these numbers continue to rise [1]. And though pancreatic cancer accounts for about 3% of new cancer diagnoses in the United States (US) it accounts for 8% of cancer-related deaths [2]. Immunotherapy has come to the forefront as a treatment option that is often less toxic with longer disease control rates in many cancer types. In pancreatic cancer, responses to immunotherapy have been limited. This is thought to be due to the complex tumor microenvironment of this type of tumor. In this chapter, we will review the components of the tumor microenvironment and how they have been evaluated in clinical trials as possible targets for therapy as well as early phase and several key phase III clinical trial results.

Developing effective immunotherapy in pancreatic cancer has proven to be a challenge riddled with numerous obstacles. Diagnostic tissue retrieval and organoid formation as well as animal models that do not translate well to human responses

K. Patel (✉)
City of Hope Department of Medical Oncology & Therapeutics Research, City of Hope Comprehensive Cancer Center Long Beach, Long Beach, CA, USA
e-mail: KruPatel@coh.org

P. Lee · J. Weng
Department of Radiation Oncology, City of Hope Orange County Lennar Foundation Cancer Center, Irvine, CA, USA

L. Melstrom · M. Raoof · A. Lewis
Department of Surgical Oncology, City of Hope Comprehensive Cancer Center (COH), Duarte, CA, USA

V. Chung
Department of Medical Oncology & Therapeutics Research, City of Hope National Medical Center, Duarte, CA, USA



R. Salgia, P. Kulkarni (eds.), *Immunotherapies in Solid Tumors*, Cancer Treatment and Research 129, https://doi.org/10.1007/978-3-031-97242-3_11

pose room for improvement in pre-clinical data collection. Effective therapies both at a cellular level as well as clinically often with the challenge of appropriate activity in the tumor microenvironment and in tumor cells have resulted in signs of safety and efficacy in phase I and II studies but limited overall survival (OS), disease-free survival (DFS), and progression-free survival (PFS) rates in phase III trials. Physical delivery of drugs at the necessary and effective location often poses surgical and procedural challenges in good clinical outcomes. Patient enrollment, in a disease still rare and hard to diagnose, continues to also come with its own challenges. Rapid decline in performance status from tumor progression makes it nearly impossible for patients to travel to large academic centers to access clinical trials or new treatment options. As such a comprehensive team-based approach that includes basic scientists, veterinarians, a dynamic team of community and academic medical oncologists, surgeons, radiation oncologists, pharmacists, and even medical subspecialists will be our best and possibly only chance at advancing effective therapies in this very resistant and pervasive disease.

## 11.2 Tumor Microenvironment of Pancreatic Cancer

The tumor microenvironment (TME) in pancreatic cancer is composed of two types of cells: immune and non-immune cells. These cell types each play a role in the development and growth of pancreatic tumors. A deeper understanding of these cells, their interactions with the rest of the tumor microenvironment, and their role in tumor growth and resistance can provide necessary insights in developing effective therapeutic strategies against this tumor with a hostile TME. There are a number of immune cells that are involved in various roles of the tumor microenvironment and pancreatic cancer; these include T lymphocytes, natural killer (NK) cells, dendritic cells (DCs), tumor-associated macrophages (TAMs), myeloid-derived suppressor cells (MDSCs), tumor-associated neutrophils (TANs), as well as B lymphocytes. The non-immune cells consist of pancreatic cancer stem cells (PCSCs), mesenchymal stem/stromal cells (MSCs), cancer-associated fibroblasts (CAFs), pancreatic stellate cells (PSCs), and endothelial cells [3].

### 11.2.1 Immune Components

#### 11.2.1.1 Cytotoxic T Lymphocytes, T Helper Cells, and Regulatory T Cells

The cold tumor microenvironment of pancreatic cancer is distinct in this tumor type where infiltration of myeloid cells and CD8+ T cells are usually absent. Furthermore, many immune cells can play both tumor-protective and tumor-fighting roles. For example, there is some evidence that patients who had exhibited a greater percentage of CD8+ T cells or CD8+ tumor infiltrating lymphocytes (TILs) but a lesser percentage of CD4+ T cells encircling cancer or within the tumor tissue had a better survival rate [4, 5].

Interleukin-17A (IL-17A) is an example of an interleukin produced by CD4+ TILs that is associated with an aggressive form of pancreatic ductal adenocarcinoma (PDAC) [6]. Recent studies have shown that IL-17A affects the transcription of cancer-associated fibroblasts (CAF) [7]. The induction of CAF's is promoted by T cells that produce IL-17A and contributes to the progression of PDAC. The promotion of tumorigenesis is then facilitated by the upregulation of B7–H4 through IL-17 receptor signaling in the pancreatic epithelium [8, 9]. The role of TH17 and IL-17A and pancreatic cancer is not yet fully understood with evidence suggesting both tumor protumorigenic and antitumorigenic effects [6]. TH17 cells play a key role in maintaining mucosal barriers and contributing to pathogen clearance at mucosal surfaces [10]. There have also been increased quantities of interleukin-17 produced by CD4-positive T cells in aggressive forms of pancreatic cancer [6].

It had long been thought that T cell infiltration is limited in PDAC due to the inhibitory environment shaped by fibroblasts and desmoplastic stroma [11, 12]. However, the presence of desmoplastic elements might not be a large influence on the accumulation of T cells, thus revealing a separate spatial arrangement of T cells in PDAC [13]. There has been some evidence that extreme Kras-driven immunosuppression may result in neoepitope-specific T cells that are not triggered, fail to expand, fail to infiltrate the tumor, or all the above [14, 15].

Regulatory T cells (Tregs) influence cancer progression and immune responses in the tumor microenvironment [16]. They do this through various mechanisms including production of suppressive cytokines such as TGF-β, IL-10, and IL-35 and the engagement of inhibitory immune checkpoints and enzymes, such as cytotoxic T-lymphocyte-associated protein 4 (CTLA-4), PD-1, LAG-3, TIM-3, T cell immunoreceptor with Ig and ITIM domains (TIGIT), CD39, CD73, and IDO [3]. Tregs play a part in controlling the immune response as PDAC advances from a premalignant state to a cancerous stage. The presence of elevated Tregs is linked to a more unfavorable prognosis in PDAC [17].

#### 11.2.1.2 Natural Killer Cells

NK cells play a role in monitoring and controlling tumor growth and tumor immunosurveillance [18]. Both preclinical and clinical studies have demonstrated a link between decreased NK cell activity and an increased susceptibility to cancer as well as a higher chance of cancer spread and metastasis [19, 20].

The function of NK cells is inhibited in the microenvironment of human PDAC by activated pancreatic stellate cells [21]. In pancreatic cancer, the orchestration of anti-tumor immune responses through CXCL8 (IL-8) cytokines by radiotherapy is reliant on NK cells. Radiation triggers CXCL8 release and NK cell migration toward irradiated tumors. In xenografted mice, the use of high-dose radiotherapy in conjunction with adoptive NK cell transfer resulted in enhanced tumor control compared to using either treatment alone, indicating that combining NK cells with radiotherapy is a logical approach for cancer therapy [22].

#### 11.2.1.3 Dendritic Cells

DCs, which are crucial for effective anti-tumor T cell responses, are scarce in the pancreatic tumor environment and are usually found at the tumor edges. Increasing the numbers and/or activity of scarce DCs in PDAC is a distinct strategy that could improve cytotoxic or immune-based therapies that by themselves are poorly effective in the treatment of this disease [23].

It is suggestive that the pancreatic tumors themselves influence immune function as surgical removal of pancreatic tumors has been found to enhance the function of dendritic cells [24].

There have been some indications that cDC1s, cDC2s, and pDCs, as major human blood DC subsets, are components of the PDAC immune landscape. In addition, tumor-infiltrating DCs are associated with the survival of PDAC patients and that their density and spatial organization play an important role for the clinical outcome. PDAC-infiltrating cDC1s and pDCs may represent independent prognostic markers for improved survival [25].

One study looked at whether indirect presentation (the cross-priming mechanism) could contribute to effective in vivo priming of tumor-specific CD8+ T cells that are capable of eradicating cancer in patients. A clinical trial of vaccination with granulocyte-macrophage–colony-stimulating factor–transduced pancreatic cancer lines found that vaccination with an allogeneic pancreatic tumor vaccine induces mesothelin-specific (MSLN) CD8+ T cells [26].

#### 11.2.1.4 Tumor-Associated Macrophages

Tumor-associated macrophages (TAMs) in pancreatic cancers are monocytes that are in circulation and are drawn toward the tumor microenvironment and then transformed into macrophages [27]. They are a key component of the cancer microenvironment, and influence tumor growth and progression. TAMs can have a dual supportive and inhibitory influence on cancer, depending on the stage of the disease, the tissue involved, and the host microbiota. These cells can limit the antitumor activity of conventional chemotherapy and radiotherapy by orchestrating a tumor-promoting repair response to tissue damage, and by providing a protective niche for cancer stem cells. Conversely, TAMs contribute to the antitumor activity of selected chemotherapeutic agents, such as doxorubicin (under certain conditions), and of monoclonal antibody therapies via antibody-dependent cellular cytotoxicity (ADCC) and phagocytosis (ADCP). Therapeutic strategies targeting macrophages as tumor-promoting factors, and/or aimed at macrophage activation and re-education are undergoing clinical assessment; such strategies have the potential to complement cytoreductive, antiangiogenic, and immune-checkpoint-inhibitor treatments [28].

Subpopulation M1, macrophages and M2 macrophages play opposite roles in tumor development. M1 macrophages are considered proinflammatory cytokines and have antineoplastic impacts and M2 macrophages have anti-inflammatory signals and may exacerbate tumor development [29].

Exosomes from tumor cells package assorted proteins and chemokines with immunomodulatory capability, including CSF-1, CCL2, and TGF-β, to promote

M2-like characterization of TAMs [30]. In post-resection patients of PDAC, CCL2/CCR2 chemokine signals can be prognostic of reduced survival [31]. The polarization of TAMs acts as a key link in the tumor microenvironment and exerts significant roles in PDAC progression thus vesicle transport as the major intercellular communication approach can be better applied to improve the conversion rate of TAMs, superior to single antibody or receptor blockade, being the future development direction [32].

#### 11.2.1.5 Myeloid-Derived Suppressor Cells

There are two types of myeloid-derived suppressor cells (MDSCs). M-MDSCs which closely resemble monocytes while PMN-MDSCs are more equivalent to neutrophils. PMN-MDSCs make up more than 80% of the MDSCs in the tumor microenvironment. The main characteristic that defines MDSCs is their ability to inhibit immune responses, including those mediated by T cells, B cells, and natural killer (NK) cells. M-MDSCs and PMN-MDSCs share key biochemical features that enable their suppression of immune responses, including the upregulation of signal transducer and activator of transcription 3 (STAT3) expression, induction of ER stress, expression of arginase 1, and expression of S100A8/A9 [33].

One study looked at the role of MDSC in pancreatic cancer and the effects of targeting MDSC therapeutically. Treatment with zoledronic acid, potent amino bisphosphonate previously shown to target MDSC, impaired intratumoral MDSC accumulation resulting in delayed tumor growth rate, prolonged median survival, and increased recruitment of T cells to the tumor [34].

Pancreatic ductal adenocarcinoma (PDAC) is an aggressive cancer with poor survival rates and often carries oncogenic *KRAS* mutation. Downstream of mutant KRAS, the transcription regulator Yes-associated protein (YAP) is essential for neoplastic progression of PDAC. The abundance of YAP mRNA, which encodes Yes-associated protein (YAP), a protein regulated by the Hippo pathway during tissue development and homeostasis, was increased in human PDAC tissue compared with that in normal pancreatic epithelia [35]. The interaction between YAP/TAZ (downstream effectors of the Hippo pathway) and TEAD (transcriptional enhanced associate domain) proteins facilitate the cancer-promoting functions of YAP. Thus, small-molecule inhibitors like GNE-7883 and IAG933, which block the interactions between YAP/TAZ and TEAD, can disrupt oncogenic YAP/TAZ signaling in RAS-altered tumors like PDAC and overcome KRAS G12C inhibitor resistance [36, 37].

Cancer-associated conditions, including hypoxia, nutrient deficiency, acidity, endoplasmic reticulum stress, and long-term production of inflammatory mediators, promote the generation of myeloid-derived suppressor cells (MDSCs). MDSCs support the progression of most cancer entities by suppressing antitumor immune responses, stimulating angiogenesis, and fostering metastasis through a variety of mechanisms. MDSCs contribute to primary and acquire resistance to cancer immunotherapy; thus, combinatorial therapeutic targeting of these cells might improve patient outcomes. Other cancer treatments, such as chemotherapy, radiotherapy, targeted therapies, or hormone therapies, can have distinct and disparate effects on MDSCs and should be studied further [38].

A robust understanding of MDSCs may help us discover more ways to create cytotoxic approaches to therapy as well as increase the capabilities of T cells and NK cells in fighting this disease with therapeutic options.

#### 11.2.1.6 Tumor-Associated Neutrophils

Neutrophils are traditionally known as the first line of defense against infection and injury. Tumor-associated neutrophils (TANs), much like macrophages, can have varying roles in the tumor microenvironment primarily promoting but, in some circumstances, suppressing cancer growth [3, 39].

As one of the first cells to enter a damaged site from the circulation, the rapid recruitment of large numbers of neutrophils into the tissue is key for their protective function [40]. Notably, this process is co-opted in pathological settings such as cancer, where persistent neutrophil infiltration into the tumor has been consistently associated with poorer patient outcomes [41].

Neutrophils can be drawn in by factors secreted by tumor cells such as IL-1, CD200, CXCR2 ligands (like CXCL1, CXCL2, CXCL5, and CXCL8) [42], granulocyte-macrophage colony-stimulating factor (GM-CSF), granulocyte colony-stimulating factor (G-CSF), and various other substances. N1 TANs exert an antitumor activity, by direct or indirect cytotoxicity. N2 TANs, on the other hand, promote immunosuppression, tumor expansion, angiogenesis, and metastasis by causing DNA instability and releasing cytokines and chemokines [43]. Recently, a new type of TANs called T3 neutrophils has been discovered. These T3 neutrophils stimulate angiogenesis, thus improving the ability of pancreatic tumors to survive in low-oxygen and nutrient-deficient environments [39].

The growth of pancreatic cancer at primary and secondary sites is reduced and the effectiveness of immune checkpoint blockade (ICB) treatment with anti-PD-1 is enhanced through the inhibition of TANs by lorlatinib [44].

#### 11.2.1.7 B Lymphocytes in Tumor Microenvironment

B cells in the TME of PDAC are mainly plasma cells and memory B cells that highly express CD27 [45]. IL-1β and type I interferons upregulate CXCL13, inducing more regulatory B cell (Breg) recruitment to exert immunosuppressive functions [46, 47]. Bregs could stimulate STAT3 signaling in themselves and CD8+ T cells through IL-35. This resulted in two outcomes: (a) the transcriptional regulator *BCL-6* is upregulated in naive B cells, which disrupts B cell differentiation into plasma cells; (b) the function of cytotoxic T lymphocytes (CTLs) is inhibited [48, 49]. A recent study found that the resistance to stimulators of interferon gene (STING) agonists in PDAC is due to its induction of IL-35+ B cell expansion. Systemic anti-IL-35 and STING agonists can synergistically inhibit Breg amplification and enhance the efficacy of NK cells [50]. In addition, a phase III trial explored the effect of ibrutinib, a Bruton's tyrosine kinase inhibitor, in inhibiting the immunosuppressive B cells. However, ibrutinib/nab-paclitaxel/gemcitabine did not improve OS or PFS in patients with PDAC compared with controls [51].

### 11.2.2 Non-immune Cells

While non-immune cells and pancreatic cancer often create a protective barrier and mechanism against chemotherapy and immunotherapy treatment to cancer cells, they can also play an important role in drug delivery, identification, and can be used in a variety of therapeutic approaches to this tumor. Non-immune cells in the tumor microenvironment include pancreatic cancer stem cells (PCSCs), mesenchymal stem/stromal cells (MSCs), cancer-associated fibroblasts (CAFs), pancreatic stellate cells (PSCs), and endothelial cells.

#### 11.2.2.1 Pancreatic Cancer Stem Cells

PCSCs have the ability to self-renew and initiate tumorigenesis. That can contribute to the initiation of metastasis and recurrence of PDAC and are also responsible for resistance to chemotherapy and radiation. They can activate multiple signaling pathways which include irregular signaling via mechanisms such as Hedgehog, Wnt, Notch, JAK-STAT, Nodal/Activin, and Hippo which enables PCSCs to preserve their self-renewal ability, develop resistance to chemotherapy and radiation, enhance their capacity to induce tumors, and spread to other parts of the body [52].

The cell-autonomous E2F1/4-pRb/RBL2 axis balances non-cell-autonomous signaling in healthy ductal cells but becomes deregulated upon KRAS mutation. PCSCs have been shown to be involved in PDAC resistance to chemotherapy, displaying increased prevalence within the tumor after treatment with gemcitabine [53]. This axis, thus, may be an axis requiring further investigation and understanding as a possibility for therapeutic targeting.

#### 11.2.2.2 Mesenchymal Stem Cells/Stromal Cells

Mesenchymal stem cells (MSC) have a characteristic tendency to home to tumor sites [54]. As such MSCs are easy to obtain, thus they may have clinical applications for tissue injuries and may be an attractive candidate as drug delivery vehicles. They have also been modified to deliver prodrugs, oncolytic viruses, antiangiogenic agents, pro-apoptotic proteins, growth factor antagonist interference, or interleukins [55].

#### 11.2.2.3 Cancer-Associated Fibroblasts

The emergence of single-cell RNA sequencing (scRNAseq) technology has revealed the existence of transcriptionally diverse cancer-associated fibroblast (CAF) populations among many solid tumors [56]. CAFs with an inflammatory gene expression signature have been defined as inflammatory CAFs (iCAF), while CAFs with an extracellular matrix rich gene expression signature resembling smooth muscle actin ($\alpha$SMA) high myofibroblasts were named myofibroblastic CAFs (myCAF) [57]. In primary PDAC tumors, besides iCAF and myCAF, an additional antigen presenting CAF (apCAF) subpopulation has been described [58]. In murine PDAC liver metastasis, three distinct metastasis-associated fibroblast (MAF) populations have been described, resembling transcriptional phenotypes of iCAF, myCAF, and a mesothelial-like CAF (mesCAF) subtype [59]. However, there is emerging evidence that CAF subtypes with similar transcriptional phenotypes may have functionally distinct roles in different organs. In PDAC, the depletion of αSMA+ myofibroblastic CAFs in the pancreas accelerates disease progression, while depletion of αSMA+ myofibroblastic MAFs in the liver reduces metastatic disease progression, highlighting organ-specific functional discrepancies among myofibroblasts [60].

#### 11.2.2.4 Pancreatic Stellate Cells

The interaction between PSCs and pancreatic cancer cells promotes tumor progression. PSCs release several growth factors including matrix metalloproteinases (MMPs), which provoke the proliferation, migration, and invasion of pancreatic tumor cells. PSCs serve as a significant source of MMP-2 and they hasten the advancement of the tumor in a murine xenograft model [61]. Also, TGF-β1 secreted by PSCs promotes stemness and tumorigenicity in pancreatic cancer cells through L1CAM downregulation [62].

#### 11.2.2.5 Endothelial Cells

Tumors stimulate angiogenesis, promoting tumor growth and metastasis [63]. Studies reveal that high expression of the endothelial cell marker CD31, and genes involved in vascular stability correlate with better prognosis and improved survival in PDAC. This suggests that a subset of patients with highly vascular PDAC may benefit from antiangiogenic therapies [64]. Endothelial cells and their expression of cell adhesion molecules regulate cell trafficking. PDAC tumors with decreased leukocyte infiltration show reduced endothelial cell adhesion molecules, and these tumors display activation of hypoxia pathways that may in turn influence endothelial cell biology. These observations highlight the interdependent relationships between vascularity, fibrosis, and cellular recruitment [63].

Certepetide (formerly LSTA1 or CEND-1), an iRGD-based therapy, is a novel cyclic peptide that can increase the penetration of anti-cancer drugs to tumors through selective targeting of tumor endothelial cell receptors that activates a novel uptake pathway. It improves targeted penetration of co-administered drugs into tumor and stroma, leading to potentially increased anti-neoplastic activity. ASCEND is a randomized phase II trial designed to investigate the impact of adding certepetide to gemcitabine/nabpaclitaxel. The addition of certepetide is safe and despite showing no improvement in 6-mo PFS, a possible signal of benefit in OS and ORR, including the 4 complete responses was observed, warranting further investigation. A further cohort of the ASCEND study evaluating the addition of a second dose of certepetide is ongoing [103].

Additionally, LSTA-1 administration promotes CD8+ immune cell tumor infiltration, potentially enabling immunotherapy as a treatment modality. The preliminary results of iLSTA study suggested that the combination of gemcitabine and nab-paclitaxel with LSTA-1 and durvalumab is safe and potentially induces tumor-infiltrating lymphocytes and RECIST response in locally advanced pancreatic adenocarcinomas [104].

## 11.3 Immunotherapeutic Approaches to PDAC: A Team-Based Approach

Given the complexities in pancreatic cancer and the tumor microenvironment surrounding it, the understanding and then therapeutic approaches to this disease have required numerous experts and studies. Recent advances in tissue imaging capabilities, single-cell analytics, and disease modeling have shed light on organizing principles that shape the stromal complexity of PDAC tumors.

Clinical outcomes may be correlated with spatial distance among TME immune cells in PDAC. Comprehensive spatial analysis with HALO software was used to measure mean cell distance between CD8+ T cells and other cells. Longer survival was seen when CD8+ T cells were closer to FAK+ tumor cells, CXCR4+ TANs, and CAFs and further away from M2 and M1 macrophages [105].

These insights into the functional and spatial dependencies that coordinate cancer cell biology and the relationships that exist between cells and extracellular matrix components present in tumors are expected to unveil therapeutic vulnerabilities [63].

When considering immunotherapeutic approaches, a large variety of mechanisms have been studied with some advancement in both understanding of the complex interactions as well as some improvements in patient outcomes. We will review these approaches including oncolytic virus therapy (OVT), adoptive cell transfer therapy, immune checkpoint-oriented immunotherapy, cancer vaccines, strategies based on targeting myeloid cells and CAFs, gut microbiome modulating immune checkpoint blockade, and immune modulation with radiation therapy.

### 11.3.1 Oncolytic Virus Therapy

OVT represents an innovative form of immunotherapy where an oncolytic virus, upon infiltrating and lysing a cancerous cell, initiates an immune reaction by discharging tumor antigens into the circulatory system [65]. Oncolytic viruses possess desirable qualities and specificity that make them an attractive strategy for treatment. Their ability to invade cancer cells is made possible by the genetic composition of these viruses [66]. A phase I/II trial demonstrated that the combination of intratumoral injections of LOAd703, an oncolytic adenovirus with transgenes encoding trimerized, membrane-bound (TMZ)-CD40L and the CD137 receptor (4-1BB ligand), with standard nab-paclitaxel/gemcitabine chemotherapy was both safe and feasible for patients with unresectable or metastatic PDAC. The treatment met the target response rate at the highest dose level, with an ORR of 44% and a disease control rate of 94% [67]. Moreover, a study found that the combination of pelareorep, non-genetically modified reovirus derived from the Type 3 Dearing strain that selectively infects and replicates in tumor cells and pembrolizumab showed modest efficacy in unselected patients, with a clinical benefit rate of 42% among the 12 patients. Notably, the treatment led to significant immunological changes, including a decrease in VDAC1 expression in peripheral CD8+ T cells and on-treatment peripheral CD4+ Treg levels in patients who responded to the treatment [68].

There are ongoing trials with talimogene laherparepvec (T-VEC), administered endoscopically, and a new technology called ONCOTECH, which combines oncolytic adenoviruses (OAs) with T cells to enhance the delivery of viruses to tumors. These advanced approaches working with gastroenterologists as well as our scientific colleagues have created innovative solutions to reaching this complex tumor [69].

### 11.3.2 Adoptive Cell Transfer Therapy

Adoptive cell transfer therapy takes advantage of the patient's own immune cells and obtains, replicates, and alters these cells usually in vitro to augment their efficiency to focus on cancer cells and then transfers these cells back to patients for treatment. Modified T cells possess the ability to discern tumor cells through their unique molecular features [70].

#### 11.3.2.1 Tumor-Infiltrating Lymphocyte Therapy

Tumor-infiltrating lymphocytes (TILs) have been identified in primary tumor tissue, tumor-bearing lymph nodes, and metastases of numerous cancer types. TILs are defined as lymphocytes within and around cancer cells and have been associated with a survival benefit [71].

According to a study, it was found that functional expanded TILs from tumors in the pancreas possess the capability to identify antigens associated with pancreatic cancer [72]. Based on a meta-analysis, the long-term oncological prognosis of patients with PDAC is significantly associated with specific categories of TILs, specifically CD8+ T cells [5].

Successful techniques for increasing the production and reactivity of TILs encompass inhibiting the PD-1 receptor, stimulating 4-1BB, and augmenting CD8+ T cell levels [72]. Yet traditional expansion methods, including rapid expansion with OKT3, lack selectivity and may exacerbate TIL exhaustion [73]. STIL-101, leverages prior TIL programs to promote sustained anti-tumor immune responses. Using PepSeq technology [74], an advanced proteomics platform, we can rapidly screen extensive DNA-encoded peptide libraries against a patient‘s HLA class-II proteins. Alongside in-silico HLA class-I binding models, this method prioritizes potential neoantigens to selectively expand neoantigen-reactive TILs, enhancing response rates and durability by broadening the tumor-specific T cell repertoire. In xenograft studies, STIL-101 has demonstrated the ability to reduce or limit tumor growth in various types, including melanoma and pancreatic cancer [75].

#### 11.3.2.2 Genetically Modified T Cells Therapy

These include TCR engineered T cell therapy, CAR-T cell therapy, CAR-NK cell therapy and cytokine-induced killer (CIK) cell therapy. These therapies focus on a specified target often within the TME and require T or NK cell infiltration into the tumor. In "cold" tumors such as PDAC data has been limited to pre-clinical models such as mice, tumor tissue, and xenograft as well as small subsets of patients. There are numerous ongoing trials targeting Her2, CD22, CD7, Claudin 18.2, CEA, and MSLN. One phase II trial using CIK cells as a second-line therapy in gemcitabine-refractory advanced pancreatic cancer demonstrated a median overall survival (mOS) of 6.2 months [76]. In advanced pancreatic cancer, gemcitabine-resistant patients who underwent CIK cell therapy in combination with S-1, an oral fluoropyrimidine derivative, demonstrated a mOS of 6.6 months, surpassing the mOS of patients solely treated with S-1 alone (6.1 months). Following CIK cell therapy, the DCR rate was 29.8% in the chemotherapy group and 68.0% in the combined therapy group [77].

These limited responses highlight the challenges involved in the TME and creating effective therapies. Re-evaluating not only targets, but combinations, and sequencing of treatment options will be key in advancing how these novel tools are used. Addressing many of these challenges will require surgeons, interventional radiologists, gastroenterologists, basic scientists, pharmacists, radiation oncologists, and medical oncologists optimizing combined efforts to change survival outcomes.

### 11.3.3 Immune-Checkpoint Oriented Therapy

These therapies include inhibitory immune checkpoints such as PD1/PDL1, CTLA4, LAG-3, TIGIT, VISTA, and CD39/CD73 axis as well as bispecific antibodies. Given the success of some of these therapies in several other tumor types as well as their availability as approved drugs, ICB with PD1/PDL1 and CTLA4 have been of high interest in treatment approaches. Single-agent PD1/PDL1 therapy has had very limited efficacy with one trial terminating due to this. Most trials combine therapies with either multiple immune targets, chemotherapy, or radiation therapy. Much of the safety data has been completed, however, efficacy studies are ongoing [3].

Treatments with bispecific antibodies have also been limited to partial responses. This again highlights the aggressive nature of the TME and challenges in the drug delivery of these multi-targeted agents.

### 11.3.4 Cancer Vaccines

Cancer vaccines and their combinations have completed safety data collection with promising efficacy trends. These trends tend to be consistent with our understanding of using a multi-pronged approach to PDAC therapy to battle the aggressive TME with better DFS and OS in combination arms than in single-agent therapy. A list of cancer vaccine trials is included in Table 11.1.

#### 11.3.4.1 Whole Tumor Vaccines

The most promising data in whole tumor vaccines thus far were in combination with PD1 antagonist and CD137 antagonist antibodies. Median DFS was 13.90 months, 14.98 months, and 33.51 months for Cy-GVAX along (Arm A),

**Table 11.1** Whole tumor vaccines

<table>
<tr><th>Study title</th><th>Interventions</th><th>Primary outcome measures</th><th>Enrollment</th></tr>
<tr><td>A Trial of Boost Vaccinations of Pancreatic Tumor Cell Vaccine</td><td>BIOLOGICAL: PANC 10.05 pcDNA-1/GM-Neo and PANC 6.03 pcDNA-1 neo vaccine.</td><td>Disease-free overall survival. Safety as measured by local and systemic toxicity according to NCI CTCAE v 3.0, total of 13 years with 6 months between vaccines.</td><td>71</td></tr>
<tr><td>Adjuvant GVAX Vaccine Therapy in Patients With Pancreatic Cancer</td><td>BIOLOGICAL: GVAX pancreas vaccine</td><td>Number of Patients Experiencing a Grade 3 or Above Treatment-Related Toxicity, When calculating the incidences of adverse events, each adverse event (as defined by NCI CTCAE v3) will be counted only once for a given subject, 14 years</td><td>56</td></tr>
<tr><td>Vaccine Study for Surgically Resected Pancreatic Cancer</td><td>BIOLOGICAL: HyperAcute(R)-Pancreatic Cancer Vaccine</td><td>The primary objective of this Phase II trial is to assess disease-free survival (DFS) at one (1) year following initiation of treatment as the primary endpoint of the study in subjects treated with the HyperAcuteÂ®-Pancreatic Cancer Vaccine, 1 year</td><td>73</td></tr>
<tr><td>Immunotherapy and SBRT Study in Borderline Resectable Pancreatic Cancer</td><td>DRUG: mFOLFIRINOX|BIOLOGICAL: Algenpantucel-L Immunotherapy|RADIATION: SBRT|DRUG: Gemcitabine</td><td>Progression Free Survival, The primary objective of this study is to assess progression-free survival after treatment with a regimen of mFOLFIRINOX with algenpantucel-L immunotherapy followed by SBRT in subjects who have borderline resectable pancreatic cancer, 18 months (assuming enrollment period of 1 year)</td><td>10</td></tr>
<tr><td>Pancreatic Tumor Cell Vaccine (GVAX), Cyclophosphamide, SBRT, and FOLFIRINOX in Patients With Resected Adenocarcinoma of the Pancreas</td><td>DRUG: Cyclophosphamide|BIOLOGICAL: GVAX Pancreas Vaccine|RADIATION: Stereotactic Body Radiation|DRUG: FOLFIRINOX</td><td>Dose-Limiting Toxicities, The number of participants experiencing grade 3–4 diarrhea, neutropenia, and thrombocytopenia within the first 2 cycles (8 weeks) of treatment, regardless of attribution. The rates of each of these toxicities were considered unacceptable if they were 40%, 60%, and 40%, respectively. A decision rule similar to the traditional 3 + 3 design was used to determine whether it was safe to continue on to the next cohort, 8 weeks|Grade 3 or Higher Cy/GVAX-related Adverse Events, Number of participants with grade 3 or above adverse event attributed to Cy or the GVAX pancreas vaccine. Each adverse event (as defined by NCI CTCAE v4.0) was counted only once for a given subject, 116 months</td><td>19</td></tr>
</table>

<table>
<tr><td>GVAX Pancreas Vaccine (With CY) in Combination With Nivolumab and SBRT for Patients With Borderline Resectable Pancreatic Cancer</td><td>DRUG: Cyclophosphamide|DRUG: Nivolumab|DRUG: GVAX Pancreas Vaccine|RADIATION: Stereotactic Body Radiation (SBRT)</td><td>CD8+ T Cell Density in Tumor Tissue, Mean CD8+ T cell density \[log (cells per mm\^2)\], found in resected surgical tissue by immunohistochemistry (IHC), evaluated at time of surgery, approximately 2 months from first dose of study drug</td><td>31</td></tr>
<tr><td>Vaccine Therapy Combined With Adjuvant Chemoradiotherapy in Treating Patients With Resected Stage I or Stage II Adenocarcinoma (Cancer) of the Pancreas</td><td>BIOLOGICAL: GVAX pancreatic cancer vaccine</td><td>Overall Survival, Overall survival in patients treated with adjuvant chemoradiotherapy in sequence with the irradiated allogeneic GM-CSF transfected pancreatic tumor cell lines. Overall survival is defined as time from surgery until death, regardless of cause. Participants were followed for the duration of the study, an average of 2 years|Disease-free Survival, Disease-free Survival in Patients Treated With Adjuvant Chemoradiotherapy in Sequence With the Irradiated Allogeneic GM-CSF Transfected Pancreatic Tumor Cell Lines. DFS is defined as time from surgery until clinical evidence of disease (e.g., CT scan) or death due to any cause. Participants were followed for the duration of the study, an average of 2 years</td><td>60</td></tr>
<tr><td>Vaccine Therapy, Chemotherapy, and GM-CSF in Treating Patients With Advanced Pancreatic Cancer</td><td>BIOLOGICAL: allogeneic tumor cell vaccine|BIOLOGICAL: recombinant interferon alfa|BIOLOGICAL: sargramostim|DRUG: cyclophosphamide</td><td></td><td></td></tr>
<tr><td>Study With CY, Pembrolizumab, GVAX Pancreas Vaccine, and SBRT in Patients With Locally Advanced Pancreatic Cancer</td><td>DRUG: Cyclophosphamide|DRUG: GVAX Pancreatic Cancer Vaccine|DRUG: Pembrolizumab|RADIATION: SBRT</td><td>Distant Metastasis Free Survival (DMFS), DMFS is defined as the duration of time from start of treatment to identification of distant metastases on imaging or death, whichever occurs first. Estimation based on the Kaplan-Meier curve, 62 months</td><td>58</td></tr>
<tr><td>FOLFIRINOX Followed by Ipilimumab With Pancreatic Tumor Vaccine in Treatment of Metastatic Pancreatic Cancer</td><td>DRUG: Ipilimumab|BIOLOGICAL: Vaccine|DRUG: FOLFIRINOX</td><td>Overall Survival (OS), Overall Survival is the time between the date of randomization on study and death, 4 years</td><td>83</td></tr>
<tr><td>Vaccine Treatment for Surgically Resected Pancreatic Cancer</td><td>BIOLOGICAL: HyperAcute-Pancreatic Cancer Vaccine</td><td>To assess the side effects, dose-limiting toxicity and maximum tolerated dose, 6 months</td><td>7</td></tr>
</table>

(continued)

**Table 11.1** (continued)

| Study title | Interventions | Primary outcome measures | Enrollment |
|---|---|---|---|
| Vaccine Therapy With or Without Cyclophosphamide in Treating Patients Undergoing Chemotherapy and Radiation Therapy for Stage I or Stage II Pancreatic Cancer That Can Be Removed by Surgery | BIOLOGICAL: GVAX pancreatic cancer vaccine\|DRUG: cyclophosphamide | Safety as Measured by Number of Participants With Treatment-related Grade 3 or 4 Local and Systemic Toxicity as Defined by NCI CTCAE v3.0, 7 years\|Amount of T-regulatory Cells (Tregs) and CD4+ and CD8+ Effector T Cells, After Neoadjuvant GVAX Pancreatic Cancer Vaccination, up to 8 years\|Change in the Number and Function of Peripheral Mesothelin-specific CD8+ T Cells and CD4+, FoxP3+, and GITR+ Tregs, Change in the number and function of peripheral mesothelin-specific CD8+ T cells and CD4+, FoxP3+, and GITR+ Tregs after each GVAX pancreatic cancer vaccination when administered alone or in combination with a single dose or metronomic doses of cyclophosphamide, up to 8 years | 87 |
| Investigation of a Therapeutic Vaccine (ACIT-1) in Cancer | BIOLOGICAL: ACIT-1 | Toxicity, Toxicity based on the National Cancer Institute Common Terminology Criteria for Adverse Events (NCI CTCAE) v4.03. From start of treatment to 20 weeks | 34 |
| Platform Study of Neoadjuvant and Adjuvant Immunotherapy for Patients With Resectable Adenocarcinoma of the Pancreas | DRUG: Cyclophosphamide\|BIOLOGICAL: GVAX pancreatic cancer\|DRUG: Nivolumab\|DRUG: Urelumab\|DRUG: BMS-986253 | IL17A expression, median IL17A expression in lymphoid aggregates from resected tumor (Arms A and B only), 4 years\|Intratumoral CD8+ CD137+ cells, Fold change of intratumoral CD8+ CD137+ cells before and after neoadjuvant therapy (Arms B and C only), 4 years\|Intratumoral granzyme B+ PD-1+ CD137+ cells, Percent change of intratumoral granzyme B+ PD-1+ CD137+ cells in surgical (post-treatment) tissue compared to baseline (pre-treatment) biopsy (Arm D only), 4 years\|Pathologic Response, Percent of patients with a response grade of 0–2 (0 = complete response 1 = marked response, 2 = moderate response) at time of surgery, 4 years | 76 |
| Trial of Neoadjuvant and Adjuvant Nivolumab and BMS-813160 With or Without GVAX for Locally Advanced Pancreatic Ductal Adenocarcinomas | RADIATION: Stereotactic Body Radiation (SBRT)\|DRUG: Nivolumab\|DRUG: CCR2/CCR5 dual antagonist\|DRUG: GVAX | Number of Participants experiencing study drug-related toxicities, Number of participants who experienced study drug-related toxicities as defined by CTCAE v5.0, 3 years\|Percentage of participants treated with immunotherapy who achieve an immune response, Percentage of participants who have/>80% increase of infiltration of CD8+ CD137+ T cells into the pancreatic ductal adenocarcinoma after treatment with immunotherapy compared to baseline before treatment, 3 years | 46 |

nivolumab with Cy-GVAX (Arm B), and urelumab, nivolumab, and Cy-GVAX (Arm C) respectively. Median OS was 23.59 months, 27.01 months, and 35.55 months for Arms A, B, and C, respectively. There were limited patients with only 2 completing the trial and extended-treatment phase [78]. Patient enrollment, especially for trials limited to large academic centers, continues to be a challenge due to both the limited incidence as well as the rapidly progressive nature of PDAC and correlating decline in performance status and ability for patients to travel. As such, opening trials at a larger number of institutions and providing access to patients in communities near home will aid in our understanding of this disease and create power studies that can discern the nuanced differences in treatment approaches as well as the differences in the disease itself. Table 11.1 lists whole tumor vaccine trials in pancreatic cancer.

#### 11.3.4.2 Dendritic Cell Vaccines

DCs that were isolated from the patient's peripheral blood were loaded with tumor-associated antigens (TAAs) or tumor-derived mRNA. After the administration of these vaccines, the modified DCs proceed to the lymph nodes, where they transmit antigens to T lymphocytes and concurrently induce co-stimulatory signals [79]. In a study, DCs were gathered from patients who had stage III/IV pancreatic cancer through the employment of apheresis. Afterward, these collected DCs underwent the process of being pulsed with MUC-1 peptide. The injection of MUC-1-pulsed DCs in these patients exhibited both safety and efficacy, successfully triggering an immune response toward the MUC-1 [80].

A retrospective multicenter analysis was conducted on 255 patients with pancreatic cancer. These patients were receiving standard chemotherapy and a DC vaccine. This study showed that in patients with pancreatic cancer who received a DC vaccine, a positive erythema reaction at the site of DC vaccine injection was linked to better survival [81].

The administration of lymphokine-activated killer (LAK) cell therapy significantly extended the survival of patients with advanced pancreatic cancer who underwent DC vaccine-based immunotherapy along with gemcitabine. Nevertheless, the use of immunotherapy on its own enhanced the quantity of cancer antigen–targeting CTLs while decreasing the presence of Tregs [82]. MUC and LAK phase 1 studies showed that these vaccines were well tolerated with no grade 3 or 4 toxicities, but a small number of pts enrolled. Table 11.2 lists dendritic cell vaccine trials in pancreatic cancer. As efficacy studies are planned, consideration for larger cohorts and more geographic involvement may help power future data collection.

#### 11.3.4.3 Peptide Vaccines

One phase II trial with vaccine candidate GV1001 showed promising median survival data in patients who were responders. However, when combined with chemotherapy in phase III trials there was no significant improvement in OS [83]. This complex interplay between immune activation and chemotherapy will prove a new challenge as we attempt to combine therapy options and efficacy.

**Table 11.2** Dendritic cell vaccines

<table>
<tr><th>Study title</th><th>Interventions</th><th>Primary outcome measures</th><th>Enrollment</th></tr>
<tr><td>DC1 Vaccine + Chemokine Modulatory Regimen (CKM) as Adjuvant Treatment of Peritoneal Surface Malignancies</td><td>BIOLOGICAL: DC vaccine| DRUG: Celecoxib| DRUG: Interferon Alfa-2b|BIOLOGICAL: rintatolimod</td><td>Recommended Phase 2 Dose (RP2D) (Phase 1), Number of patients treated at each of the three possible dose levels of Interferon Î± (5 MU/m\^2, 10 MU/m\^2 or 20 MU/m\^2) during the Phase 1 portion of the study. Up to 24 weeks|Adverse Events Possibly, Probably or Definitely Related to Study Treatment, Number of participants with adverse events (by Grade) that were possibly, probably or definitely related to the combined study immunotherapy regimen (Î±DC1 vaccines + CKM) per CTCAE v 4.0 (Common Terminology Criteria for Adverse Events), Up to 24 weeks</td><td>64</td></tr>
</table>

| | | | |
|---|---|---|---|
| First-in-human Interleukin-15-transpresenting Wilms' Tumor Protein 1-targeting Autologous Dendritic Cell Vaccination in Cancer Patients | BIOLOGICAL: IL15-transpresenting WT1-targeted Dendritic Cell Vaccine | Feasibility of leukapheresis, Proportion of patients in the intention-to-treat population that had a successful leukapheresis. Upon completion of leukapheresis, on average 4 weeks after inclusion (baseline)\|Feasibility of IL15/IL15Ra/WT1 DC vaccine production, Proportion of patients in the intention-to-treat population that had successful vaccine production (i.e., production of at least 6 IL-15-transpresenting WT1-targeting DC vaccines meeting all quality control measurements). Upon completion of vaccine production and quality testing (i.e., from leukapheresis until 4 weeks after), on average 8 weeks after inclusion (baseline)\|Feasibility of study treatment scheme, Proportion of patients in the intention-to-treat population who complete the study treatment schedule of 6 IL-15-transpresenting WT1-targeting DC vaccines. Study treatment scheme (i.e., from administration of first to 6th vaccine (+- 10 weeks))\|Feasibility of DC vaccine administration (administration of 1st vaccine), Proportion of efficacy evaluable patients (i.e., having received at least 1 vaccine + no major protocol violation) in the intention-to-treat population. At administration of first vaccine\|Safety of IL15/IL15Ra/WT1 DC vaccine administration: Related (Severe) Adverse Events ((S)AEs), Proportion of patients of the safety population that experienced (S)AEs possibly, probably or definitely related to IL15/IL15Ra/WT1 DC vaccination, over the entire study duration (i.e., from inclusion (baseline) to end of follow-up, which lasts until 90 days after the last DC vaccine), on average 7 months\|Safety of IL15/IL15Ra/WT1 DC vaccine administration: total (S)AEs (number), Number of (S)AEs in the safety population (i.e., having received at least 1 DC vaccine), over the entire study duration (i.e., from inclusion (baseline) to end of follow-up, which lasts until 90 days after the last DC vaccine), on average 7 months\|Safety of IL15/IL15Ra/WT1 DC vaccine administration: total (S)AEs (grade), Grade of (S)AEs in the safety population, over the entire study duration (i.e., from inclusion (baseline) to end of follow-up, which lasts until 90 days after the last DC vaccine), on average 7 months | 10 |

(continued)

**Table 11.2** (continued)

| Study title | Interventions | Primary outcome measures | Enrollment |
|---|---|---|---|
| Direct Tumor Injection KLH-Pulsed Dendritic Cells in Unresectable Pancreatic Cancer | BIOLOGICAL: KLH-pulsed autologous dendritic cell vaccine | Overall Survival, Patients will be followed until death | 24 |
| Ability of a Dendritic Cell Vaccine to Immunize Melanoma or Epithelial Cancer Patients Against Defined Mutated Neoantigens Expressed by the Autologous Cancer | BIOLOGICAL: Peptide loaded dendritic cell vaccine | Percentage of Patients Who Had a Clinical Response (Complete Response (CR) + Partial Response (PR)) to Treatment, Response was assessed by the RECIST v1.1. Complete Response is disappearance of all target lesions. Any pathological lymph nodes (whether target or non-target) must have reduction in short axis to \<10 mm. Partial Response is at least a 30% decrease in the sum of the diameters of target lesions, taking as reference the baseline sum of diameters, up to 6 months | 1 |
| Vaccine Therapy and Biological Therapy in Treating Patients With Advanced Cancer | BIOLOGICAL: aldesleukin\|BIOLOGICAL: mutant p53 peptide pulsed dendritic cell vaccine\|BIOLOGICAL: ras peptide cancer vaccine\|BIOLOGICAL: sargramostim\|BIOLOGICAL: therapeutic autologous lymphocytes\|BIOLOGICAL: therapeutic tumor infiltrating lymphocytes | | |

Another peptide cancer vaccine, KIF20A-66, was also examined in a phase I/II trial and found to be well-tolerated. The mOS and median progression-free survival (mPFS) were reported as 142 days and 56 days, respectively [84].

Recently, the phase 1 study of ELI-002 2P in patients with KRAS-mutated pancreatic cancer demonstrated promising results. ELI-002 2P is a cancer vaccine that specifically targets lymph nodes and consists of three components. These components include modified G12D and G12R mKRAS long peptides, which have been modified with amphiphiles, and an amphiphile-modified TLR9 agonist CpG-7909 DNA. The therapy was well-tolerated, induced significant T cell responses, and resulted in biomarker clearance and improved relapse-free survival. Direct ex vivo mKRAS-specific T cell responses were observed in 21 of 25 patients (84%; 59% both CD4+ and CD8+); tumor biomarker responses were observed in 21 of 25 patients (84%); biomarker clearance was observed in six of 25 patients (24%; three pancreatic and three colorectal); and the median RFS was 16.33 months. Efficacy correlated with T cell responses above or below the median fold increase over baseline (12.75-fold): median tumor biomarker reduction was −76.0% versus −10.2%, and the median RFS was not reached versus 4.01 months. ELI-002 2P was safe and induced considerable T cell responses in patients with immunotherapy-recalcitrant KRAS-mutated tumors [85]. Table 11.3 reviews peptide vaccine trials in pancreatic cancer.

#### 11.3.4.4 DNA Vaccines

Several studies have shown that DNA vaccines targeting tumor-associated antigens (TAAs) can effectively prolong survival in mice with PDAC. Table 11.4 lists DNA vaccine trials in pancreatic cancer. Targeting α-Enolase (ENO1) with a DNA vaccine has been particularly effective [86]. In addition, combining this DNA vaccine with chemotherapy using gemcitabine has shown improved efficacy against multiple TAAs, including ENO1, glyceraldeheyde-3-phosphate dehydrogenase (G3P), keratin, type II cytoskeletal 8 (K2C8), and far upstream binding protein 1 (FUBP1) [87]. Another DNA vaccine targeting mucin 1-variable number tandem repeat (MUC1-VNTRn) has demonstrated strong cytotoxic effects in both in vivo and in vitro experiments [88]. Furthermore, a chimeric DNA vaccine that targets human fibroblast activation protein alpha (FAPα) and survivin has been shown to reduce immunosuppressive cells and increase TILs, thereby creating a more favorable TME for immune responses against pancreatic tumors [89].

#### 11.3.4.5 RNA Vaccines

Many of these trials are ongoing or have not yet released their full data yet however these personalized vaccines encode tumor-specific antigens (TSAs) and shown some promising activity. Table 11.5 demonstrates RNA vaccine trials in pancreatic cancer with the corresponding enrollment numbers. An mRNA vaccine called autogene cevumeran was generated using uridine mRNA-lipoplex nanoparticles. After the surgical procedure, a combination therapy that included atezolizumab, the mRNA vaccine (with a maximum of 20 neo-antigens per patient), and chemotherapy was conducted. The results indicated that vaccine-enhanced T cells, which

**Table 11.3** Peptide vaccine trials

<table>
<tr><th>Study title</th><th>Interventions</th><th>Primary outcome measures</th><th>Enrollment</th></tr>
<tr><td>Open Label Immunotherapy Trial of Inoperable Pancreatic Cancer</td><td>BIOLOGICAL: V3-P</td><td>Effect of V3-P on tumor burden, Changes in CA19.9 tumor marker induced by daily dose of oral vaccine V3-P in an open label trial in patients with inoperable pancreatic cancer, 3 months</td><td>30</td></tr>
<tr><td>Comparing Neoadjuvant/ Adjuvant GVAX vs a mKRASvax Given With Anti-PD-1 and Anti-CD137 for Surgically Resectable Pancreatic Cancer</td><td>DRUG: AGEN2373|DRUG: Balstilimab|DRUG: Cyclophosphamide|DRUG: GVAX|DRUG: AGEN2373 (RP2D)|DRUG: Balstilimab|DRUG: mKRASvax</td><td>Dose Limiting Toxicities in Phase I participants, Phase I participants will be evaluated for dose limiting toxicities (DLTs) during the first 14 day cycle and 14 days post-operatively for the purpose of determining the recommended phase II dose of AGEN2373 when given concurrently with balstilimab and cancer vaccination, 1 month|Number of participants experiencing Grade 3 or Higher study drug-related toxicities, Number of participants experiencing study drug-related adverse events Grade 3 or higher as defined by CTCAE v5.0, 2 years|Number of participants who form Intratumoral tertiary lymphoid structures (TLS), Number of participants who form at least one tertiary lymphoid structure (TLS) following one cycle of study drugs. The presence of at least 50 CD20+ B cells and 50 CD3+ T cells in a â‰¥50 ÂµM area of surgical tissue is considered "positive" for TLS, 2 weeks</td><td>38</td></tr>
<tr><td>Antiangiogenic Peptide Vaccine Therapy With Gemcitabine in Treating Patient With Pancreatic Cancer (Phase1/2)</td><td>BIOLOGICAL: VEGFR1-1084, VEGFR2-169|DRUG: Gemcitabine</td><td>Toxicities as assessed by NCI-CACAE ver3), 3 months</td><td>17</td></tr>
</table>

<table>
<tr><td>QUILT-3.070:Pancreatic Cancer Vaccine: Subjects With Pancreatic Cancer Who Have Progressed on or After Standard-of-care Therapy</td><td>DRUG: Aldoxorubicin HCl|BIOLOGICAL: ALT-803|BIOLOGICAL: ETBX-011|BIOLOGICAL: GI-4000|BIOLOGICAL: haNK for infusion|BIOLOGICAL: avelumab|BIOLOGICAL: bevacizumab|DRUG: Capecitabine|DRUG: Cyclophosphamide|DRUG: Fluorouracil|DRUG: Leucovorin|DRUG: nab-Paclitaxel|DRUG: lovaza|DRUG: Oxaliplatin|PROCEDURE: SBRT</td><td>Number of Participants With Treatment-emergent Adverse Events (AEs) and Serious AEs (SAEs), Graded Using the National Cancer Institute (NCI) Common Terminology Criteria for Adverse Events (CTCAE) Version 4.03. Phase 1b primary endpoint, 30 days after last dose, up to 8 months</td><td>4</td></tr>
<tr><td>QUILT-3.039: NANT Pancreatic Cancer Vaccine: Combination Immunotherapy in Subjects With Pancreatic Cancer Who Have Progressed on or After Standard-of-care Therapy</td><td>DRUG: Cyclophosphamide|DRUG: Oxaliplatin|DRUG: Capecitabine|DRUG: 5-Fluorouracil|DRUG: Leucovorin|DRUG: nab-paclitaxel|BIOLOGICAL: bevacizumab|BIOLOGICAL: avelumab|BIOLOGICAL: ALT-803|BIOLOGICAL: aNK for Infusion|BIOLOGICAL: ETBX-011|BIOLOGICAL: GI-4000</td><td>Number of Participants With Adverse Events, 30 days after last dose, up to 2 years</td><td>3</td></tr>
</table>

(continued)

**Table 11.3** (continued)

| Study title | Interventions | Primary outcome measures | Enrollment |
|---|---|---|---|
| QUILT-3.060: NANT Pancreatic Cancer Vaccine: Molecularly Informed Integrated Immunotherapy in Subjects With Pancreatic Cancer Who Have Progressed on or After Standard-of-care Therapy | BIOLOGICAL: ALT-803IBIOLOGICAL: ETBX-011IBIOLOGICAL: GI-4000IBIOLOGICAL: haNK for infusionIBIOLOGICAL: avelumabIBIOLOGICAL: bevacizumabIDRUG: CapecitabineIDRUG: CyclophosphamideIDRUG: FluorouracilIDRUG: LeucovorinIDRUG: nab-PaclitaxelIDRUG: lovazaIDRUG: OxaliplatinIPROCEDURE: SBRT | Number of Participants With Treatment-emergent Adverse Events (AEs) and Serious AEs (SAEs), Graded Using the National Cancer Institute(NCI) Common Terminology Criteria for Adverse Events (CTCAE) Version 4.03, 30 days after last dose, up to 2 years (up to 1 year in each treatment phase) or until they experience confirmed progressive disease or unacceptable toxicity, withdrawn consent, or if the Investigator feels it is no longer in their best interest. | 6 |
| QUILT-3.088: NANT Pancreatic Cancer Vaccine | DRUG: GemcitabineIDRUG: Nab-paclitaxelIDRUG: Aldoxorubicin HCIIBIOLOGICAL: ALT-803IBIOLOGICAL: ETBX-011IBIOLOGICAL: ETBX-021IBIOLOGICAL: ETBX-051IBIOLOGICAL: ETBX-061IBIOLOGICAL: GI-4000IBIOLOGICAL: GI-6207IBIOLOGICAL: GI-6301IBIOLOGICAL: haNKIDRUG: AvelumabIDRUG: BevacizumabIDRUG: CapecitabineIDRUG: CyclophosphamideIDRUG: 5-FluorouracilIDRUG: LeucovorinIDRUG: Oxaliplatin | Progression-Free Survival, Compare the efficacy of the NANT Pancreatic Cancer Vaccine regimen vs standard-of-care (SoC) therapy as first-line treatment for patients with metastatic pancreatic cancer as assessed by progression-free survival (PFS) using RECIST Version 1.1, 12 months | 0 |

| | | | |
|---|---|---|---|
| Survivin Peptide Vaccination for Patients With Advanced Melanoma, Pancreatic, Colon and Cervical Cancer | BIOLOGICAL: Survivin peptide vaccine | Progression-free survival\|Overall survival\|Immunological response | 70 |
| Antigen-specific Cancer Immunotherapy (TG01) and Gemcitabine as Adjuvant Therapy in Resected Pancreatic Cancer | BIOLOGICAL: TG01\|BIOLOGICAL: TG01 | Patients' Safety During Study, Assess the safety (number and nature of Adverse events and laboratory data occurring during study (before, during and after chemotherapy is given) in subjects treated with the Pancreatic Cancer ASCI, 2 years\|Patients' Immune Response, Assess the Immune response (DTH responses and Proliferative T cell responses) up to 2 years of treatment, During the 2 years of treatment | 32 |
| A Phase II Trial of CG 8020 and CG 2505 in Patients With Nonresectable or Metastatic Pancreatic Cancer | BIOLOGICAL: CG 8020 and CG 2505 | Safety\|Efficacy measured by clinical benefit response\|Progression-free survival\|Overall survival | 50 |
| Temozolomide and Survivin Long Peptide Vaccine (SurVaxM) for the Treatment of Patients With Progressing Metastatic Neuroendocrine Tumors | PROCEDURE: Biospecimen Collection\|PROCEDURE: Computed Tomography\|BIOLOGICAL: Incomplete Freund's Adjuvant\|PROCEDURE: Magnetic Resonance Imaging\|BIOLOGICAL: Sargramostim\|BIOLOGICAL: SVN53-67/M57-KLH Peptide Vaccine\|DRUG: Temozolomide | Progression-free survival (PFS) (Part 1), Summarized using frequencies and relative frequencies. At 6 months\|Incidence of adverse events (Part 1), Defined using National Cancer Institute (NCI) Common Terminology Criteria for Adverse events (CTCAE) version (v) 5.0. Adverse events will be summarized by attribution and grade using frequencies and relative frequencies. Up to 1 year\|PFS (Part 2), Clinical benefit compared between treatment arms. PFS will be summarized by study arm using frequencies and relative frequencies, at 6 months | 132 |
| Vaccine Therapy in Treating Patients With Cancer of the Gastrointestinal Tract | BIOLOGICAL: carcinoembryonic antigen peptide 1-6D\|BIOLOGICAL: incomplete Freund's adjuvant\|BIOLOGICAL: sargramostim | Production of CAP 1-6D T cells\|Production of cytotoxic T cells\|Antitumor response\|Frequency and severity of toxic effects | 7 |
| Study of CAP1-6D in Patients With Locally Advanced or Surgically Resected Pancreatic Adenocarcinoma | BIOLOGICAL: modified CEA peptide (10mcg)\|BIOLOGICAL: modified CEA peptide (100mcg)\|BIOLOGICAL: modified CEA peptide (1000mcg) | Maximum T Cell Response From Baseline, T cell frequency (spots per 10\^4 CD8+ cells) was measured by ELISPOT (Enzyme-linked immunosorbent spot) assay. Blood was collected for this assay at baseline and every 4 weeks for the first 8 cycles. After the eighth cycle, a blood sample was collected at the time of disease progression. The maximum T cell response was calculated as: peak value on treatment—baseline value. | |

(continued)

**Table 11.3** (continued)

<table>
<tr><th>Study title</th><th>Interventions</th><th>Primary outcome measures</th><th>Enrollment</th></tr>
<tr><td>Study of CAP1-6D in Patients With Locally Advanced or Surgically Resected Pancreatic Adenocarcinoma</td><td>BIOLOGICAL: modified CEA peptide (10mcg)|BIOLOGICAL: modified CEA peptide (100mcg)|BIOLOGICAL: modified CEA peptide (1000mcg)</td><td>Maximum T Cell Response From Baseline, T cell frequency (spots per 10\^4 CD8+ cells) was measured by ELISPOT (Enzyme-linked immunosorbent spot) assay. Blood was collected for this assay at baseline and every 4 weeks for the first 8 cycles. After the eighth cycle, a blood sample was collected at the time of disease progression. The maximum T cell response was calculated as: peak value on treatment—baseline value. A positive value indicates an increase from baseline, T cell response collected at baseline and every 4 weeks on treatment</td><td>23</td></tr>
<tr><td>Vaccine Therapy Plus Biological Therapy in Treating Adults With Metastatic Solid Tumors</td><td>BIOLOGICAL: aldesleukin|BIOLOGICAL: ras peptide cancer vaccine|BIOLOGICAL: sargramostim|DRUG: DetoxPC</td><td></td><td></td></tr>
<tr><td>A Study of a Personalized Cancer Vaccine Targeting Shared Neoantigens</td><td>BIOLOGICAL: GRT-C903|BIOLOGICAL: GRT-R904|BIOLOGICAL: nivolumab|BIOLOGICAL: ipilimumab</td><td>Incidence of adverse events (AEs), serious adverse events (SAEs), and dose-limiting toxicities (DLTs), Initiation of study treatment through 100 days post-last dose (up to approximately 27 months)|Objective Response Rate (ORR) in Phase 2 using RECIST v1.1, Initiation of study treatment until disease progression (up to approximately 27 months)|Identify the recommended Phase 2 dose (RP2D) of GRT-C903 and GRT-R904, Up to approximately 6 months</td><td>39</td></tr>
<tr><td>A Study of ELI-002 7P in Subjects With KRAS/NRAS Mutated Solid Tumors</td><td>DRUG: ELI-002 7P</td><td>Phase 1: Evaluate the safety of ELI-002 7P, Safety will be assessed by the incidence of adverse events (AEs) and clinically significant changes in laboratory tests and vital signs, 28 days after the first dose of ELI-002 7P|Phase 2: Compare ELI-002 7P versus standard of care (SOC; observation) in DFS (disease free survival), DFS is assessed by the investigator through computed tomography (CT) imaging or magnetic resonance imaging (MRI) with contrast and using iRECIST criteria, After the last radiographic assessment at Visit 26 (Week 150)</td><td>158</td></tr>
</table>

**Table 11.4** DNA vaccines

| Study title | Interventions | Primary outcome measures | Enrollment |
|---|---|---|---|
| Vaccine Therapy, Cyclophosphamide, and Cetuximab in Treating Patients With Metastatic or Locally Advanced Pancreatic Cancer | DRUG: Cetuximab\|BIOLOGICAL: Pancreatic tumor vaccine\|DRUG: Cyclophosphamide | Safety of Combining the Pancreatic Tumor Vaccine in Sequence With Cyclophosphamide and Erbitux. Safety is Defined as the Number of Treatment-related Grade 3 or 4 Adverse Events Observed in Greater Than 5% of the Patient Population, 7 months | 60 |
| Efficacy and Safety of BC-819 and Gemcitabine in Patients With Locally Advanced Pancreatic Adenocarcinoma | BIOLOGICAL: Biological/Vaccine: BC-819 | Progression-free Survival (PFS), To compare the effect of intratumoral endoscopic ultrasound injection of BC-819 administered with intravenous gemcitabine on progression-free survival. PFS was defined as the time from the date of consent until objective tumor progression or death. Median PFS by Kaplan-Meier analysis was used for evaluation. The target tumor lesion was identified and the longest diameter of the target lesion was measured according to Response Evaluation Criteria in Solid Tumors (RECIST) 1.1 guidelines. For disease evaluations after treatment, scans conducted at baseline that were used for tumor measurements were repeated, 24 months | 12 |

**Table 11.5** RNA vaccines

| Study title | Interventions | Primary outcome measures | Enrollment |
| --- | --- | --- | --- |
| Cvac as Maintenance Treatment Patients With Resected Stage I or Stage II Adenocarcinoma (Cancer) of the Pancreas | BIOLOGICAL: CVac | Assessment of safety and tolerability of CVac. (Adverse events, vital signs, 12 lead ECG, relevant changes in physical examination), Safety analyses will be performed on the Safety Population. Safety and tolerability will be summarized using descriptive statistics and or listed and assessed by adverse events, vital signs, 12 lead ECG, relevant changes in physical examination, 10–12 months | 0 |
| QUILT-3.080: NANT Pancreatic Cancer Vaccine | DRUG: Aldoxorubicin HCl\|BIOLOGICAL: ALT-803\|BIOLOGICAL: ETBX-011\|BIOLOGICAL: ETBX-021\|BIOLOGICAL: ETBX-051\|BIOLOGICAL: ETBX-061\|BIOLOGICAL: GI-4000\|BIOLOGICAL: GI-6207\|BIOLOGICAL: GI-6301\|BIOLOGICAL: haNK for infusion\|BIOLOGICAL: bevacizumab\|DRUG: Capecitabine\|DRUG: Cyclophosphamide\|DRUG: Fluorouracil\|DRUG: Leucovorin\|DRUG: nab-Paclitaxel\|DRUG: Oxaliplatin\|BIOLOGICAL: Avelumab\|PROCEDURE: SBRT | Number of Participants With Treatment-emergent Adverse Events (AEs) and Serious AEs (SAEs), Graded Using the National Cancer Institute (NCI) Common Terminology Criteria for Adverse Events (CTCAE) Version 4.03, Up to 230 days | 3 |
| QUILT-3.040: ETBX-011 (Ad5 [E1-, E2b-]-CEA(6D)) Vaccine in Combination With ALT-803 (Super-agonist IL-15) in Subjects Having CEA-Expressing Cancer | BIOLOGICAL: ETBX-011\|BIOLOGICAL: ALT-803 | Number of Participants With Dose-Limiting Toxicities, 9 weeks | 3 |

accounted for as much as 10% of the total T cells in the bloodstream, experienced re-expansion through a vaccine booster. These re-expanded cells consisted of durable, polyfunctional CD8+ T cells that targeted pancreatic cancer neo-antigens. After a median follow-up period of 18 months, patients who exhibited vaccine-enhanced T cells demonstrated a significantly prolonged median recurrence-free survival when compared to the control group [90].

#### 11.3.4.6 Viral/Bacterial/Yeast-Based Vaccines

Early data in this controversial treatment approach have brought promising preclinical and early phase results. Table 11.6 reviews viral, bacterial, and yeast vaccine trials. One of the widely recognized cancer vaccines of this kind is CRS207, which is a live attenuated strain of Listeria monocytogenes engineered to express MSLN. Enhanced mesothelin-specific CD8 T cell responses were associated with longer OS, regardless of treatment arm [91].

Utilization of an exogenous immunization antigen, administered via Salmonella bacteria acting as a vector showed eradication of pancreatic tumors in PDAC mouse models [92]. VXM01, an oral tumor vaccine using attenuated Salmonella with a VEGFR-2 expression plasmid, was tested in a phase I trial with advanced pancreatic cancer patients. VXM01 was well tolerated, with no dose-limiting toxicities and significant increases in VEGFR2-specific T effector responses. Vaccinated patients showed reduced tumor perfusion and elevated serum biomarkers indicative of anti-angiogenic activity [93].

Pelareorep (pela) is a non-genetically modified, intravenously administered reovirus that selectively infects cancer cells. It stimulates the expansion of pre-existing tumor-infiltrating lymphocyte (TIL) clones, and it makes tumors visible to the immune system by upregulating interferon-induced gene expressions including PD-L1, CXCL9, CXCL10, and CXCL11. PD-L1 upregulation also provides a basis for potential synergy between pela and immune checkpoint inhibitors. Pela combined with gemcitabine/nab-paclitaxel/atezolizumab showed promising tumor responses in mPDAC [102].

#### 11.3.4.7 Stem-Cell-Based Vaccines

The fact that cancer cells and embryonic tissues have several similar cellular and molecular characteristics suggests that we can potentially utilize iPSCs to stimulate anti-tumor responses within cancer vaccines. In murine breast cancer, mesothelioma, and melanoma mouse model's tumor prevention has been successful [94]. Cancer vaccine derived from iPSCs stimulates a defensive immune response in a PDAC mouse model [95]. Table 11.7 lists a stem cell-based vaccine trial.

### 11.3.5 Gut Microbiome

Studies have shown that the number of tumor microbiome species present within tumor samples was significantly higher in the long-term survivor patients compared to short-term survivor patients on validation cohorts at MD Anderson Cancer Center

**Table 11.6** Viral, bacterial, and yeast vaccines

| Study title | Interventions | Primary outcome measures | Enrollment |
|---|---|---|---|
| Tg01 Vaccine/Qs-21 Stimulon With Or Without Balstilimab As Maintenance Therapy Following Adjuvant Chemotherapy In Patients With Resected Pancreatic Cancer | BIOLOGICAL: TG01 VaccineIDRUG: QS-21IDRUG: Balstilimab | Molecular disease control rate, To assess 6-month molecular disease control rate in each cohort as defined by ctDNA stability, decrease, or clearance, 6 months | 24 |
| Safety and Efficacy of the Therapeutic Vaccine GI-4000 in Combination With Gemcitabine Versus Placebo for the Treatment of Non-metastatic, Post-resection Pancreas Cancer | BIOLOGICAL: GI-4000IDRUG: Gemcitabine | Recurrence-free time and survival, 5 years | 176 |

| | | | |
|---|---|---|---|
| Safety and Efficacy Study of Mix Vaccine in Pancreatic Carcinoma Patient | BIOLOGICAL: MV\|OTHER: Standard Treatment | efficacy as measured by modified Response Evaluation Criteria In Solid Tumors (RECIST) criteria version 1.1, 2 years | 20 |
| Analyzing Childhood Recall Antigens in Patients With Pancreatic Cancer | DRUG: Gemcitabine\|BIOLOGICAL: TT vaccine booster | Change in CD4 T Cell Responses Before TT Booster, The relative difference in CD4 T cell counts before and after administration of the TT booster vaccine (Day 8) will be compared. The number of cells per microliter (cells/ÂµL) will be determined. The proportion of at least threefold increase will be reported along with its 95% CI. The actual magnitude of change will be examined by taking a log scale of CD4 counts and report a mean of change on CD4 on its log scale along with its 95% CI. Day 1\|Change in CD4 T Cell Responses Before TT Booster, The relative difference in CD4 T cell counts before and after administration of the TT booster vaccine (Day 8) will be compared. The number of cells per microliter (cells/ÂµL) will be determined. The proportion of at least threefold increase will be reported along with its 95% CI. The actual magnitude of change will be examined by taking a log scale of CD4 counts and report a mean of change on CD4 on its log scale along with its 95% CI. Day 8\|Change in CD4 T Cell Responses After TT Booster, The relative difference in CD4 T cell counts before and after administration of the TT booster vaccine (Day 8) will be compared. The number of cells per microliter (cells/ÂµL) will be determined. The proportion of at least threefold increase will be reported along with its 95% CI. The actual magnitude of change will be examined by taking a log scale of CD4 counts and report a mean of change on CD4 on its log scale along with its 95% CI. Day 15\|Change in CD4 T Cell Responses After TT Booster, The relative difference in CD4 T cell counts before and after administration of the TT booster vaccine (Day 8) will be compared. The number of cells per microliter (cells/ÂµL) will be determined. The proportion of at least threefold increase will be reported along with its 95% CI. The actual magnitude of change will be examined by taking a log scale of CD4 counts and report a mean of change on CD4 on its log scale along with its 95% CI, Day 28 | 10 |

(continued)

**Table 11.6** (continued)

| Study title | Interventions | Primary outcome measures | Enrollment |
|---|---|---|---|
| Immunotherapy Combined With Radiation and Influenza Vaccine for Pancreatic Cancer | DRUG: Nivolumab\|DRUG: Ipilimumab\|BIOLOGICAL: Influenza vaccine\|RADIATION: SBRT | Objective response rate (ORR), ORR in all patients using Investigator assessments, 12 months | 19 |
| Study of CRS-207, Nivolumab, and Ipilimumab With or Without GVAX Pancreas Vaccine (With Cy) in Patients With Pancreatic Cancer | DRUG: Cyclophosphamide\|DRUG: Nivolumab\|DRUG: Ipilimumab\|DRUG: GVAX Pancreas Vaccine\|DRUG: CRS-207\|DRUG: CRS-207 | Objective Response Rate (ORR) Using Response Evaluation Criteria for Solid Tumors (RECIST 1.1), Objective Response Rate (ORR) is defined as the number of patients achieving a complete response (CR) or partial response (PR) based on RECIST 1.1 criteria. CR = disappearance of all target lesions, PR is =\>30% decrease in sum of diameters of target lesions. Participants who discontinue due to toxicity or clinical progression prior to post-baseline tumor assessments will be considered as non-responders. Participants who discontinue for other reasons prior to their first dose of study drug will not be included in the analysis, 18 months | 61 |
| Epacadostat, Pembrolizumab, and CRS-207, With or Without CY/GVAX Pancreas in Patients With Metastatic Pancreas Cancer | DRUG: Epacadostat\|DRUG: Pembrolizumab\|BIOLOGICAL: CRS-207\|DRUG: Cyclophosphamide\|BIOLOGICAL: GVAX Pancreas Vaccine | Maximum Tolerated Dose (MTD) of Epacadostat, Dose escalation (part I of the trial only) to determine the maximum tolerated dose (MTD) in mg BID. Epacadostat (100, 300, or 600 mg) was taken by mouth twice a day, every day, 9 weeks\|6 Month Survival, Number of subjects who are alive 6 months or longer after the date of first treatment, 6 months | 41 |

| | | | |
|---|---|---|---|
| Safety and Efficacy of Combination Listeria/GVAX Immunotherapy in Pancreatic Cancer | BIOLOGICAL: GVAX Pancreas\|BIOLOGICAL: CRS-207\|DRUG: Cyclophosphamide | Overall Survival (OS) in Subjects Receiving Test Treatments (FAS), For all treated subjects, OS was defined as the time between the date of randomization and the date of death or censoring, and was estimated using Kaplan-Meier (KM) methods with 95% confidence intervals (CIs). Subjects without documentation of death at the time of the final analysis were censored using the date the subject was last known to be alive. Per the study protocol, following an Interim Analysis (IA), subjects in the Cy/GVAX arm were offered rollover to Cy/GVAX + CRS-207 arm. 3 subjects rolled over to the Cy/GVAX + CRS-207 arm (rollover subjects). These rollover subjects were censored at the day prior to the first rollover treatment dose date, and were included for analysis in the Cy/GVAX arm. Additionally, 2 subjects originally treated per the Cy/GVAX + CRS-207 arm discontinued treatment and entered follow-up, but following IA were re-treated per the Cy/GVAX + CRS-207 arm regimen. Data from these "re-treated subjects" were included in the Cy/GVAX + CRS-207 arm analysis. Subjects were followed from the date of randomization to the date of death or discontinuation, whichever came first, assessed up to 60 months. | 93 |

(continued)

**Table 11.6** (continued)

<table>
<tr><th>Study title</th><th>Interventions</th><th>Primary outcome measures</th><th>Enrollment</th></tr>
<tr><td>Cyclophosphamide Plus Vaccine Therapy in Treating Patients With Advanced Cancer</td><td>BIOLOGICAL: allogeneic tumor cell vaccine|BIOLOGICAL: autologous tumor cell vaccine|BIOLOGICAL: recombinant interferon alfa|BIOLOGICAL: recombinant interferon gamma|BIOLOGICAL: sargramostim|DRUG: cyclophosphamide</td><td>Clinical response (patients with evaluable disease)|Duration of response (patients with evaluable disease)|Survival (patients with evaluable disease)|Time to recurrence (patients without evaluable disease)|Survival (patients without evaluable disease)</td><td>40</td></tr>
<tr><td>Vaccine Therapy, Interleukin-2, and Sargramostim in Treating Patients With Advanced Tumors</td><td>BIOLOGICAL: ALVAC-CEA vaccine|BIOLOGICAL: aldesleukin|BIOLOGICAL: sargramostim| BIOLOGICAL: vaccinia-CEA vaccine</td><td></td><td>24</td></tr>
<tr><td>GVAX Pancreas Vaccine (With CY) and CRS-207 With or Without Nivolumab</td><td>BIOLOGICAL: CRS-207|BIOLOGICAL: CRS-207|DRUG: nivolumab|BIOLOGICAL: GVAX|DRUG: CY</td><td>Overall Survival (OS), OS will be measured from date of randomization until death or end of follow-up (OS will be censored on the date the subject was last known to be alive for subjects without documentation of death at the time of analysis), 2 years and 7 months</td><td>93</td></tr>
</table>

| | | | |
|---|---|---|---|
| Safety and Efficacy of Combination Listeria/GVAX Pancreas Vaccine in the Pancreatic Cancer Setting | BIOLOGICAL: GVAX Pancreas Vaccine\|BIOLOGICAL: CRS-207\|DRUG: Chemotherapy\|DRUG: cyclophosphamide | Primary Cohort: Overall Survival (OS) Censored at 138 Deaths (ITT Set), OS was estimated using Kaplan-Meier (KM) methods with 95% confidence intervals (CIs), with censoring at the date when 138 deaths were reached in the Primary Cohort in the FAS. Subjects without documentation of death at the time of final analysis were censored as of the date the subject was last known to be alive on/prior to the primary analysis data cut. Subjects were followed from date of randomization to the date of death by any cause, whichever came first, assessed up to 32 months. Analysis conducted when 138 deaths reached in the Primary Cohort in the FAS.\|Primary Cohort: OS (All Data, FAS), For all treated subjects, OS was calculated using KM methods with 95% CIs. Subjects without documentation of death at the time of the analysis were censored as of the date the subject was last known to be alive on/prior to the final analysis data cut. Subjects followed for survival from date of randomization until lost to follow-up, withdrawal of consent, or death, whichever came first, assessed up to 32 months.\|2nd-line Cohort: OS (All Data, FAS), For all treated subjects, OS was calculated using KM methods with 70% CIs. Subjects without documentation of death at the time of the analysis were censored as of the date the subject was last known to be alive on/prior to the final analysis cut. 70% CIs were selected to provide an 80% probability to rule out differences in median survival less than −2.4 months between the 2nd-line Cohort: Chemotherapy arm and the 2nd-line Cohort: Cy/GVAX + CRS-207 and 2nd-line Cohort: CRS-207 arms, based upon the assumptions made in the statistical analysis plan (SAP). Subjects followed for survival from date of randomization until lost to follow-up, withdrawal of consent, or death, whichever came first, assessed up to 32 months | 303 |

(continued)

**Table 11.6** (continued)

| Study title | Interventions | Primary outcome measures | Enrollment |
|---|---|---|---|
| Anti-CD38 Antibody With KRAS Vaccine and Anti-PD-1 Antibody in Subjects With Pancreatic Ductal Adenocarcinoma and Refractory Non-Small Cell Lung Cancer | DRUG: Daratumumab \|BIOLOGICAL: KRAS vaccine\|DRUG: Nivolumab | Objective Response Rate (ORR) (Efficacy), Evaluation of response by ORR by irRECIST criteria. Response classification will follow the irRECIST criteria and will be defined as PR or CR. Patients who are lost to follow-up without a valid response assessment will be classified as NR (non-responder, progression). The ORR will be computed for all patients with at least one cycle of the study drug, every 8 weeks, approximately 2 years | 54 |
| A Phase I/II Study With CEA(6D) VRP Vaccine in Patients With Advanced or Metastatic CEA-Expressing Malignancies | BIOLOGICAL: AVX701\|BIOLOGICAL: AVX701\|BIOLOGICAL: AVX701\|BIOLOGICAL: AVX701\|BIOLOGICAL: AVX701 | determine the safety of immunization with CEA(6D) VRP, 2.5 years | 28 |
| A Vaccine (Ad5.F35-hGCC-PADRE) for the Treatment of Gastrointestinal Adenocarcinoma | BIOLOGICAL: Adenovirus 5/F35-Human Guanylyl Cyclase C-PADRE | Incidence of adverse events (AEs), AEs classified by System Organ Class, preferred term, severity, and relationship to study treatment, and graded in accordance with the document entitled "Common Terminology Criteria for Adverse Events" (CTCAE), National Cancer Institute version 5 issued by the United States Department of Health and Human Services. Injection-site reactions including, but not necessarily limited to, local skin erythema, induration, pain and tenderness at administration site. Clinically-significant changes in safety laboratory tests. The percentage of subjects with AEs and DLTs will be summarized along with corresponding 95% confidence intervals for each treatment arm and overall. 13 weeks\|Antigen-specific T cell response to guanylyl cyclase C (GCC), Will be measured by enzyme-linked immunosorbent spot (ELISpot) assay. The immune parameters will be summarized via percentages of responders and mean/median values, along with corresponding 95% confidence intervals, by treatment arm and measurement time. Antibody and T cell data will be summarized by positive response rates (each subject recorded as yes/no) and exact 2-sided 95% confidence intervals. For this study, a statistically significant increase in GCC-specific T cell response at Weeks 5, 9, or 13 compared with baseline will be considered a response at that time. Significance of the change from baseline will be assessed using the modified distribution-free resampling (DFR) method. Will estimate response rates across disease types. 13 weeks | 81 |

**Table 11.7** Stem cell-based vaccines

| Study title | Interventions | Primary outcome measures | Enrollment |
|---|---|---|---|
| Safety Study of Cancer Stem Cell Vaccine to Treat Pancreatic Cancer | BIOLOGICAL: cancer stem cell vaccine | The primary study purpose to determine the safety of immunization with cancer stem cells vaccine by the number of participants with adverse events, up to 3 months | 40 |

in Johns Hopkins Hospital. The increased number of species is defined as alpha diversity of the tumor microbiome [106]. When class levels of bacteria were evaluated, long-term survivor tumors exhibited predominance of alpha protein, spinobacteria, and flavobacteria. And the short term survivors were dominated by clostridia and bacterioid class levels.

The gut microbiome cross talks with the tumor microbiome thus this is one mechanism that we can use to shape the immune tumor microenvironment [107]. Recent studies have shown that gut microbiome composition can improve the outcome of cancer immunotherapy such as anti-CTLA4 and anti-PD-L1 by influencing the immune system [108].

An exploratory study suggested an association between microbial composition and treatment response, with Firmicutes potentially being associated with an improved treatment response, and Proteobacteria with a worsened response [109].

### 11.3.6 Immune Modulation with Radiation Therapy

In other tumor types, there has been a growing interest in the use of radiotherapy and immunotherapy combinations. Radiation therapy may act synergistically with immunotherapy by releasing tumor-associated antigens, priming cytotoxic T-cells, and damaging tumor-supporting stroma [110]. The optimal immunostimulatory radiation fractionation regimen is unknown, however, lymphocytes are exquisitely sensitive to radiation. Thus, conventional fractionation regimens delivered over 5–6 weeks can result in significant lymphopenia, which may dampen the effectiveness of immunotherapy [111]. Although historically pancreas radiotherapy required conventional fractionation due to close tumor proximity to bowel, modern radiotherapy techniques such as stereotactic body radiation therapy permit highly conformal treatments in 5 fractions and may provide new opportunities for combination studies with immunotherapy. The SMART (Stereotactic MR-guided Adaptive/Ablative Radiation therapy) trial and approach used five-fraction MRI-guided high-dose radiation therapy and showed promising results. In this study, patients received ablative doses—50 Gy in 5 fractions—with daily online adaptation to account for interfractional changes in anatomy and improve normal tissue sparing. The study enrolled 136 patients across multiple institutions. The results demonstrated that SMART was well tolerated with only 8.8% grade 3 or higher acute GI toxicity possibly or probably attributed to SMART. One-year local control and overall survival from diagnosis were 90.0% and 93.9%, respectively [112]. In a recent study evaluating the role of consolidative radiotherapy for oligometastatic pancreatic cancer, defined as less than or equal to five metastatic sites, radiation therapy has shown a benefit. The EXTEND trial is a multicenter phase II basket trial where 41 patients with oligometastatic pancreatic adenocarcinoma were randomized to standard-of-care systemic therapy compared to systemic therapy and the addition of metastases-directed therapy (MDT). At the median follow-up time of 17 months, median PFS was 10.3 months with MDT vs. 2.5 months with standard of care ($p = 0.030$). This study suggests that there is a subset of favorable metastatic pancreatic adenocarcinoma patients such that radiation therapy may induce systemic immunity in combination with systemic therapy [113].

## 11.4 Immune Signatures in PDAC

Immunotherapy treatments have been met with challenges in eliciting the great responses that these agents have shown in other malignancies such as melanoma and even lung cancer. A recent meta-analysis looking at early-phase trials of immunotherapy showed limited activity in the disease. 4 phase I (23.5%), 2 phase Ib (11.8%), 1 phase Ib/II (5.9%), and 5 phase II (29.4%), 1 retrospective study (5.9%) and 4 prospective studies (23.5%) were included. The median age of the patients was 61 years and 55.6% (398/716) were male. Immunotherapies included were GVAX, tremelimumab, Mesothelin-specific Chimeric Antigen Receptor T cells, durvalumab, pembrolizumab, canerpaturev, sotigalimab, nivolumab, CO-1.01, allogeneic natural killer cell immunotherapy, anti-EGFR chimeric antigen receptor-modified T cells, bispecific antibody armed T cells, and clivatuzumab tetraxetan. The pooled overall response rate was calculated at 16% demonstrating some measurable activity [101].

Immune evasion leads to a poor response to immune checkpoint inhibitors and a poor survival in PDAC. Identifying the key immune escape-related genes which are significantly associated with a PDAC patient's prognosis is an important method to assess and improve the effect of immunotherapy. In addition, molecular biomarkers based on immune escape-related genes have improved prognosis estimation for PDAC in daily clinical practice [96].

One study integrated 27 prognostic immune escape genes to establish an immune escape-related gene prognosis index (IEGPI) score and validated the expression of PTPN2, CEP55, and JAK2 in cell lines, which showed a good prediction in the prognosis of PDAC and immunotherapy response. The IEGPI might represent a potential prognostic biomarker as well as therapeutic targets of immunotherapy in the future. The higher the IEGPI score is, the higher the level of immune escape is, the worse the killing effect of the body's immune system on tumor cells is, and the worse the prognosis is. However, when patients received immunotherapy, patients with higher IEGPI score were more sensitive to immunotherapy. Because immunotherapy alters the tumor microenvironment, these individuals have a higher CR/PR ratio and better prognosis. Therefore, IEGPI score also can be used to screen clinical PDAC patients for immunotherapy, allowing them to achieve a better prognosis [96].

Scores like IEGPI will be an important part in identifying features of each patient's tumor that can be a predictor for response in different treatment modalities. Then selecting the appropriate treatment for each patient can help improve outcomes in each patient based on their tumor behavior and expected response.

## 11.5 Distinct PDAC Behavior Based on Metastasis to Lung Only vs Liver

Isolated pulmonary metastatic disease has significantly better prognosis than patients with liver metastases [98]. This clinical distinction is not unique to PDACs. Similar prognostic contrast has been noted for melanomas and lung cancers, and patients with liver metastases have poorer survival outcomes when treated with PD-1 immune checkpoint therapy when compared with patients who have disease involvement in other visceral sites including lung [99].

These differences have generally been attributed to clonal heterogeneity of the tumor itself, as well as tissue-specific features of the tumor microenvironment (TME) [100]. A deeper understanding of the distinctive features within different metastatic TMEs has the potential to inform future therapeutic strategies and/or identify novel targets for therapy against metastatic PDAC [97].

## 11.6 Team-Based Future Directions for Approaching Challenges, Treatment Strategies, and Drug Development in PDAC

Our ongoing understanding of PDAC and its TME is rapidly evolving. The components that play a large role not only in disease development but PDAC's ability to withstand a large variety of treatment strategies demonstrate this disease's ability to behave in the aggressive nature that we see in patients clinically even today. Even in early-stage disease PDAC patients, recurrence rates are high, and adjuvant therapy continues to have limited efficacy.

With some early evidence vaccines in the right combination and the right patient may have the ability to offer longer-term control of disease. This is crucial in creating a pathway to longer remissions and possible cures in patients with pancreatic cancer. Certainly, it will be important to remember the large benefit in early disease detection at diagnosis with effective adjuvant therapy options for patients in the early stages of PDAC. This gives at least a portion of pancreatic cancer patients the chance for sustainable disease control with possible long-term remission rates.

As we consider the best approaches to treatment in PDAC patients with metastatic disease and a more aggressive disease course, being able to identify which patients may respond best to which therapies and being selective in how we treat patients may offer some improved therapeutic approaches in this complex disease.

Developing strategies to best understand and utilize immune signatures for treatment as well as predicting immune escape mechanisms to guide multiple lines of therapy will be crucial in offering the correct treatments and sequences in a very aggressive disease course.

Collaborating with experts in basic science and drug development to best guide how we can approach each patient in trial by identifying the appropriate patients for the appropriate treatment may be key in developing drugs in a manner that captures their true efficacy in a very complex disease process. As each therapy may be specific to a certain disease pattern, being able to accurately identify these unique signatures with preclinical data that will translate to expected cancer patient responses will help focus therapy and expedite appropriate and effective therapeutic options. Partnering with veterinarians, statisticians, and even experts in artificial intelligence will offer necessary approaches to understanding this complex and rapidly changing disease.

Working together with gastroenterologists and even community practitioners to identify patients with pancreatic cancer early will create a pathway to offer many more patients a chance at longer-term remissions. Furthermore, treating patients early, effectively, and close to home will offer PDAC patients the best chance at a sense of normalcy as well as offer scientists the optimal power in data collection.

Having strong academic institution leadership to its surrounding communities and nationwide will help advance both our understanding of PDAC, its responses on numerous therapies, and allow us to best capture efficacy as well as the null hypothesis early and effectively. With basic science and early phase safety data collection happening at large academic institutions and integrating community practices in phase II and III trials, scientific breakthroughs may be more easily brought to patients and clinical data collection can happen with increasing access for patients and enrollment numbers for higher power data collection in a generally rare disease. Figure 11.1 demonstrates how these trials can be implemented with the larger circles demonstrating further outreach of trials opening at more centers allowing access to more patients. At City of Hope, where the largest academic center is surrounded by community network sites, we have been able to meaningfully bring trials to patients and expand collaboration to offer trials to newly diagnosed patients and patients who may not otherwise have access to an academic center. Not only does this bring treatment options to patients early in drug development, but it helps in enrolling more patients for higher-powered studies and more rapid and meaningful data collection.

As we develop new therapy options with combined modalities including radiation, surgery, and even significant immune responses, medical oncologists will partner with each of these experts and even hematologists to manage cytokine release syndrome and offer PDAC patients a variety of treatment approaches based on their disease pattern.

These powerful partnerships in PDAC research and patient care may be our best chance at creating therapies that can be tested appropriately and brought to patients swiftly with improved responses and hope for effective disease control.

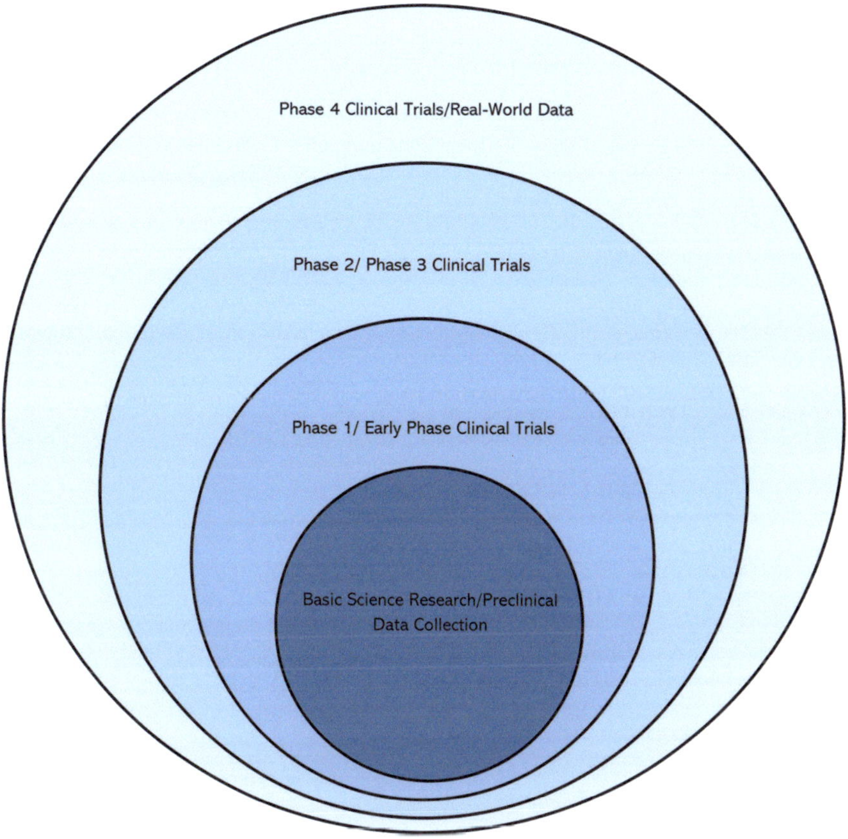


**Fig. 11.1** Interactions between academic institutions and surrounding communities can help advance our understanding of pancreatic cancer its responses to therapies

**Acknowledgments** Data for tables was collected from clinicaltrials.gov.

## References

1. American Cancer Society. Key statistics for pancreatic cancer [Internet]. www.cancer.org. 2024. Available from: https://www.cancer.org/cancer/types/pancreatic-cancer/about/key-statistics.html
2. National Cancer Institute. Cancer of the pancreas—cancer stat facts [Internet]. SEER. National Cancer Institute; 2018. Available from: https://seer.cancer.gov/statfacts/html/pancreas.html
3. Farhangnia P, Khorramdelazad H, Nickho H, Delbandi AA. Current and future immunotherapeutic approaches in pancreatic cancer treatment. J Hematol Oncol. 2024;17(1):40.
4. Carstens JL, Correa de Sampaio P, Yang D, Barua S, Wang H, Rao A, et al. Spatial computation of intratumoral T cells correlates with survival of patients with pancreatic cancer. Nat Commun. 2017;8(1):15095.

5. Orhan A, Vogelsang RP, Andersen MB, Madsen MT, Hölmich ER, Raskov H, et al. The prognostic value of tumour-infiltrating lymphocytes in pancreatic cancer: a systematic review and meta-analysis. Eur J Cancer [Internet]. 2020 [cited 2023 Jan 2];132(0959–8049):71–84. Available from: https://www.sciencedirect.com/science/article/pii/S0959804920301544
6. Alam MS, Gaida MM, Bergmann F, Lasitschka F, Giese T, Giese NA, et al. Selective inhibition of the p38 alternative activation pathway in infiltrating T cells inhibits pancreatic cancer progression. Nat Med [Internet]. 2015 [cited 2025 Apr 6];21(11):1337–43. Available from: https://pmc.ncbi.nlm.nih.gov/articles/PMC4636461/
7. Mucciolo G, Curcio C, Roux C, Li WY, Capello M, Curto R, et al. IL17A critically shapes the transcriptional program of fibroblasts in pancreatic cancer and switches on their protumorigenic functions. Proc Natl Acad Sci. 2021;118(6):e2020395118.
8. Simon F, Lutz V, Brichkina A, Neuhaus F, Ruckenbrod T, Hupfer A, et al. IL-17A-producing CD8+T cells promote PDAC via induction of inflammatory cancer-associated fibroblasts. Gut. 2023;72(8):1510–22.
9. Castro-Pando S, Howell RM, Li L, Mascaro M, Faraoni EY, Roux OL, et al. Pancreatic epithelial IL17/IL17RA signaling drives B7-H4 expression to promote tumorigenesis. Cancer Immunol Res [Internet]. 2024 [cited 2025 Apr 7];12(9):1170–83. Available from: https://aacrjournals.org/cancerimmunolres/article/12/9/1170/747082/Pancreatic-Epithelial-IL17-IL17RA-Signaling-Drives
10. Saravia J, Chapman NM, Chi H. Helper T cell differentiation. Cell Mol Immunol [Internet]. 2019 [cited 2020 Aug 20];16(7):634–43. Available from: https://www.nature.com/articles/s41423-019-0220-6
11. Ene-Obong A, Clear AJ, Watt J, Wang J, Fatah R, Riches JC, et al. Activated pancreatic stellate cells sequester CD8+ T cells to reduce their infiltration of the juxtatumoral compartment of pancreatic ductal adenocarcinoma. Gastroenterology. 2013;145(5):1121–32.
12. Balachandran VP, Łuksza M, Zhao JN, Makarov V, Moral JA, Remark R, et al. Identification of unique neoantigen qualities in long-term survivors of pancreatic cancer. Nature. 2017;551(7681):512–6.
13. Balli D, Rech AJ, Stanger BZ, Vonderheide RH. Immune cytolytic activity stratifies molecular subsets of human pancreatic cancer. Clin Cancer Res. 2017;23(12):3129–38.
14. Vonderheide Robert H. Tumor-promoting inflammatory networks in pancreatic neoplasia: another reason to loathe Kras. Cancer Cell. 2014;25(5):553–4.
15. Pylayeva-Gupta Y, Lee K, Hajdu Cristina H, Miller G, Bar-Sagi D. Oncogenic Kras-induced GM-CSF production promotes the development of pancreatic neoplasia. Cancer Cell. 2012;21(6):836–47.
16. Vignali DAA, Collison LW, Workman CJ. How regulatory T cells work. Nat Rev Immunol [Internet]. 2008;8(7):523–32. Available from: https://www.nature.com/articles/nri2343
17. Hiraoka N, Onozato K, Kosuge T, Hirohashi S. Prevalence of FOXP3+ regulatory T cells increases during the progression of pancreatic ductal adenocarcinoma and its premalignant lesions. Clin Cancer Res [Internet]. 2006 [cited 2019 Dec 11];12(18):5423–34. Available from: https://clincancerres.aacrjournals.org/content/12/18/5423?ijkey=1f82553a4f1cf3c621cb809eadb7c83921b342b5&keytype2=tf_ipsecsha
18. Laskowski TJ, Biederstädt A, Rezvani K. Natural killer cells in antitumour adoptive cell immunotherapy. Nat Rev Cancer. 2022;22(10):557–75.
19. Guerra N, Tan YX, Joncker NT, Choy A, Gallardo F, Xiong N, et al. NKG2D-deficient mice are defective in tumor surveillance in models of spontaneous malignancy. Immunity [Internet]. 2008 [cited 2019 Dec 12];28(4):571–80. Available from: https://www.ncbi.nlm.nih.gov/pmc/articles/PMC3528789/
20. López-Soto A, Gonzalez S, Smyth MJ, Galluzzi L. Control of metastasis by NK cells. Cancer Cell. 2017;32(2):135–54.
21. Huang Q, Huang M, Meng F, Sun R. Activated pancreatic stellate cells inhibit NK cell function in the human pancreatic cancer microenvironment. Cell Mol Immunol. 2018;16(1):87–9.
22. Walle T, Kraske JA, Liao B, Lenoir B, Timke C, von Bohlen Und Halbach E, et al. Radiotherapy orchestrates natural killer cell dependent antitumor immune responses through CXCL8. Sci

Adv [Internet]. 2022 [cited 2023 Mar 14];8(12):eabh4050. Available from: https://pubmed.ncbi.nlm.nih.gov/35319989/
23. Hegde S, Krisnawan VE, Herzog BH, Zuo C, Breden MA, Knolhoff BL, et al. Dendritic cell paucity leads to dysfunctional immune surveillance in pancreatic cancer. Cancer Cell. 2020;37(3):289–307.e9.
24. Takahashi K, Hideyoshi Toyokawa, Takai S, Sohei Satoi, Hiroaki Yanagimoto, Naoyoshi Terakawa, et al. Surgical influence of pancreatectomy on the function and count of circulating dendritic cells in patients with pancreatic cancer. Cancer Immunol Immunother [Internet]. 2005 [cited 2025 Apr 7];55(7):775–84. Available from: https://pmc.ncbi.nlm.nih.gov/articles/PMC11029902/
25. Plesca I, Benešová I, Beer C, Sommer U, Müller L, Wehner R, et al. Clinical significance of tumor-infiltrating conventional and plasmacytoid dendritic cells in pancreatic ductal adenocarcinoma. Cancers [Internet]. 2022;14(5):1216. Available from: https://pmc.ncbi.nlm.nih.gov/articles/PMC8909898/
26. Thomas A, Santarsiero LM, Lutz ER, Armstrong TD, Chen YC, Huang L, et al. Mesothelin-specific CD8+ T cell responses provide evidence of in vivo cross-priming by antigen-presenting cells in vaccinated pancreatic cancer patients. J Exp Med. 2004;200(3):297–306.
27. Gordon S, Taylor PR. Monocyte and macrophage heterogeneity. Nat Rev Immunol. 2005;5(12):953–64.
28. Mantovani A, Marchesi F, Malesci A, Laghi L, Allavena P. Tumour-associated macrophages as treatment targets in oncology. Nat Rev Clin Oncol. 2017;14(7):399–416.
29. Zeng W, Li F, Jin S, Ho PC, Liu PS, Xie X. Functional polarization of tumor-associated macrophages dictated by metabolic reprogramming. J Exp Clin Cancer Res [Internet]. 2023;42(1). Available from: https://www.ncbi.nlm.nih.gov/pmc/articles/PMC10517486/
30. Park JE, Dutta B, Tse SW, Gupta N, Tan CF, Low JK, et al. Hypoxia-induced tumor exosomes promote M2-like macrophage polarization of infiltrating myeloid cells and microRNA-mediated metabolic shift. Oncogene. 2019;38(26):5158–73.
31. Sanford DE, Belt BA, Panni RZ, Mayer A, Deshpande AD, Carpenter D, et al. Inflammatory monocyte mobilization decreases patient survival in pancreatic cancer: a role for targeting the CCL2/CCR2 axis. Clin Cancer Res [Internet]. 2013 [cited 2021 Feb 23];19(13):3404–15. Available from: https://www.ncbi.nlm.nih.gov/pmc/articles/PMC3700620/
32. Yang S, Liu Q, Liao Q. Tumor associated macrophages in pancreatic ductal adenocarcinoma: origin, polarization, function, and reprogramming. Front Cell Dev Biol [Internet]. 2021 [cited 2022 Jan 16];8:607209. Available from: https://www.ncbi.nlm.nih.gov/pmc/articles/PMC7829544/
33. Veglia F, Sanseviero E, Gabrilovich DI. Myeloid-derived suppressor cells in the era of increasing myeloid cell diversity. Nat Rev Immunol. 2021;21(8):485–98.
34. Porembka MR, Mitchem JB, Belt BA, Hsieh CS, Lee HM, Herndon J, et al. Pancreatic adenocarcinoma induces bone marrow mobilization of myeloid-derived suppressor cells which promote primary tumor growth. Cancer Immunol Immunother. 2012;61(9):1373–85.
35. Zhang W, Nandakumar N, Shi Y, Manzano M, Smith A, Graham G, et al. Downstream of mutant KRAS, the transcription regulator YAP is essential for neoplastic progression to pancreatic ductal adenocarcinoma. Sci Signal. 2014;7(324):ra42.
36. Hagenbeek TJ, Zbieg JR, Hafner M, Mroue R, Lacap JA, Sodir NM, et al. An allosteric pan-TEAD inhibitor blocks oncogenic YAP/TAZ signaling and overcomes KRAS G12C inhibitor resistance. Nat Cancer [Internet]. 2023 [cited 2023 Oct 25];4(6):812–28. Available from: https://www.nature.com/articles/s43018-023-00577-0
37. Chapeau EA, Sansregret L, Galli GG, Chène P, Wartmann M, Mourikis TP, et al. Direct and selective pharmacological disruption of the YAP–TEAD interface by IAG933 inhibits Hippo-dependent and RAS–MAPK-altered cancers. Nat Can. 2024;5(7):1102–20.
38. Lasser SA, Ozbay Kurt FG, Arkhypov I, Utikal J, Umansky V. Myeloid-derived suppressor cells in cancer and cancer therapy. Nat Rev Clin Oncol [Internet]. 2024;21(2):147–64. Available from: https://www.nature.com/articles/s41571-023-00846-y#:~:text=MDSCs%20support%20the%20progression%20of%20most%20cancer%20entities

39. Ng M, Kwok I, Tan L, Shi C, Cerezo-Wallis D, Tan Y, et al. Deterministic reprogramming of neutrophils within tumors. Science. 2024;383(6679)
40. Ng LG, Ostuni R, Hidalgo A. Heterogeneity of neutrophils. Nat Rev Immunol. 2019;19(4):255–65.
41. Gentles AJ, Newman AM, Liu CL, Bratman SV, Feng W, Kim D, et al. The prognostic landscape of genes and infiltrating immune cells across human cancers. Nat Med. 2015;21(8):938–45.
42. Chao T, Furth EE, Vonderheide RH. CXCR2-dependent accumulation of tumor-associated neutrophils regulates T-cell immunity in pancreatic ductal adenocarcinoma. Cancer Immunol Res. 2016;4(11):968–82.
43. Masucci MT, Minopoli M, Carriero MV. Tumor associated neutrophils. Their role in tumorigenesis, metastasis, prognosis and therapy. Front Oncol. 2019;9:1146.
44. Nielsen SR, Strøbech JE, Horton ER, Jackstadt R, Laitala A, Bravo MC, et al. Suppression of tumor-associated neutrophils by lorlatinib attenuates pancreatic cancer growth and improves treatment with immune checkpoint blockade. Nat Commun [Internet]. 2021;12(1):3414. Available from: https://www.nature.com/articles/s41467-021-23731-7
45. Luo W, Wen T, Qu X. Tumor immune microenvironment-based therapies in pancreatic ductal adenocarcinoma: time to update the concept. J Exp Clin Cancer Res. 2024;43(1):8.
46. Takahashi R, Macchini M, Sunagawa M, Jiang Z, Tanaka T, Valenti G, et al. Interleukin-1β-induced pancreatitis promotes pancreatic ductal adenocarcinoma via B lymphocyte-mediated immune suppression. Gut [Internet]. 2021;70(2):330–41. Available from: https://pubmed.ncbi.nlm.nih.gov/32393543/
47. Denton AE, Innocentin S, Carr EJ, Bradford BM, Lafouresse F, Mabbott NA, et al. Type I interferon induces CXCL13 to support ectopic germinal center formation. J Exp Med. 2019;216(3):621–37.
48. Mirlekar B, Wang Y, Li S, Zhou M, Entwistle S, De Buysscher T, et al. Balance between immunoregulatory B cells and plasma cells drives pancreatic tumor immunity. Cell Rep Med. 2022;3(9):100744.
49. Mirlekar B, Michaud D, Lee SS, Kren NP, Harris CD, Greene KG, et al. B cell–derived IL35 drives STAT3-dependent CD8+ T-cell exclusion in pancreatic. Cancer. 2020;8(3):292–308.
50. Li S, Mirlekar B, Johnson BM, June Brickey W, Wrobel JA, Yang N, et al. STING-induced regulatory B cells compromise NK function in cancer immunity. Nature. 2022;610(7931):373–80.
51. Tempero M, Oh DY, Tabernero J, Reni M, Van Cutsem E, Hendifar A, et al. Ibrutinib in combination with nab-paclitaxel and gemcitabine for first-line treatment of patients with metastatic pancreatic adenocarcinoma: phase III RESOLVE study. Ann Oncol [Internet]. 2021 [cited 2022 May 23];32(5):600–8. Available from: https://pubmed.ncbi.nlm.nih.gov/33539945/
52. Bubin R, Romans Uljanovs, Ilze Strumfa. Cancer stem cells in pancreatic ductal adenocarcinoma. 2023 [cited 2023 Jun 8];24(8):7030–0. Available from: https://www.ncbi.nlm.nih.gov/pmc/articles/PMC10138709/
53. Chang CH, Liu F, Militi S, Hester S, Nibhani R, Deng S, et al. The pRb/RBL2-E2F1/4-GCN5 axis regulates cancer stem cell formation and G0 phase entry/exit by paracrine mechanisms. Nat Commun. 2024;15(1):3580.
54. Ullah M, Liu DD, Thakor AS. Mesenchymal stromal cell homing: mechanisms and strategies for improvement. iScience. 2019;15:421–38.
55. Lim S, Khoo B. An overview of mesenchymal stem cells and their potential therapeutic benefits in cancer therapy (Review). Oncol Lett. 2021;22(5):785.
56. Chhabra Y, Weeraratna AT. Fibroblasts in cancer: unity in heterogeneity. Cell. 2023;186(8):1580–609.
57. Elyada E, Bolisetty M, Laise P, Flynn WF, Courtois ET, Burkhart RA, et al. Cross-species single-cell analysis of pancreatic ductal adenocarcinoma reveals antigen-presenting cancer-associated fibroblasts. Cancer Discov. 2019;9(8):1102–23.
58. Huang H, Wang Z, Zhang Y, Pradhan RN, Ganguly D, Chandra R, et al. Mesothelial cell-derived antigen-presenting cancer-associated fibroblasts induce expansion of regulatory T cells in pancreatic cancer. Cancer Cell. 2022;40(6):656–673.e7.

59. Bhattacharjee S, Hamberger F, Ravichandra A, Miller M, Nair A, Affo S, et al. Tumor restriction by type I collagen opposes tumor-promoting effects of cancer-associated fibroblasts. J Clin Invest. 2021;131(11):e146987.
60. Raymant M, Astuti Y, Alvaro-Espinosa L, Green D, Quaranta V, Bellomo G, et al. Macrophage-fibroblast JAK/STAT dependent crosstalk promotes liver metastatic outgrowth in pancreatic cancer. Nat Commun. 2024;15(1):3593.
61. Schneiderhan W, Diaz F, Fundel M, Zhou S, Siech M, Hasel C, et al. Pancreatic stellate cells are an important source of MMP-2 in human pancreatic cancer and accelerate tumor progression in a murine xenograft model and CAM assay. J Cell Sci. 2007;120(3):512–9.
62. Cave DD, Di Guida M, Costa V, Sevillano M, Ferrante L, Heeschen C, et al. TGF-β1 secreted by pancreatic stellate cells promotes stemness and tumourigenicity in pancreatic cancer cells through L1CAM downregulation. Oncogene [Internet]. 2020;39(21):4271–85. Available from: https://www.nature.com/articles/s41388-020-1289-1
63. Sherman MH, Beatty GL. Tumor microenvironment in pancreatic cancer pathogenesis and therapeutic resistance. Annu Rev Pathol Mech Dis. 2023;18(1):123–48.
64. Rhim AD, Oberstein PE, Thomas DH, Mirek ET, Palermo CF, Sastra SA, et al. Stromal elements act to restrain, rather than support, pancreatic ductal adenocarcinoma. Cancer Cell [Internet]. 2014 [cited 2021 Dec 9];25(6):735–47. Available from: https://pubmed.ncbi.nlm.nih.gov/24856585/
65. Nisar M, Paracha RZ, Adil S, Qureshi SN, Janjua HA. An extensive review on preclinical and clinical trials of oncolytic viruses therapy for pancreatic cancer. Front Oncol. 2022;12:875188.
66. Lou E. Oncolytic herpes viruses as a potential mechanism for cancer therapy. Acta Oncol (Stockholm, Sweden) [Internet]. 2003;42(7):660–71. Available from: https://pubmed.ncbi.nlm.nih.gov/14690152/
67. Musher BL, Rowinsky EK, Smaglo BG, Abidi W, Othman M, Patel K, et al. LOAd703, an oncolytic virus-based immunostimulatory gene therapy, combined with chemotherapy for unresectable or metastatic pancreatic cancer (LOKON001): results from arm 1 of a non-randomised, single-centre, phase 1/2 study. Lancet Oncol [Internet]. 2024 [cited 2025 Apr 8];25(4):488–500. Available from: https://www.thelancet.com/journals/lanonc/article/PIIS1470-2045(24)00079-2/abstract
68. Mahalingam D, Chen S, Xie P, Loghmani H, Heineman T, Kalyan A, et al. Combination of pembrolizumab and pelareorep promotes anti-tumour immunity in advanced pancreatic adenocarcinoma (PDAC). Br J Cancer [Internet]. 2023 [cited 2025 Apr 8];129(5):782–90. Available from: https://pmc.ncbi.nlm.nih.gov/articles/PMC10449917/
69. Chen Y, Chen X, Bao W, Liu G, Wei W, Ping Y. An oncolytic virus–T cell chimera for cancer immunotherapy. Nat Biotechnol. 2024;42(12):1876–87.
70. Rosenberg SA, Restifo NP, Yang JC, Morgan RA, Dudley ME. Adoptive cell transfer: a clinical path to effective cancer immunotherapy. Nat Rev Cancer [Internet]. 2008;8(4):299–308. Available from: https://www.ncbi.nlm.nih.gov/pmc/articles/PMC2553205/
71. Fridman WH, Pagès F, Sautès-Fridman C, Galon J. The immune contexture in human tumours: impact on clinical outcome. Nat Rev Cancer [Internet]. 2012;12(4):298–306. Available from: https://www.nature.com/articles/nrc3245
72. Hall M, Liu H, Malafa MP, Centeno BA, Hodul PJ, Pimiento JM, et al. Expansion of tumor-infiltrating lymphocytes (TIL) from human pancreatic tumors. J Immunother Cancer. 2016;4(1):61.
73. Levin N, Kim SP, Marquardt CA, Vale NR, Rosenberg SA. Neoantigen-specific stimulation of tumor-infiltrating lymphocytes enables effective TCR isolation and expansion while preserving stem-like memory phenotypes. J ImmunoTher Cancer [Internet]. 2024;12(5). Available from: https://www.researchgate.net/publication/381027736_Neoantigen-specific_stimulation_of_tumor-infiltrating_lymphocytes_enables_effective_TCR_isolation_and_expansion_while_preserving_stem-like_memory_phenotypes
74. Henson SN, Elko EA, Swiderski PM, Liang Y, Engelbrektson AL, Piña A, et al. PepSeq: a fully in vitro platform for highly multiplexed serology using customizable DNA-barcoded

peptide libraries. Nat Protocols [Internet]. 2022 [cited 2025 Apr 8];18(2):396–423. Available from: https://www.nature.com/articles/s41596-022-00766-8
75. Chung V, Soldi R, Ghosh-Halder T, Huang P, Chih S, Lin M, et al. Clinical development of STL-101, a personalized Til therapy for treatment of advance solid tumors 1 [Internet]. [cited 2025 Apr 8]. Available from: https://jitc.bmj.com/content/jitc/12/Suppl_2/A781.full.pdf
76. Chung MJ, Park JY, Bang S, Park SW, Song SY. Phase II clinical trial of ex vivo-expanded cytokine-induced killer cells therapy in advanced pancreatic cancer. Cancer Immunol Immunother [Internet]. 2014 [cited 2025 Apr 8];63(9):939–46. Available from: https://pmc.ncbi.nlm.nih.gov/articles/PMC11029701/
77. Wang Z, Liu Y, Li R, Shang Y, Zhang Y, Zhao L, et al. Autologous cytokine-induced killer cell transfusion increases overall survival in advanced pancreatic cancer. J Hematol Oncol [Internet]. 2016 [cited 2021 Nov 19];9:6. Available from: https://www.ncbi.nlm.nih.gov/pmc/articles/PMC4740990/
78. Heumann T, Judkins C, Li K, Lim SJ, Hoare J, Parkinson R, et al. A platform trial of neoadjuvant and adjuvant antitumor vaccination alone or in combination with PD-1 antagonist and CD137 agonist antibodies in patients with resectable pancreatic adenocarcinoma. Nat Commun [Internet]. 2023 [cited 2023 Jul 17];14(1):3650. Available from: https://www.nature.com/articles/s41467-023-39196-9
79. McCormick KA, Coveler AL, Rossi GR, Vahanian NN, Link CJ, Gabriela Chiorean E. Pancreatic cancer: update on immunotherapies and algenpantucel-L. Hum Vaccin Immunother. 2015;12(3):563–75.
80. Rong Y, Qin X, Jin D, Lou W, Wu L, Wang D, et al. A phase I pilot trial of MUC1-peptide-pulsed dendritic cells in the treatment of advanced pancreatic cancer. Clin Exp Med [Internet]. 2012;12(3):173–80. Available from: https://pubmed.ncbi.nlm.nih.gov/21932124/
81. Kobayashi M, Shimodaira S, Nagai K, Ogasawara M, Takahashi H, Abe H, et al. Prognostic factors related to add-on dendritic cell vaccines on patients with inoperable pancreatic cancer receiving chemotherapy: a multicenter analysis. Cancer Immunol Immunother [Internet]. 2014 [cited 2025 Apr 8];63(8):797–806. Available from: https://pmc.ncbi.nlm.nih.gov/articles/PMC11028555/
82. Kimura Y, Tsukada J, Tomoda T, Takahashi H, Imai K, Shimamura K, et al. Clinical and immunologic evaluation of dendritic cell–based immunotherapy in combination with gemcitabine and/or S-1 in patients with advanced pancreatic carcinoma. Pancreas. 2012;41(2):195–205.
83. Bernhardt SL, Gjertsen MK, Trachsel S, Møller M, Eriksen JA, Meo M, et al. Telomerase peptide vaccination of patients with non-resectable pancreatic cancer: a dose escalating phase I/II study. Br J Cancer. 2006;95(11):1474–82.
84. Asahara S, Takeda K, Yamao K, Maguchi H, Yamaue H. Phase I/II clinical trial using HLA-A24-restricted peptide vaccine derived from KIF20A for patients with advanced pancreatic cancer. J Transl Med [Internet]. 2013;11:291. Available from: https://pubmed.ncbi.nlm.nih.gov/24237633/
85. Pant S, Wainberg ZA, Weekes CD, Furqan M, Kasi PM, Devoe CE, et al. Lymph-node-targeted, mKRAS-specific amphiphile vaccine in pancreatic and colorectal cancer: the phase 1 AMPLIFY-201 trial. Nat Med [Internet]. 2024 [cited 2024 Feb 3]:1–12. Available from: https://www.nature.com/articles/s41591-023-02760-3
86. Cappello P, Rolla S, Chiarle R, Principe M, Cavallo F, Perconti G, et al. Vaccination with ENO1 DNA prolongs survival of genetically engineered mice with pancreatic cancer. Gastroenterology. 2013;144(5):1098–106.
87. Mandili G, Curcio C, Bulfamante S, Follia L, Ferrero G, Mazza E, et al. In pancreatic cancer, chemotherapy increases antitumor responses to tumor-associated antigens and potentiates DNA vaccination. J ImmunoTher Cancer [Internet]. 2020;8(2):e001071. Available from: https://jitc.bmj.com/content/8/2/e001071
88. Gong YF, Zhou QB, Liao YD, Mai C, Chen TJ, Tang YQ, et al. Optimized construction of MUC1-VNTRn DNA vaccine and its anti-pancreatic cancer efficacy. Oncol Lett [Internet].

2017 [cited 2025 Apr 8];13(4):2198–206. Available from: https://pmc.ncbi.nlm.nih.gov/articles/PMC5403551/
89. Geng F, Dong L, Bao X, Guo Q, Guo J, Zhou Y, et al. CAFs/tumor cells co-targeting DNA vaccine in combination with low-dose gemcitabine for the treatment of Panc02 murine pancreatic cancer. Mol Ther Oncolytics. 2022;26:304–13.
90. Rojas LA, Sethna Z, Soares KC, Olcese C, Pang N, Patterson E, et al. Personalized RNA neoantigen vaccines stimulate T cells in pancreatic cancer. Nature [Internet]. 2023;618(7963):1–7. Available from: https://www.nature.com/articles/s41586-023-06063-y
91. Le DT, Wang-Gillam A, Picozzi V, Greten TF, Crocenzi T, Springett G, et al. Safety and survival with GVAX pancreas prime and listeria monocytogenes–expressing mesothelin (CRS-207) boost vaccines for metastatic pancreatic cancer. J Clin Oncol [Internet]. 2015;33(12):1325–33. Available from: https://www.ncbi.nlm.nih.gov/pmc/articles/PMC4397277/pdf/zlj1325.pdf
92. Raman V, Howell LM, Shoshana HCL, Wetherby VE, Minter LM, et al. Intracellular Salmonella delivery of an exogenous immunization antigen refocuses CD8 T cells against cancer cells, eliminates pancreatic tumors and forms antitumor immunity. Front Immunol. 2023;14:1228532.
93. Schmitz-Winnenthal FH, Hohmann N, Niethammer AG, Friedrich T, Lubenau H, Springer M, et al. Anti-angiogenic activity of VXM01, an oral T-cell vaccine against VEGF receptor 2, in patients with advanced pancreatic cancer: a randomized, placebo-controlled, phase 1 trial. Onco Targets Ther. 2015;4(4):e1001217.
94. Kooreman NG, Kim Y, de Almeida PE, Termglinchan V, Diecke S, Shao NY, et al. Autologous iPSC-based vaccines elicit anti-tumor responses in vivo. Cell Stem Cell [Internet]. 2018;22(4):501–513.e7. Available from: https://www.cell.com/action/showPdf?pii=S1934-5909%2818%2930016-X
95. Ouyang X, Liu Y, Zhou Y, et al. Antitumor effects of iPSC-based cancer vaccine in pancreatic cancer. Stem Cell Rep [Internet]. 2021; Available from: https://www.sciencedirect.com/science/article/pii/S2213671121001995?via%3Dihub
96. Lu H, Zheng LY, Wu LY, Chen J, Xu N, Mi SC. The immune escape signature predicts the prognosis and immunotherapy sensitivity for pancreatic ductal adenocarcinoma. Front Oncol [Internet]. 2022 [cited 2025 Apr 15];12. Available from: https://pmc.ncbi.nlm.nih.gov/articles/PMC9486201/
97. Ho WJ, Erbe R, Danilova L, Phyo Z, Bigelow E, Stein-O'Brien G, et al. Multi-omic profiling of lung and liver tumor microenvironments of metastatic pancreatic cancer reveals site-specific immune regulatory pathways. Genome Biol. 2021;22(1):154.
98. Kruger S, Haas M, Burger PJ, Ormanns S, Modest DP, Westphalen CB, et al. Isolated pulmonary metastases define a favorable subgroup in metastatic pancreatic cancer. Pancreatology [Internet]. 2016;16(4):593–8. Available from: https://www.sciencedirect.com/science/article/abs/pii/S1424390316300096?via%3Dihub
99. Tazdait M, Mezquita L, Lahmar J, Ferrara R, Bidault F, Ammari S, et al. Patterns of responses in metastatic NSCLC during PD-1 or PDL-1 inhibitor therapy: comparison of RECIST 1.1, irRECIST and iRECIST criteria. Eur J Cancer [Internet]. 2018 [cited 2020 Feb 26];88:38–47. Available from: https://www.sciencedirect.com/science/article/pii/S0959804917313576
100. Oliver AJ, Lau PKH, Unsworth AS, Loi S, Darcy PK, Kershaw MH, et al. Tissue-dependent tumor microenvironments and their impact on immunotherapy responses. Front Immunol. 2018;9:70.
101. Shahzad M, Vyas A, Dave P, Irfan S, Khan A, Chaudhry A, et al. Clinical outcomes of immunotherapy in metastatic pancreatic carcinoma: a systematic review and meta-analysis. J Clin Oncol. 2025;43(4 Suppl):688.
102. Seufferlein T, Arnold D, Burkhart N, Reinacher-Schick AC, Ungerechts G, Martens UM, et al. GOBLET study: results of the safety run-in for first-line metastatic pancreatic ductal adenocarcinoma (PDAC) patients treated with pelareorep + modified FOLFIRINOX +/− atezolizumab. J Clin Oncol. 2025;43(4 Suppl):730.

103. Dean AP, Sjoquist K, Gebski V, Karapetis CS, Lomma C, Burge ME, et al. AGITG ASCEND: randomised, double-blind phase II study of certepetide or placebo added to gemcitabine plus nab-paclitaxel in patients with untreated metastatic pancreatic ductal adenocarcinoma: initial results. J Clin Oncol. 2025;43(4 Suppl):728.
104. Dean AP, Johansson M, Yusoff I, Rao S, Sparrow S, Kumarasinghe P, et al. Immunotherapy engagement in pancreatic adenocarcinoma: provisional results of iLSTA study—durvalumab, LSTA1 (certepetide), gemcitabine, and nab-paclitaxel for locally advanced pancreatic ductal adenocarcinoma. J Clin Oncol. 2025;43(4 Suppl):746.
105. Ebia M, Abbas AA, Dotson S, Elmadbouh OHM, Davelaar J, Hendifar AE, et al. CD8+ T cell proximity analysis of the tumor microenvironment (TME) in patients with pancreatic ductal adenocarcinoma (PDAC) and associated clinical outcomes. J Clin Oncol. 2025;43(4 Suppl):754.
106. Riquelme E, Zhang Y, Zhang L, Montiel M, Zoltan M, Dong W, et al. Tumor microbiome diversity and composition influence pancreatic cancer outcomes. Cell [Internet]. 2019;178(4):795–806.e12. Available from: https://www.ncbi.nlm.nih.gov/pmc/articles/PMC7288240/pdf/nihms-1537195.pdf
107. Kharofa J, Haslam D, Wilkinson R, Weiss A, Patel S, Wang K, et al. Analysis of the fecal metagenome in long-term survivors of pancreas cancer. Cancer. 2023;129(13):1986–94.
108. Zhang M, Liu J, Xia Q. Role of gut microbiome in cancer immunotherapy: from predictive biomarker to therapeutic target. Exp Hematol Oncol. 2023;12(1):84.
109. Dean AP, Comito OR, Yusoff I, Rao S, Johansson M, Navadgi S, et al. Potential effect of the gut microbiome on tumour response to anti-cancer treatment in patients diagnosed with pancreatic ductal adenocarcinoma. J Clin Oncol. 2025;43(4 Suppl):757.
110. Bernstein MB, Krishnan S, Hodge JW, Chang JY. Immunotherapy and stereotactic ablative radiotherapy (ISABR): a curative approach? Nat Rev Clin Oncol. 2016;13(8):516–24.
111. Ko EC, Formenti SC. Radiation therapy to enhance tumor immunotherapy: a novel application for an established modality. Int J Radiat Biol. 2019;95(7):936–9.
112. Chuong MD, Lee P, Low DA, Kim J, Mittauer KE, Bassetti MF, et al. Stereotactic MR-guided on-table adaptive radiation therapy (SMART) for borderline resectable and locally advanced pancreatic cancer: a multi-center, open-label phase 2 study. Radiother Oncol. 2024;191:110064.
113. Ludmir EB, Sherry AD, Fellman BM, Liu S, Bathala T, Haymaker C, et al. Addition of metastasis-directed therapy to systemic therapy for oligometastatic pancreatic ductal adenocarcinoma (EXTEND): a multicenter, randomized phase II trial. J Clin Oncol. 2024;42(32):3795–805.

# Advancing Prostate Cancer Treatment: Innovations and Challenges in Immunotherapy

12

Gargi Singhal, Pankaj Garg, Atish Mohanty, Sudarsan Vishnu Kollimuttathuillam, Deric Wheeler, Bamidele A. Adesunloye, and Sharad S. Singhal

## Abbreviations

| | |
|---|---|
| ADT | Androgen Deprivation Therapy |
| AI | Artificial Intelligence |
| ATM | Ataxia Telangiectasia Mutated |
| BRCA1/2 | Breast Cancer 1 and 2 (genes) |
| CAR-T | Chimeric Antigen Receptor T-Cell |
| CTLA-4 | Cytotoxic T-Lymphocyte-Associated Protein 4 |
| DNA | Deoxyribonucleic Acid |
| ddMMR | Deficient Mismatch Repair |
| GVAX | Granulocyte-Macrophage Colony-Stimulating Factor-Based Vaccine |
| ICIs | Immune Checkpoint Inhibitors |

G. Singhal
Undergraduate Medical Sciences, S.N. Medical College Agra, Agra, Uttar Pradesh, India

P. Garg
Department of Chemistry, GLA University, Mathura, Uttar Pradesh, India

A. Mohanty · S. S. Singhal (✉)
Department of Medical Oncology & Therapeutics Research, Beckman Research Institute of City of Hope, Comprehensive Cancer Center and National Medical Center, Duarte, CA, USA
e-mail: ssinghal@coh.org

S. V. Kollimuttathuillam
Department of Medical Oncology, City of Hope, Irvine, CA, USA

D. Wheeler
Department of Human Oncology, School of Medicine and Public Health, University of Wisconsin, Madison, WI, USA

Carbone Cancer Center, University of Wisconsin, Madison, WI, USA

B. A. Adesunloye
City of Hope, Newnan, GA, USA



R. Salgia, P. Kulkarni (eds.), *Immunotherapies in Solid Tumors*, Cancer Treatment and Research 129, https://doi.org/10.1007/978-3-031-97242-3_12

| | |
|---|---|
| IL | Interleukin |
| irAEs | Immune-Related Adverse Events |
| LAG3 | Lymphocyte Activation Gene-3 |
| MDSCs | Myeloid-Derived Suppressor Cells |
| MSI | Microsatellite Instability |
| NK Cells | Natural Killer Cells |
| PARP | Poly (ADP-Ribose) Polymerase |
| PD-1 | Programmed Death-1 |
| PD-L1 | Programmed Death-Ligand 1 |
| TCR | T-Cell Receptor |
| TAA | Tumor-Associated Antigens |
| TAMs | Tumor-Associated Macrophages |
| TIM-3 | T-Cell Immunoglobulin and Mucin-Domain Containing-3 |
| TILs | Tumor-Infiltrating Lymphocytes |
| TIGIT | T-cell Immunoreceptor with Ig and ITIM Domains |
| TME | Tumor Microenvironment |
| Tregs | Regulatory T cells |
| TSA | Tumor-Specific Antigens |

## 12.1 Introduction

Prostate cancer (PCa) is among the world's most prevalent malignancies in male patients, even though there exist geographic and racial disparities in incidences and mortality rates. It is the second most prevalent type of cancer and the number one cancer killer in men. PCa generally runs an indolent course but can be rapidly aggressive in the late stages, with metastasis affecting patient survival and quality of life [1]. Surgery, irradiation, and androgen deprivation therapy (ADT) have been proven effective; however, these treatments are most effective at localized disease stages. These approaches have been proven less adequate in the relapse of latent, advanced, or castration-resistant prostate cancer (CRPC), wherein the therapeutic options are constrained and therefore the survival rate of the patient is less favorable [2].

Immunotherapy is one of the biggest advancements in the world of cancer and has shifted the landscape in different cancers, such as melanoma, lung, and bladder cancers over the last few years. Although immunotherapy has not been as successful in PCa as compared with other cancer types, research is still ongoing to explore and improve its utility [3]. Immunologically, PCa has certain associated factors that make immunotherapies less effective, such as low tumor mutational burden (TMB) and immunosuppressive features with few infiltrating immune cells [4]. Novel approaches such as cancer vaccines, immune checkpoint inhibitors (ICIs), and adoptive cell therapies are giving an initial indication of successful outcomes when used in conjunction with other treatment modalities, including ADT or radiotherapy [5].

This chapter is written to introduce the readers to the present state and future prospect of immunotherapy in PCa. Here, we outline the immunological profile of

PCa, overview known and novel immuno-therapeutic strategies, and assess their implementation in clinical trials. Further, the chapter focuses on prospects and outlooks, including challenges, opportunities, and future developments in the rapidly growing field of PCa treatment. This chapter highlights the importance of immunotherapy in changing the approach to managing PCa to generate good prognoses and better treatment outcomes for patients [6].

## 12.2 Immunological Landscape of PCa

PCa is truly regarded as an immunogenic malignancy, which concludes that the cross-interactions between the cancer cells and the tumor microenvironment (TME) still needs further explorations. The TME in PCa is made of cellular and non-cellular components, such as immune cells, stromal cells, endothelial cells, and ECM, which can influence the progression of disease and its therapy intervention. Unlike most other tumors, which are considered "hot", or possessing a preponderance of infiltrating immune cells and a favorable environment that encourages antitumor immunity, PCa is considered as "cold" [7].

Of the immune cells commonly identified within the prostate TME, T cells, macrophages, and natural killer (NK) cells are especially important. T cells and particularly CD8+ cytotoxic T cells, which are prime for direct tumor cell lysis, can be present either at low levels or have an altered function at the site of the prostate tumor. On the other hand, regulatory T cells (Tregs) are reported to be present in high numbers and reduce the functions of effector T cells, thus down-regulating the immune response. Among them, tumor-associated macrophages (TAMs), which are mainly in M2 state, play a crucial role in immune evasion by supporting angiogenesis, tissue remodeling, and suppression of the anti-tumor immune response. Finally, NK cells capable of exhibiting antitumor activity may become impaired by immunosuppressive signals in the TME [8, 9].

PCa cells utilize several immunosuppressive tactics to escape the surveillance of the immune system. These include inhibition of cytokines that have pro-inflammatory effects (e.g., TGF-β and IL-10) and modulation of immune-checkpoint molecules, namely PD-L1. Moreover, an acidotic and hypoxic TME affects the responsiveness of the immune effector cells as well [10]. The second major reason for immune evasion in PCa is the low neoantigen burden of the tumor. In contrast with other highly mutated cancers, such as melanoma, a limited number of prostate tumor-specific neoantigens are generated, which are more likely to be recognized by the immune system [11]. Tumor cells also reduce their antigenicity through antigen masking, down-regulation of major histocompatibility complex (MHC) class II molecules, and also by recruiting immunosuppressive cell populations to the tumor site [12].

As a result, knowledge and comprehension of the immunological nature of the prostate and TME are important for devising the immunotherapies. Thus, immunization and enhancement of immunogenicity in Pca can respond to challenges such as immune suppression and low immunogenicity to allow for altering PCa to an immunologically manageable disease with improved therapeutic impacts.

## 12.3 Established Immunotherapy Modalities in PCa

Immunotherapy has created a glimmer of hope in the management of cancer, and among all the malignancies, PCa, which was traditionally considered as immune refractory, has experienced a new ray of hope in this field. Other therapeutic approaches of immunotherapy include cancer vaccines, ICIs, adoptive cell therapies, and cytokine therapies; all these approaches are employed with the aim of improving the immunity-mediated killing of cancer cells. Indeed, each modality has demonstrated a different degree of success, but sustained developments bear the singular intention of countering the barriers of the PCa microenvironment [13].

### 12.3.1 Cancer Vaccines

PCa vaccines as a type of immunotherapy can be regarded as the first generation of treatment at the cellular level.

- **Sipuleucel-T**: Sipuleucel, being the first cancer vaccine accredited by the FDA, particularly for patients with metastatic castration-resistant prostate cancer (mCRPC), is an autologous cellular immunotherapy medication. It entails an isolation of the patient's peripheral blood mononuclear cells, mainly the antigen-presenting cells (APCs), which are then activated ex vivo by the use of recombinant fusion protein (PAP-GM-CSF) [14]. These cells, upon reinfusion, elicit an immunogenicity against prostate-specific antigen (PSA) positive tumor cells. In clinical trials, the beneficial effect on survival has been confirmed and the median overall survival of patients has been reported to be increased by about 4 months. Despite its efficacy, Sipuleucel-T is not commonly used because of logistic difficulties, high cost, and relatively moderate effectiveness [15].
- **DNA-Based Vaccines**: PROSTVAC, an allogeneic viral vector-based vaccine targeted at the PSA, has its value proven in terms of eliciting constructive T-cell reactions. PROSTVAC activates T cell and improves immune recognition by incorporating poxvirus vectors, which deliver PSA and immune costimulatory molecules. Initial phases demonstrated enhanced mCRPC patient survival, but subsequent phase III trials failed to attain the primary goals; thus, there is an urgent need for pursuing combination strategies to overcome resistance [16, 17].
- **Peptide Vaccines**: GVAX is a cellular vaccine made from genetically engineered PCa cells that release granulocyte-macrophage colony-stimulating factor (GM-CSF) to promote immune reactions. Early in vivo studies showed favorable immunogenicity; however, clinical trials combined with docetaxel showed only moderate gains because of issues such as insufficient activation of T cells and immune-checkpoint blockade [18, 19].
- **Limitations and Challenges**: Nonetheless, cancer vaccines including prostate-specific membrane antigen (PSMA) have some drawbacks like low immunogenicity, tumor heterogeneity, and immunosuppressive property of the prostate

TME. For enhanced outcomes, synergistic therapies with ICIs, cytokines, or radiation therapy are being experimented with [20].

### 12.3.2 Immune Checkpoint Inhibitors (ICIs)

ICIs change the standard of care in a number of cancers by waking up T cells that have been rendered inactive by inhibitory signals. Nevertheless, their use in PCa has been hampered by the fact that PCa tumor exhibits a generally low mutation rate and immunosuppressive TME [21].

- **CTLA-4 Inhibitors**: This includes a class of cytotoxic T-lymphocyte-associated protein 4 (CTLA-4) inhibitors, including ipilimumab and antagonists of the anti-stimulatory signals that dampen immune response [22]. Some studies carried out on ipilimumab in patients with PCa initially proved only moderate effectiveness; however, special effects were observed in cases with low disease burden or after combinatorial radiation therapy [23].
- **PD-1/PD-L1 Inhibitors**: Targets of ICIs include programmed death-1 (PD-1) like pembrolizumab and programmed death-ligand 1 (PD-L1) inhibitors. In mCRPC patients, clinical trials have produced only a limited response, particularly in those with a "Deficient Mismatch Repair" (dMMR) or high microsatellite instability (MSI). These inhibitors, therefore, encounter difficulties because of marginal responses in PCa [24].
- **Challenges**: The inherent ability of PCa to suppress the immune system and the low immunogenicity of the cancer tissue compromises the effectiveness of ICIs. To overcome these barriers current research focuses on combinatorial treatments where ICIs are combined with target therapies, radiation, or vaccines [25].

### 12.3.3 Adoptive Cell Therapies (ACT)

- ACT entail modifying the patient's immune system to make their cells better at identifying cancerous cells. In the PCa, this is an emerging field with great potential [26].
- **CAR-T Cell Therapies**: Chimeric antigen receptor (CAR)-T cell therapies have transformed the treatment pedagogy of hematologic malignancies but face obstacles in treating solid malignancies such as PCa. CAR-T cells have been designed for targeting PSMA. The efficacy of trials is modest mainly due to the suppressive nature of the TME and off-target toxicities [27].
- **TCR-Based Therapies**: T-cell receptor (TCR)-based therapies can recognize intracellular tumor antigens on the surface of antigen-presenting cells via MHC molecules. Antigens on the surface of tissue and cancer cells have been examined; for instance, NY-ESO-1 antigens present in PCa cells. As with any outlined therapy, TCR-based therapies face challenges in the form of antigen heterogeneity and immune evasion mechanisms [28] (Fig. 12.1 and Table 12.1).

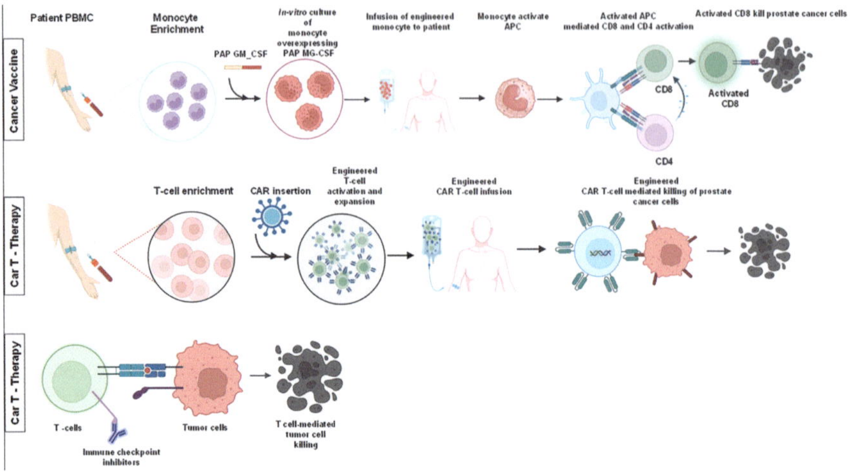


**Fig. 12.1** Mechanisms of immunotherapy in PCa. Schematic representation of the key immunotherapy strategies used in PCa treatment. This includes cancer vaccines (e.g., Sipuleucel-T), which stimulate the immune system to target PCa cells, checkpoint inhibitors (e.g., PD-1/PD-L1 inhibitors), which block immune checkpoints and enhance anti-tumor immunity, and adoptive T-cell therapies, where T cells are engineered to recognize and kill PCa cells. Each therapy's mechanism is outlined within the context of the immune response and PCa cell targeting

### 12.3.4 Cytokine-Based Immunotherapies

Cytokine treatments include the introduction of agents that affect the functional activity of the immune system to encompass greater scaling of the immune cells.

- **IL-2 and IL-12**: Interleukin-2 (IL-2) promotes T-cell growth, NK cell activation, T-cell cytotoxicity, and Th-1 response [29]. In PCa, these cytokines have proven to be ineffective if used singly because their toxicity is systemic, and the cytokines' half-life is short [30].
- **Combination Strategies**: Cytokines, when used with ICIs or cancer vaccines, have higher efficacy in terms of the preclinical data. For example, to enhance the efficacy of PD-1 inhibitors, IL-12 has been used and demonstrates the possibility to overcome resistance in the prostate TME [31].

Cytokine-based therapies are still considered as promising. New delivery systems are being sought, and cytokine toxicity has been mitigated. Altogether, both of the described established immunotherapy modalities reveal further advancements in overcoming the peculiarities of PCa. Despite the limitations that exist in various forms of cancer treatment methods, future prospects look bright because of the development of combination therapies and delivery systems [32].

**Table 12.1** Established and emerging immunotherapy strategies for PCa treatment

| Immunotherapy modality | Description | Examples/therapies | Mechanism of action | Challenges | References |
|---|---|---|---|---|---|
| Cancer vaccines | Stimulate the immune system to recognize and attack prostate cancer cells. | Sipuleucel-T, PROSTVAC, GVAX | Induces antigen-specific immune responses. | Limited efficacy, challenges in overcoming TME suppression | [16, 18, 20] |
| Immune checkpoint inhibitors | Block inhibitory signals that suppress immune cell activity, allowing enhanced anti-tumor response. | CTLA-4 inhibitors, PD-1/PD-L1 inhibitors | Enhances T-cell-mediated immune responses by blocking inhibitory signals. | Low response rates, TME resistance | [21, 49, 55] |
| Adoptive cell therapies | Transfer ex vivo expanded immune cells back into the patient to target cancer cells. | CAR-T cell therapies, TCR-based therapies | Reprogramming and expanding immune cells to target cancer-specific antigens. | Limited efficacy in solid tumors, TME-related challenges | [13, 54, 82] |
| Cytokine-based immunotherapies | Use cytokines to stimulate immune cell activity and increase immune response to tumors. | IL-2, IL-12, combination with checkpoint inhibitors | Boosts immune cell proliferation and activation. | Toxicity, limited clinical success | [29–31] |
| Oncolytic viruses | Viruses engineered to selectively infect and kill cancer cells, while stimulating immune responses. | Clinical trials for oncolytic viral therapies in prostate cancer | Direct tumor cell destruction and immune stimulation. | Safety, delivery issues, limited evidence | [35–37] |
| Neoantigen-based therapies | Target cancer-specific antigens unique to tumor cells, personalized to each patient's cancer. | Personalized vaccines, T-cell therapies | Targets specific mutations in tumor cells, generating a personalized immune response. | Difficulty in identifying neoantigens, tumor heterogeneity | [11, 38, 40] |
| Bispecific antibodies | Engineered antibodies that can simultaneously bind to two different targets, enhancing immune response. | Emerging studies in prostate cancer | Bridges T cells and tumor cells, enhancing immune activation. | Complexity in design and manufacturing | [41–43] |

## 12.4 Emerging Immunotherapy Approaches

The drawbacks of conventional immunotherapy in PCa have led to the emergence of new approaches designed to modulate immune tolerance and improve targeting of the tumor. New strategies like oncolytic viruses, neoantigens based on individualized immunotherapy, and bispecific antibodies present new opportunities to counter the issues characterized with PCa physiology. From the mechanistic perspective, current experimental therapies have focused on improving tumor specificity, immune engagement, and creating long-term therapeutic outcomes in patients [33].

### 12.4.1 Oncolytic Viruses

- Oncolytic viruses are viruses that have been modified genetically or are naturally occurring and preferentially kill tumor cells, while leaving the rest of the body tissues intact. Both types directly act on cancer cells, while also mobilizing the body's immune system, and are considered ideal for the treatment of PCa [34].
- **Mechanisms of Action and Clinical Relevance**: Oncolytic viruses are toxic to tumor cells wherein they replicate, lyse, and subsequently offer tumor antigens. This process not only kills cancer cells, but also induces a very powerful antitumor immune response mediated by dendritic cells, T cells, and other immune effector cells at the tumor site. Similar to the way oncolytic viruses infect tumor cells, these viruses can be designed to release immune-stimulating factors, including cytokines or ICIs [35].
- **Case Studies in PCa**: CG0070 (modified adenovirus that produces a GM-CSF) and ProstAtak (HSV-TK) have been used as oncolytic viruses for the treatment of PCa in early-phase trials [36]. To date, these viruses have shown to be safe and have moderate antitumor activity when combined with ICIs or radiotherapy. Oncolytic viruses are not fully developed yet but are expected to become a revolutionary approach in future treatments of PCa [37].

### 12.4.2 Neoantigen-Based Personalized Immunotherapy

Neoantigens are proteins, developed because of genetic mutations and present specifically on tumor cells, and are excellent candidates for immunotherapy. Unlike normal antigens, neoantigens are expressed on tumor cells but not on normal tissues, so there is minimal crossfire reported on normal cells and thus specificity in immunotherapy [38].

- **Development of Personalized Vaccines and T-Cell Therapies**: Personalized vaccines are developed mathematically through neoantigen prediction algorithms from patients' tumor samples and are produced and deployed to the patients. The development of these vaccines generates a strong T-cell response to the tumor; however, their treatment for use in PCa is still limited. Salutations to the use of next-generation sequencing and development of molecular biology and bioinformatics techniques that the therapy for neoantigen is constantly growing [39]. Furthermore, neoantigen-specific T-cell therapies include identifying and activating the T cells from a particular patient, identifying neoantigens, and then reinfusing the altered cells. These therapies are most effective for patients with higher genomic or molecular alterations like DNA damage repair abnormalities in prostate tumors. Initial evidence indicates that patient-tailored neoantigen-guided treatments could provide a survival benefit to specific groups of patients [40] (Table 12.1).

### 12.4.3 Bispecific Antibodies and Immune Engagers

Bispecific antibodies are constructed as two distinct antigens, a tumor antigen and a T-cell receptor, allowing the labeling of cancer cells and bringing immune cells closer to the tumor, thus promoting tumor cell killing [41].

- **Mechanisms and Emerging Data in PCa**: The most developed type of constructs is bispecific T-cell engagers (BiTEs). In the case of PCa, BiTEs against both PSMA and CD3 on T cells are being investigated. These molecules attract only cytotoxic T cells to bind to the tumor mass, resulting in a sustained focal immune response and tumor cell apoptosis [42].

Initial reports of bispecific antibodies in clinical trials of PCa did not reveal any severe toxicities; however, future research is directed toward enhancing pharmacokinetic properties of bispecific antibodies and minimizing off-target effects. Other combinational strategies include involvement with ICIs or CAR-T therapies, which remain under investigation. These novel immunotherapy approaches offer room for improvement for PCa therapies. Also, their association with new approaches and individual plans enhances a number of therapeutic options for treating this complex disease [43].

## 12.5 Challenges in Immunotherapy for PCa

PCa remains an intractable model for immunotherapy because of its specific biological and immunological peculiarities, even with the recent developments of immunotherapy treatments. The immunosuppressive tumor microenvironment, lack of ideal therapeutic biomarkers, and managing immune-related adverse events (irAEs) as complementary issues; all endure as the main challenges that need to be addressed to enhance the effectiveness of treatment [44].

### 12.5.1 Immunosuppressive TME: Factors That Hinder Therapeutic Effects

The PCa TME is highly immunosuppressive, representing a major challenge to the success of immunotherapy approaches. High TME density is defined by the dense stroma surrounded by a cancer cell landmass, low TMB, and a high number of Tregs, MDSCs, and TAMs. Together these elements suppress the activation and function of cytotoxic T cells, which are all important in antitumor immunity [45]. Moreover, synthesized inhibitory cytokines, like transforming growth factor-(TGF-β) and interleukin-10(IL-10), are produced by prostate tumors in order to inhibit immune activation. These concerns present immense challenges that can only be mitigated by non-traditional strategies such as an aberrant focus on stromal factors or by reprogramming the immune milieu, or by a unique combination of immunotherapy and treatments that directly or indirectly target the TME (for instance, radiation or other targeted therapies) [46] (Fig. 12.2).

### 12.5.2 Predicting Biomarkers of Responsiveness to Therapy and Drug Resistance

The understanding of criteria by which biomarkers can be trusted is critical for the prognosis of patients who may undergo immunotherapy, and critical for the evasion of resistance. In PCa treatment, the absence of biomarkers has been a key reason why survival rates and treatment methods for a given patient have not been clearly determined [47]. For instance, dMMR and MSI are genetically rare in patients with PCa but are clinically linked with improved ICI sensitivity. On the other hand, biomarkers of resistance include low PD-L1 expression and TILs, and high levels of immunosuppressive cytokines that led to poor overall survival. Genomic, proteomic, and transcriptomic strategies for identifying new biomarkers, including tumor neoantigens and immune-gene signatures, that could be potentially used in tailoring immunotherapy for PCa are being developed [48].

### 12.5.3 Managing Immune-Related Adverse Events (irAEs)

Immune-related adverse events (irAEs) are critically imponderable, affecting the applicability of immunotherapy. These adverse events are the outcome of immune triggering against normal tissues and involve all organ systems, such as the integumentary, gastrointestinal, hepatobiliary pulmonary, and endocrine systems. While mild irAEs can be effectively treated with corticosteroids or immunosuppressive drugs, severe irAEs imply cessation of treatment, and therefore, observable limitations to effectiveness [49]. In PCa characterized by low immunogenicity, at the onset of treatment, irAEs might also occur as a result of a heightened immune response triggered by combination therapies. Optimization of approaches and methods for early identification and

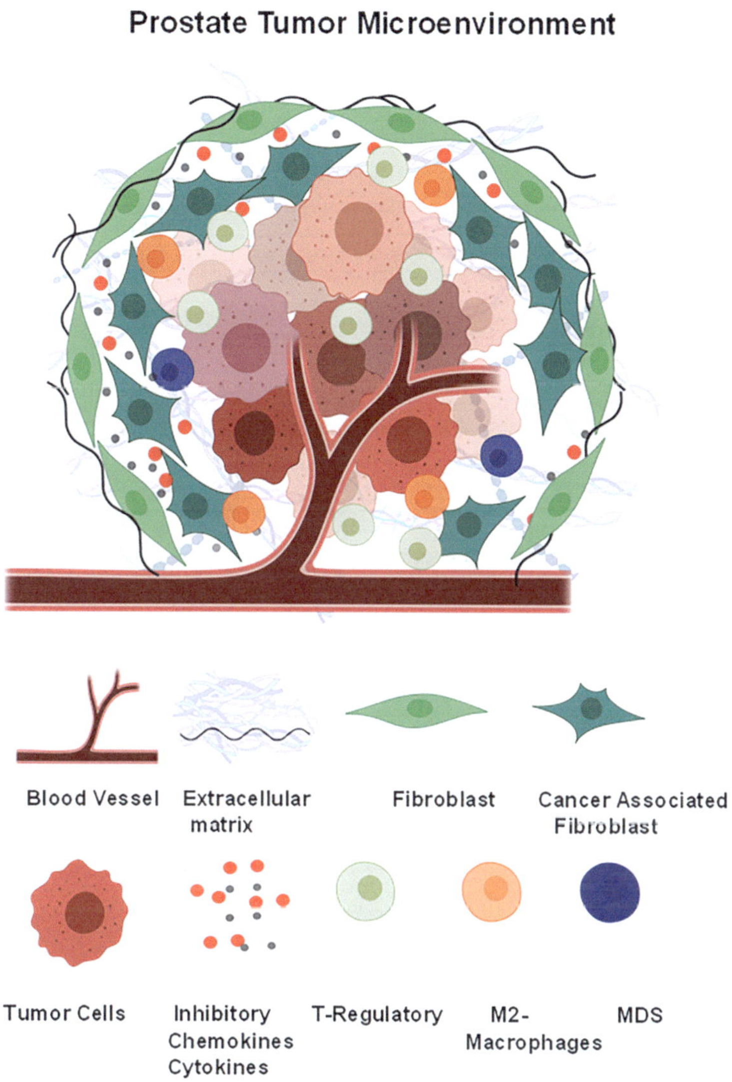


**Fig. 12.2** TME in PCa and immunotherapy. Illustration of the PCa TME and its interactions with immune cells, including T cells, dendritic cells, macrophages, and myeloid-derived suppressor cells (MDSCs). This figure highlights immune suppression within the TME via factors such as TGF-β, IL-10, and other cytokines, which inhibit the effective immune response against cancer. The role of immunotherapy in overcoming these immune barriers and enhancing therapeutic efficacy is also depicted

management of irAEs is essential for the manipulation of immunotherapy. The principles include patient education and multimodality involvement of oncologists, immunologists, and various other specialists [50]. Overcoming these challenges will lead to the advancement in knowledge of the underlying immunological theories, development of appropriate biomarkers to enhance patient enrollment, and more effective strategies in the prevention of aberrant effects. These are important approaches that need to be addressed to make progress toward the attainment of ideal immunotherapy régimes within PCa [51].

## 12.6 Combination Strategies

Combination therapies hold the potential of addressing the shortcomings of single immunotherapy in PCa. Combination strategies are applied to cancer treatments in the hopes of increasing the antitumor effects and patient survival, and to deal with mechanisms that are responsible for drug resistance. The combination of immunotherapy with hormone therapy (ADT), radiation, and molecular therapy, such as PARP inhibitors, has exhibited preclinical and clinical benefits [52] (Fig. 12.3 and Table 12.2).

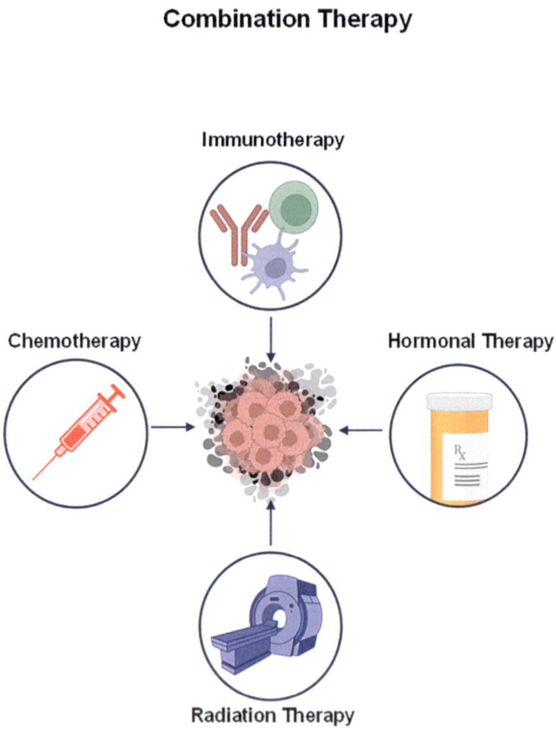


**Fig. 12.3** Combination therapies for PCa immunotherapy. Schematic depicting the potential benefits of combination therapies in PCa treatment. Immunotherapy (e.g., ICIs, cancer vaccines, adoptive T-cell therapies) is shown in combination with radiotherapy, hormonal therapy, and chemotherapy to enhance anti-tumor immune responses, modulate the TME, and reduce immune resistance. The synergistic effects of combining these treatments are represented to emphasize their potential to improve therapeutic outcomes in PCa patients

**Table 12.2** Key challenges and strategies for overcoming barriers in PCa immunotherapy

| Immunotherapy challenge | Challenge description | Impact on treatment | Impact on patient outcome | Potential solutions/ strategies | References |
|---|---|---|---|---|---|
| Immunosuppressive tumor microenvironment (TME) | The prostate TME inhibits immune cell function and limits the effectiveness of immunotherapies. | Suppresses immune response, reducing immune cell infiltration and activation against tumors. | Leads to poor therapeutic outcomes due to immune evasion. | Combination therapies, targeted immune modulation, oncolytic viruses | [7, 31, 45] |
| Limited predictive biomarkers | Difficulty in identifying biomarkers to predict response to immunotherapy. | Lack of reliable biomarkers leads to ineffective patient stratification, resulting in non-responsive treatments. | Delays treatment effectiveness and risks unnecessary toxicity. | Genomic and transcriptomic profiling, AI-driven analysis for biomarker discovery | [64, 67, 70] |
| Immune-related adverse events (irAEs) | Adverse immune responses triggered by immunotherapy causing toxicity. | Causes inflammation and damage to healthy tissues like skin, liver, and intestines, leading to treatment disruption. | Reduces patients' quality of life and may necessitate halting treatment. | Monitoring strategies, immune-suppressive drugs, dose adjustments | [44, 49, 50] |
| Low response rates | Many patients exhibit poor response to immunotherapy, especially those with advanced prostate cancer. | Results in tumor progression despite treatment, necessitating alternative therapies. | Limited improvement in survival and clinical outcomes for a significant number of patients. | Personalized immunotherapy, combination therapies, TME modulation | [28, 59, 69] |
| TME resistance to immune checkpoints | Tumor cells within the TME evade immune recognition through immune checkpoint expression. | Prevents effective T-cell activation and immune response, leading to therapeutic resistance. | Results in immune escape and reduced clinical efficacy of immunotherapy. | Targeting TME-specific immune checkpoints, enhancing immune cell infiltration | [47–49] |
| Tumor heterogeneity | Variability in tumor antigens complicates the development of universal therapies. | Inconsistent expression of antigens on tumor cells limits the effectiveness of antigen-targeted immunotherapies. | Causes incomplete responses and failure of one-size-fits-all treatments. | Neoantigen-based personalized therapies, multi-target approaches | [74–76] |

### 12.6.1 Immunotherapy with Androgen Deprivation Therapy (ADT)

ADT is currently a widely used approach for the treatment of PCa, primarily for advanced and metastatic disease. ADT lowers the level of androgens, resulting in the slower growth of androgen-dependent PCa cells. Apart from the aforementioned effects, ADT has an influence on the immune system and makes the immune system susceptible to immunotherapy [53].

- **Mechanisms of Synergy**: ADT boosts the density of T cells in the TME and decreases the number of immunosuppressive Tregs; at the same time, it increases tumor antigen presentation, enhancing their recognition by the immune response. This immunomodulatory effect offers a rationale for using ADT with ICIs, cancer vaccines, or adoptive cell therapies [54].
- **Clinical Evidence**: The combination of ADT with ICIs, including pembrolizumab and nivolumab, is currently under investigation with the hope of early improvement in immune activity. Moreover, several early-phase cancer vaccine studies have shown that ADT enhances the effectiveness of cancer antigens like sipuleucel-t through the upregulation of antigen presentation [55].

### 12.6.2 Synergetic Interactions Between Radiotherapy and Immunotherapy

Radiotherapy is an effective treatment option in localized as well as advanced-stage PCa. This important fact is recognized along with the immune-modulating effect of radiotherapy, which can enhance immunotherapy [56].

- **Mechanisms of Synergy**: Radiotherapy triggers immunogenic cell death and promotes the shedding of tumor-associated antigens and maturation of dendritic cells. This process is called the abscopal effect, and it can trigger broad antitumor immunity. This process also impacts the TME so that tumors are sensitized to inhibitors of PD-1/PD-L1 or CTLA-4 by modulating them [57].
- **Clinical Evidence**: The integration of radiotherapy with ICIs has been rapidly explored in clinical trials [58]. For instance, in trials that have looked at ipilimumab (CTLA-4 inhibitor) combined with radiation therapy in mCRPC, individual variation in immune activation has been observed. Nonetheless, the best IRRT fractionation and timing are still under investigation today [59] (Fig. 12.3).

### 12.6.3 Combining Immunotherapy with Targeted Therapies (e.g., PARP Inhibitors)

Hormonal agents secondary to chemo-sensitive drug combinations, including PARP inhibitors, have been established to treat castration-sensitive PCa harboring DNA damage repair (DDR) dysfunction like BRCA1/2 mutations [60]. These targeted therapies are incorporated with immunotherapy with the intention of capitalizing on their synergistic therapeutic pathways.

- **Mechanisms of Synergy**: PARP inhibitors will necessarily target the DNA of cancer cells and bring about the generation of neoantigens and tumor antigens. These effects help stimulate the cGAS–STING signaling that increases the type I interferon response and T-cell immunity [61]. Also, PARP inhibitors can enhance the immune checkpoint molecules because they cause resistance to PD-1/PD-L1 inhibitors [62].
- **Clinical Evidence**: The first-line trials testing PARP inhibitors, such as olaparib or rucaparib combined with ICIs, demonstrate some potential in PCa patients with DDR alteration. These combinations are being investigated in mCRPC and earlier stages of the disease [63]. Additionally, animal studies indicate that such combinations can reverse immunotherapy resistance in patients with low TMB.

Combined approaches reflect a leap forward in the management of PCa and have benefits that increase when delivered in combination with other options. Further work has to be performed in order to fine-tune these strategies, establish biomarkers of response and primary resistance, and define the order that therapies should be given to produce optimal outcomes and have low toxicity [64].

## 12.7 New Developments in the Identification of Biomarkers

Biomarker discovery is one of the key ways used to forge further progress in immunotherapy for PCa. Selecting patients, particularly for drug interventions, and gauging therapeutic as well as curative outcomes are made possible by employing valid biomarkers [65]. In PCa, the understanding of immune checkpoint blockade, the development of biomarkers to predict responses to immune therapy, and the application of genomics and transcriptomics for individualized therapy have been greatly advanced [66] (Table 12.2).

### 12.7.1 Predictive Biomarkers for Immunotherapy Response

It is crucial to identify biomarkers that could be useful for the prognosis of immunotherapy responses in order to increase the level of treatment differentiation. This is especially the case in PCa, in which the response to immune-based therapies varies and therefore predictive biomarkers are still a potential tool for precise treatment [67].

- **PD-L1 Expression**: While PD-L1 has been used as a biomarker in many other cancers, its relevance for PCa has been somewhat limited by low expression levels and the immunosuppressive TME. But patients with high levels of PD-L1 may still benefit from the use of PD-1/PD-L1 inhibitors in combination therapy [68] (Fig. 12.3).

- **Tumor Mutational Burden (TMB)**: The high TMB is associated with enhanced neoantigen presentation and improved outcomes on ICIs. Low TMB characterizes PCa in a general way; however, some patients have high TMB owing to DNA MMR or MSI, which provides a good response to immunotherapy [69].
- **Immune Gene Signatures**: Recent studies revealed the potential of immune gene expression signatures that are associated with immunotherapy outcomes [70]. Finally, researchers are using specific gene sets, such as T-cell inflamed gene signatures and interferon-gamma-related pathways, to predict patients' responses to ICIs [71].
- **Circulating Biomarkers**: The technologic advancements related to ctDNA have led to an increasing interest in the use of liquid biopsies to assess treatment response without frequent invasive procedures. Among these, CTCs, exosomes, and immune cells in the blood are now probed as promising dynamic biomarkers of immunotherapeutic clinical trials [72].

## 12.8 Role of Genomic and Transcriptomic Profiling in PCa

Personalized genomics and transcriptomic profile are now rapidly changing the horoscope of personalized care in PCa [73]. These technologies allow an evaluation of tumor biology and immune interface, defining drug targets and mechanisms of resistance (Table 12.2).

- **Genomic Alterations and Neoantigens**: Molecular characterizations have identified targetable alterations in DDR genes, including BRCA1/2 and ATM, which predict heightened antigens and sensitivity to PARP and immune blockade [74]. Moreover, dysregulations of PTEN and TP53 genes are also associated with immune changes, which may monitor combination treatments [75].
- **Transcriptomic Insights**: Specifically, transcriptomic data provides information about immune infiltration, cytokine profiles, and pathway activation in the TME. For example, RNA sequencing can define the pattern indicating the activation of the immune system that correlates with sensitization to immunotherapy [76].
- **Personalized Treatment Approaches**: Genomic as well as transcriptomic data will help clinicians personalize the immunotherapy approach that is suitable for a given patient. For instance, patients who have MSI-high or dMMR alterations can be preferential candidates for ICI treatment, and patients with distinct transcriptomic patterns may require new combinations or investigational treatments [77].

The identification of biomarkers in immunotherapy signaling is beginning to open up new avenues of specific and efficient utilization of PCa treatment. Future work on the identification of novel biomarkers for the prognosis of PCa and performing the multiple layers of omics analyses will be instrumental in overcoming therapeutic barriers and delivering the best possible care for patients [78].

## 12.9 Future Perspectives

Immunotherapy for PCa is still in its juvenile phase in terms of treatment preferences; however, remarkable progress has been made relating to the development of new therapies, incorporating innovative technology, and using research and development to support in bringing all forms of cancer treatment to those in need around the globe. These future perspectives indicate an opportunity to shift the PCa perspective from treatment to a more efficient, personalized, and accessible one [79, 80].

### 12.9.1 New Advancements in Immunotherapy for PCa

Some of the promising new approaches that can be viewed as proficient in overcoming the shortcomings of existing strategies, while extending their use, are illustrated below.

- **Next-Generation Vaccines**: Current research is focused on designing the new generation of cancer vaccines with neoantigens, multi-epitope targets, and improved adjuvants. mRNA vaccines mimicking those created for SARS-CoV-2 and other system-targeting malignancies are rapidly becoming the next rational frontline, enduring optimal antitumor immune responses [81].
- **Improved Adoptive Cell Therapies**: Novel therapies such as CAR-T and TCR-based approaches along with addressing the immunosuppressive TME could improve the progression of PCa treatment. Ideas like CAR-T cells that can withstand TME suppression are being considered [82].
- **Targeting New Immune Checkpoints**: In addition to PD-1/PD-L1 and CTLA-4, other immune checkpoints like TIM-3, LAG-3, and TIGIT are explored as potential targets. These inhibitors can also enhance other therapies or offer benefits to patients for whom standard treatments are ineffective [83].
- **Oncolytic Immunotherapy**: It is becoming prevalent to use oncolytic viruses in PCa cells to promote their lysis and stimulate the immune response. These therapies work together, directly killing tumor cells with bystander effects, which enhance the immune response against the tumor [84].

### 12.9.2 Role of AI in Personalized Immunotherapy Development

Modern immunotherapies are currently on the precipice of a new wave of enhancement through the integration of artificial intelligence (AI), which is set to provide the best way to enhance the feasibility of developing treatment plans [85].

- **Patient Stratification**: Currently, there are opportunities to use AI algorithms to recognize patients who will respond to certain immunotherapies based on multiomic data. As a result, finding conclusions in genomic, transcriptomic, and proteomic data through the use of AI contribute to precision medicine decisions based on tumor bio-specificity [86].

- **Therapeutic Development**: Machine learning models are helping to expand the understanding of antigen characterization, the definition of immune checkpoint, and the discovery of optimal combination therapies. AI also contributes to the identification of T-cell targets, the adjustment of T-cell engineering, the assessment of CAR-T cell outcomes, and the design of neoantigen vaccines [87].
- **Real-Time Monitoring**: Tools derived from AI help evaluate how quickly the response to treatment is based on imaging and biomarker parameters. AI also helps to identify resistance strategies to counteract on time [88].
- **Clinical Trial Optimization**: AI applications are revolutionizing the immunotherapy trial process through predicting recruitment outcome, deciding endpoints, and analyzing trial data [89].

### 12.9.3 Global Outlook: Addressing Disparities in Immunotherapy Access

Although immunotherapy can indeed be a revolutionary immunotherapy, the issue of disparities in the distribution of healthcare is still an issue, even on an international level.

- **Economic Barriers**: The cost of vaccine therapy and cell-based therapy is high, therefore posing a major challenge in accessing immunotherapy in low- and middle-income countries (LMICs). Strategies for making immunotherapies cheaper, for the development of improved manufacturing methods, and for increased availability of generic biologics are therefore important [90].
- **Healthcare Infrastructure**: CAR-T cell therapies, for example, are complex to manufacture, and may need additional amenities such as a CAR-T production facility. Future global capacity has to be built up and healthcare workers in LMICs have to be trained [91].
- **Equitable Research Representation**: A lack of participation from certain groups is one reason to diversify and address disparities in clinical trial participation to make immunotherapies effective for all. It is therefore important to increase the participation of patients from under-represented regions [92].
- **Policy and Advocacy**: It is imperative that governments and international organizations create policies with a goal to minimize the cost and technical requirements of immunotherapy applications. Synchronized efforts of patient organizations can help to ensure that the availability and cost of these innovative procedures are more reasonable [93].

## 12.10 Conclusion

Immunotherapy can be considered as the dawn of new treatments in PCa, promising the merging of developments and ideas. This modality of treatment including cancer vaccines, ICIs, and adoptive cell therapy, has the capacity to overcome many challenges associated with traditional strategies. Furthermore, recent advancements regarding biomarkers and the use of multiple immunotherapies have refined the precision and efficacy of immunotherapy, significantly improving patient prognoses. New-generation therapies like neoantigen-based vaccines, bispecific antibodies, and oncolytic viruses are today formulating the skyline of the upcoming PCa treatment paradigm that provides deeper and more enduring remission [94].

**Vision for Integrating Immunotherapy into Standard Care**
The next step in immunotherapy is the integration with standard of care, which will define the future management of PCa. To realize this vision, continued research into the best therapeutic strategies and strategies to overcome resistance will be required. Integrating AI and multi-omics approaches will also create possibilities for a highly individualized approach to patient care in the hopes of an effective treatment [95]. Additionally, it is crucial to level the gap when it comes to immunotherapy on an international level, as the purpose is to make these therapies available to everyone. Immunotherapy can meet its potential, also known as the "meaningful model", and deliver the durable, real, and equitable benefit that advanced PCa patients seek by recognizing the emergent innovations and addressing current difficulties [5].

## 12.11 Clinical Significance

This chapter highlights the transformative potential of immunotherapy in PCa treatment, offering a paradigm shift from traditional therapies by addressing their limitations and delivering durable, targeted outcomes. It explores groundbreaking innovations, including cancer vaccines, ICIs, and adoptive cell therapies, which, when paired with biomarker-driven precision and combination strategies, significantly enhance therapeutic efficacy. Furthermore, this chapter underscores emerging approaches and global initiatives aimed at improving accessibility, paving the way for immunotherapy to become a cornerstone in the comprehensive management of PCa.

**Acknowledgments** The figures were made using https://biorender.com.

**Declaration of Competing Interest** The authors have no conflicts of interest to disclose.

**Consent for Publication** Not applicable.

**Ethics Approval** Not applicable.

**Availability of Data and Material** No new data was created or analyzed in this study. Data sharing is not applicable to this article.

**Authors Contributions** GS; PG; SSS: had the idea for the article and performed the literature search, and writing—original draft preparation. PG; AM: review and editing. All authors read and approved the final manuscript.

**Funding** The National Cancer Institute of the National Institutes of Health (P30CA33572) and the United States Department of Defense (W81XWH-22-1-0331 and HT9425-25-1-0500) both provided funding for this project. Also appreciated is financial support from City of Hope's Beckman Research Institute.

## References

1. Rawla P. Epidemiology of prostate cancer. World J Oncol. 2019;10(2):63–89. https://doi.org/10.14740/wjon1191.
2. Choi E, Buie J, Camacho J, Sharma P, de Riese WTW. Evolution of androgen deprivation therapy (ADT) and its new emerging modalities in prostate cancer: an update for practicing urologists, clinicians and medical providers. Res Rep Urol. 2022;14:87–108. https://doi.org/10.2147/RRU.S303215.
3. Garg P, Pareek S, Kulkarni P, Horne D, Salgia R, Singhal SS. Next-generation immunotherapy: advancing clinical applications in cancer treatment. J Clin Med. 2024;13(21):6537. https://doi.org/10.3390/jcm13216537.
4. Wang I, Song L, Wang BY, Rezazadeh Kalebasty A, Uchio E, Zi X. Prostate cancer immunotherapy: a review of recent advancements with novel treatment methods and efficacy. Am J Clin Exp Urol. 2022;10(4):210–33.
5. Adamaki M, Zoumpourlis V. Immunotherapy as a precision medicine tool for the treatment of prostate cancer. Cancer. 2021;13(2):173. https://doi.org/10.3390/cancers13020173.
6. Kim JE, Lee K, Kim IY. Current update on prostate cancer immunotherapy. J Urol Oncol. 2023;21(1):14–22. https://doi.org/10.22465/juo.234600100005.
7. Feng D, Xiong Q, Wei Q, Yang L. Cellular landscape of tumour microenvironment in prostate cancer. Immunology. 2023;168(2):199–202. https://doi.org/10.1111/imm.13456.
8. Novysedlak R, Guney M, Al Khouri M, Bartolini R, Koumbas Foley L, Benesova I, Ozaniak A, Novak V, Vesely S, Pacas P, Buchler T, Ozaniak Strizova Z. The immune microenvironment in prostate cancer: a comprehensive review. Oncology. 2024:1–25. Advance online publication. https://doi.org/10.1159/000541881.
9. Yang YL, Yang F, Huang ZQ, Li YY, Shi HY, Sun Q, Ma Y, Wang Y, Zhang Y, Yang S, Zhao GR, Xu FH. T cells, NK cells, and tumor-associated macrophages in cancer immunotherapy and the current state of the art of drug delivery systems. Front Immunol. 2023;14:1199173. https://doi.org/10.3389/fimmu.2023.1199173.
10. Dutta S, Ganguly A, Chatterjee K, Spada S, Mukherjee S. Targets of immune escape mechanisms in cancer: basis for development and evolution of cancer immune checkpoint inhibitors. Biology. 2023;12(2):218. https://doi.org/10.3390/biology12020218.
11. Xie N, Shen G, Gao W, et al. Neoantigens: promising targets for cancer therapy. Signal Transduct Target Ther. 2023;8:9. https://doi.org/10.1038/s41392-022-01270-x.
12. Taylor BC, Balko JM. Mechanisms of MHC-I downregulation and role in immunotherapy response. Front Immunol. 2022;13:844866. https://doi.org/10.3389/fimmu.2022.844866.

13. Schweizer MT, Drake CG. Immunotherapy for prostate cancer: recent developments and future challenges. Cancer Metastasis Rev. 2014;33(2–3):641–55. https://doi.org/10.1007/s10555-013-9479-8.
14. Cheever MA, Higano CS. PROVENGE (Sipuleucel-T) in prostate cancer: the first FDA-approved therapeutic cancer vaccine. Clin Cancer Res. 2011;17(11):3520–6. https://doi.org/10.1158/1078-0432.CCR-10-3126.
15. Madan RA, Antonarakis ES, Drake CG, Fong L, Yu EY, McNeel DG, Lin DW, Chang NN, Sheikh NA, Gulley JL. Putting the pieces together: completing the mechanism of action jigsaw for Sipuleucel-T. J Natl Cancer Inst. 2020;112(6):562–73. https://doi.org/10.1093/jnci/djaa021.
16. Cole G, McCaffrey J, Ali AA, et al. DNA vaccination for prostate cancer: key concepts and considerations. Cancer Nano. 2015;6:2. https://doi.org/10.1186/s12645-015-0010-5.
17. Yehya A, Ghamlouche F, Zahwe A, Zeid Y, Wakimian K, Mukherji D, Abou-Kheir W. Drug resistance in metastatic castration-resistant prostate cancer: an update on the status quo. Cancer Drug Resist. 2022;5(3):667–90. https://doi.org/10.20517/cdr.2022.15.
18. Zhou W, Lu X, Tian F, Luo Q, Zhou W, Yang S, Li W, Yang Y, Shi M, Zhou T. Vaccine therapies for prostate cancer: current status and future outlook. Vaccine. 2024;12(12):1384. https://doi.org/10.3390/vaccines12121384.
19. Simons JW, Sacks N. Granulocyte-macrophage colony-stimulating factor-transduced allogeneic cancer cellular immunotherapy: the GVAX vaccine for prostate cancer. Urol Oncol. 2006;24(5):419–24. https://doi.org/10.1016/j.urolonc.2005.08.021.
20. Kaczmarek M, Poznańska J, Fechner F, Michalska N, Paszkowska S, Napierała A, Mackiewicz A. Cancer vaccine therapeutics: limitations and effectiveness—a literature review. Cells. 2023;12(17):2159. https://doi.org/10.3390/cells12172159.
21. Marei HE, Hasan A, Pozzoli G, Cenciarelli C. Cancer immunotherapy with immune checkpoint inhibitors (ICIs): potential, mechanisms of resistance, and strategies for reinvigorating T cell responsiveness when resistance is acquired. Cancer Cell Int. 2023;23(1):64. https://doi.org/10.1186/s12935-023-02902-0.
22. Buchbinder E, Hodi FS. Cytotoxic T lymphocyte antigen-4 and immune checkpoint blockade. J Clin Invest. 2015;125(9):3377–83. https://doi.org/10.1172/JCI80012.
23. Reese Z, Straubhar A, Pal SK, Agarwal N. Ipilimumab in the treatment of prostate cancer. Future Oncol. 2015;11(1):27–37. https://doi.org/10.2217/fon.14.196.
24. Isaacsson Velho P, Antonarakis ES. PD-1/PD-L1 pathway inhibitors in advanced prostate cancer. Expert Rev Clin Pharmacol. 2018;11(5):475–86. https://doi.org/10.1080/17512433.2018.1464388.
25. Garg P, Malhotra J, Kulkarni P, Horne D, Salgia R, Singhal SS. Emerging therapeutic strategies to overcome drug resistance in cancer cells. Cancer. 2024;16(13):2478. https://doi.org/10.3390/cancers16132478.
26. Restifo NP, Dudley ME, Rosenberg SA. Adoptive immunotherapy for cancer: harnessing the T cell response. Nat Rev Immunol. 2012;12(4):269–81. https://doi.org/10.1038/nri3191.
27. Ho M, Zanwar S, Paludo J. Chimeric antigen receptor T-cell therapy in hematologic malignancies: successes, challenges, and opportunities. Eur J Hematol. 2024;112(2):197–210. https://doi.org/10.1111/ejh.14074.
28. Golikova EA, Alshevskaya AA, Alrhmoun S, Sivitskaya NA, Sennikov SV. TCR-T cell therapy: current development approaches, preclinical evaluation, and perspectives on regulatory challenges. J Transl Med. 2024;22(1):897. https://doi.org/10.1186/s12967-024-05703-9.
29. Trinchieri G. Interleukin-12: a proinflammatory cytokine with immunoregulatory functions that bridge innate resistance and antigen-specific adaptive immunity. Annu Rev Immunol. 1995;13:251–76. https://doi.org/10.1146/annurev.iy.13.040195.001343.
30. Zhou Y, Quan G, Liu Y, Shi N, Wu Y, Zhang R, Gao X, Luo L. The application of interleukin-2 family cytokines in tumor immunotherapy research. Front Immunol. 2023;14:1090311. https://doi.org/10.3389/fimmu.2023.1090311.

31. Kim CG, Sang YB, Lee JH, Chon HJ. Combining cancer vaccines with immunotherapy: establishing a new immunological approach. Int J Mol Sci. 2021;22(15):8035. https://doi.org/10.3390/ijms22158035.
32. Song K. Current development status of cytokines for cancer immunotherapy. Biomol Ther. 2024;32(1):13–24. https://doi.org/10.4062/biomolther.2023.196.
33. Rekoske BT, McNeel DG. Immunotherapy for prostate cancer: false promises or true hope? Cancer. 2016;122(23):3598–607. https://doi.org/10.1002/cncr.30250.
34. Jhawar SR, Thandoni A, Bommareddy PK, Hassan S, Kohlhapp FJ, Goyal S, Schenkel JM, Silk AW, Zloza A. Oncolytic viruses-natural and genetically engineered cancer immunotherapies. Front Oncol. 2017;7:202. https://doi.org/10.3389/fonc.2017.00202.
35. Kaufman HL, Kohlhapp FJ, Zloza A. Oncolytic viruses: a new class of immunotherapy drugs. Nat Rev Drug Discov. 2015;14(9):642–62. https://doi.org/10.1038/nrd4663.
36. Burke JM, Lamm DL, Meng MV, Nemunaitis JJ, Stephenson JJ, Arseneau JC, Aimi J, Lerner S, Yeung AW, Kazarian T, Maslyar DJ, McKiernan JM. A first in human phase 1 study of CG0070, a GM-CSF expressing oncolytic adenovirus, for the treatment of nonmuscle invasive bladder cancer. J Urol. 2012;188(6):2391–7. https://doi.org/10.1016/j.juro.2012.07.097.
37. Yang K, Feng S, Luo Z. Oncolytic adenovirus, a new treatment strategy for prostate cancer. Biomedicine. 2022;10(12):3262. https://doi.org/10.3390/biomedicines10123262.
38. Ebrahimi N, Akbari M, Ghanaatian M, Roozbahani Moghaddam P, Adelian S, Borjian Boroujeni M, Yazdani E, Ahmadi A, Hamblin MR. Development of neoantigens: from identification in cancer cells to application in cancer vaccines. Expert Rev Vaccines. 2022;21(7):941–55. https://doi.org/10.1080/14760584.2021.1951246.
39. Blass E, Ott PA. Advances in the development of personalized neoantigen-based therapeutic cancer vaccines. Nat Rev Clin Oncol. 2021;18(4):215–29. https://doi.org/10.1038/s41571-020-00460-2.
40. Gupta RG, Li F, Roszik J, Lizée G. Exploiting tumor neoantigens to target cancer evolution: current challenges and promising therapeutic approaches. Cancer Discov. 2021;11(5):1024–39. https://doi.org/10.1158/2159-8290.CD-20-1575.
41. Yu L, Wang J. T cell-redirecting bispecific antibodies in cancer immunotherapy: recent advances. J Cancer Res Clin Oncol. 2019;145(4):941–56. https://doi.org/10.1007/s00432-019-02867-6.
42. Das G, Ptacek J, Havlinova B, Nedvedova J, Barinka C, Novakova Z. Targeting prostate cancer using bispecific T-cell engagers against prostate-specific membrane antigen. ACS Pharmacol Transl Sci. 2023;6(11):1703–14. https://doi.org/10.1021/acsptsci.3c00159.
43. Wei J, Yang Y, Wang G, Liu M. Current landscape and future directions of bispecific antibodies in cancer immunotherapy. Front Immunol. 2022;13:1035276. https://doi.org/10.3389/fimmu.2022.1035276.
44. Sridaran D, Bradshaw E, DeSelm C, Pachynski R, Mahajan K, Mahajan NP. Prostate cancer immunotherapy: improving clinical outcomes with a multi-pronged approach. Cell Rep Med. 2023;4(10):101199. https://doi.org/10.1016/j.xcrm.2023.101199.
45. Xu P, Wasielewski LJ, Yang JC, Cai D, Evans CP, Murphy WJ, Liu C. The immunotherapy and immunosuppressive signaling in therapy-resistant prostate cancer. Biomedicine. 2022;10(8):1778. https://doi.org/10.3390/biomedicines10081778.
46. Komai T, Inoue M, Okamura T, Morita K, Iwasaki Y, Sumitomo S, Shoda H, Yamamoto K, Fujio K. Transforming growth factor-β and interleukin-10 synergistically regulate humoral immunity *via* modulating metabolic signals. Front Immunol. 2018;9:1364. https://doi.org/10.3389/fimmu.2018.01364.
47. George AP, Kuzel TM, Zhang Y, Zhang B. The discovery of biomarkers in cancer immunotherapy. Comput Struct Biotechnol J. 2019;17:484–97. https://doi.org/10.1016/j.csbj.2019.03.015.
48. Zhao P, Li L, Jiang X, et al. Mismatch repair deficiency/microsatellite instability-high as a predictor for anti-PD-1/PD-L1 immunotherapy efficacy. J Hematol Oncol. 2019;12:54. https://doi.org/10.1186/s13045-019-0738-1.
49. Yin Q, Wu L, Han L, Zheng X, Tong R, Li L, Bai L, Bian Y. Immune-related adverse events of immune checkpoint inhibitors: a review. Front Immunol. 2023;14:1167975. https://doi.org/10.3389/fimmu.2023.1167975.

50. Schneider BJ, Naidoo J, Santomasso BD, Lacchetti C, Adkins S, Anadkat M, Atkins MB, Brassil KJ, Caterino JM, Chau I, Davies. Management of immune-related adverse events in patients treated with immune checkpoint inhibitor therapy: ASCO guideline update. J Clin Oncol. 2021;39(36):4073–126. https://doi.org/10.1200/JCO.21.01440.
51. Alshammari AH, Hirotsu T, di Luccio E. Overcoming challenges in cancer care: a focus on emerging technologies. Biomedicine. 2024;12(12):2787. https://doi.org/10.3390/biomedicines12122787.
52. Qiannan G, Anning Q, Ne W, Zhenxian Z, Xiaohui Z. Unlocking immunity: innovative prostate cancer vaccine strategies. Int Immunopharmacol. 2024;142:113137.
53. Isbarn H, Boccon-Gibod L, Carroll PR, Montorsi F, Schulman C, Smith MR, Sternberg CN, Studer UE. Androgen deprivation therapy for the treatment of prostate cancer: consider both benefits and risks. Eur Urol. 2009;55(1):62–75. https://doi.org/10.1016/j.eururo.2008.10.008.
54. Obradovic AZ, Dallos MC, Zahurak ML, Partin AW, Schaeffer EM, Ross AE, Allaf ME, Nirschl TR, Liu D, Chapman CG. T-cell infiltration and adaptive Treg resistance in response to androgen deprivation with or without vaccination in localized prostate cancer. Clin Cancer Res. 2020;26(13):3182–92. https://doi.org/10.1158/1078-0432.CCR-19-3372.
55. Yu P, Zhu C, You X, et al. The combination of immune checkpoint inhibitors and antibody-drug conjugates in the treatment of urogenital tumors: a review insights from phase 2 and 3 studies. Cell Death Dis. 2024;15:433. https://doi.org/10.1038/s41419-024-06837-w.
56. Ollivier L, Labbé M, Fradin D, Potiron V, Supiot S. Interaction between modern radiotherapy and immunotherapy for metastatic prostate cancer. Front Oncol. 2021;11:744679. https://doi.org/10.3389/fonc.2021.744679.
57. Rodríguez-Ruiz ME, Vanpouille-Box C, Melero I, Formenti SC, Demaria S. Immunological mechanisms responsible for radiation-induced abscopal effect. Trends Immunol. 2018;39(8):644–55. https://doi.org/10.1016/j.it.2018.06.001.
58. Akama-Garren EH, Morris ZS, Sikora AG, Weichselbaum R, Schoenfeld JD. Prospective clinical investigation of the efficacy of combination radiation therapy with immune checkpoint inhibition. Int J Radiat Oncol Biol Phys. 2021;111(5):1165–75. https://doi.org/10.1016/j.ijrobp.2021.08.009.
59. Taghizadeh H, Marhold M, Tomasich E, Udovica S, Merchant A, Krainer M. Immune checkpoint inhibitors in mCRPC—rationales, challenges and perspectives. Onco Targets Ther. 2019;8(11):e1644109. https://doi.org/10.1080/2162402X.2019.1644109.
60. Risdon EN, Chau CH, Price DK, Sartor O, Figg WD. PARP inhibitors and prostate cancer: to infinity and beyond BRCA. Oncologist. 2021;26(1):e115–29. https://doi.org/10.1634/theoncologist.2020-0697.
61. Ding L, Kim HJ, Wang Q, Kearns M, Jiang T, Ohlson CE, Li BB, Xie S, Liu JF, Stover EH, Howitt BE, Bronson RT, Lazo S, Roberts TM, Freeman GJ, Konstantinopoulos PA, Matulonis UA, Zhao JJ. PARP inhibition elicits STING-dependent antitumor immunity in Brca1-deficient ovarian cancer. Cell Rep. 2018;25(11):2972–2980.e5. https://doi.org/10.1016/j.celrep.2018.11.054.
62. Lee EK, Konstantinopoulos PA. PARP inhibition and immune modulation: scientific rationale and perspectives for the treatment of gynecologic cancers. Ther Adv Med Oncol. 2020;12:1758835920944116. https://doi.org/10.1177/1758835920944116.
63. Fan Y, Liu Z, Chen Y, He Z. Homologous recombination repair gene mutations in prostate cancer: prevalence and clinical value. Adv Ther. 2024;41(6):2196–216. https://doi.org/10.1007/s12325-024-02844-7.
64. Terada N, Akamatsu S, Kobayashi T, Inoue T, Ogawa O, Antonarakis ES. Prognostic and predictive biomarkers in prostate cancer: latest evidence and clinical implications. Ther Adv Med Oncol. 2017;9(8):565–73. https://doi.org/10.1177/1758834017719215.
65. Garg P, Krishna M, Subbalakshmi AR, Ramisetty S, Mohanty A, Kulkarni P, Horne D, Salgia R, Singhal SS. Emerging biomarkers and molecular targets for precision medicine in cervical cancer. Biochim Biophys Acta Rev Cancer. 2024;1879(3):189106. https://doi.org/10.1016/j.bbcan.2024.189106.

66. Asif S, Teply BA. Biomarkers for treatment response in advanced prostate cancer. Cancer. 2021;13(22):5723. https://doi.org/10.3390/cancers13225723.
67. Gaudreau PO, Stagg J, Soulières D, Saad F. The present and future of biomarkers in prostate cancer: proteomics, genomics, and immunology advancements. Biomarkers Cancer. 2016;8(Suppl 2):15–33. https://doi.org/10.4137/BIC.S31802.
68. Patel SP, Kurzrock R. PD-L1 expression as a predictive biomarker in cancer immunotherapy. Mol Cancer Ther. 2015;14(4):847–56. https://doi.org/10.1158/1535-7163.MCT-14-0983.
69. Jardim DL, Goodman A, de Melo Gagliato D, Kurzrock R. The challenges of tumor mutational burden as an immunotherapy biomarker. Cancer Cell. 2021;39(2):154–73. https://doi.org/10.1016/j.ccell.2020.10.001.
70. Coleman S, Xie M, Tarhini AA, Tan AC. Systematic evaluation of the predictive gene expression signatures of immune checkpoint inhibitors in metastatic melanoma. Mol Carcinog. 2023;62(1):77–89. https://doi.org/10.1002/mc.23442.
71. Ji H, Ba Y, Ma S, Hou K, Mi S, Gao X, Jin J, Gong Q, Liu T, Wang F, Liu Z, Li S, Du J, Hu S. Construction of interferon-gamma-related gene signature to characterize the immune-inflamed phenotype of glioblastoma and predict prognosis, efficacy of immunotherapy and radiotherapy. Front Immunol. 2021;12:729359. https://doi.org/10.3389/fimmu.2021.729359.
72. Wang X, Wang L, Lin H, Zhu Y, Huang D, Lai M, Xi X, Huang J, Zhang W, Zhong T. Research progress of CTC, ctDNA, and EVs in cancer liquid biopsy. Front Oncol. 2024;14:1303335. https://doi.org/10.3389/fonc.2024.1303335.
73. Iacobas S, Iacobas DA. A personalized genomics approach of the prostate cancer. Cells. 2021;10(7):1644. https://doi.org/10.3390/cells10071644.
74. Jiang M, Jia K, Wang L, Li W, Chen B, Liu Y, Wang H, Zhao S, He Y, Zhou C. Alterations of DNA damage repair in cancer: from mechanisms to applications. Ann Transl Med. 2020;8(24):1685. https://doi.org/10.21037/atm-20-2920.
75. Chen L, Liu S, Tao Y. Regulating tumor suppressor genes: post-translational modifications. Signal Transduct Target Ther. 2020;5(1):90. https://doi.org/10.1038/s41392-020-0196-9.
76. Liu W, Puri A, Fu D, Chen L, Wang C, Kellis M, Yang J. Dissecting the tumor microenvironment in response to immune checkpoint inhibitors via single-cell and spatial transcriptomics. Clin Exp Metastasis. 2024;41(4):313–32. https://doi.org/10.1007/s10585-023-10246-2.
77. Garg P, Singhal G, Pareek S, Kulkarni P, Horne D, Nath A, Salgia R, Singhal SS. Unveiling the potential of gene editing techniques in revolutionizing cancer treatment: a comprehensive overview. Biochim Biophys Acta Rev Cancer. 2025;1880(1):189233. https://doi.org/10.1016/j.bbcan.2024.189233.
78. Zhang J, Ding X, Peng K, Jia Z, Yang J. Identification of biomarkers for immunotherapy response in prostate cancer and potential drugs to alleviate immunosuppression. Aging. 2022;14(11):4839–57. https://doi.org/10.18632/aging.204115.
79. Boettcher AN, Usman A, Morgans A, VanderWeele DJ, Sosman J, Wu JD. Past, current, and future of immunotherapies for prostate cancer. Front Oncol. 2019;9:884. https://doi.org/10.3389/fonc.2019.00884.
80. Garg P, Pareek S, Kulkarni P, Salgia R, Singhal SS. Nanoengineering solutions for cancer therapy: bridging the gap between clinical practice and translational research. J Clin Med. 2024;13(12):3466. https://doi.org/10.3390/jcm13123466.
81. Ni L. Advances in mRNA-based cancer vaccines. Vaccine. 2023;11(10):1599. https://doi.org/10.3390/vaccines11101599.
82. Milone MC, Xu J, Chen SJ, Collins MA, Zhou J, Powell DJ Jr, Melenhorst JJ. Engineering enhanced CAR T-cells for improved cancer therapy. Nat Can. 2021;2(8):780–93. https://doi.org/10.1038/s43018-021-00241-5.
83. Yu L, Sun M, Zhang Q, Zhou Q, Wang Y. Harnessing the immune system by targeting immune checkpoints: providing new hope for oncotherapy. Front Immunol. 2022;13:982026. https://doi.org/10.3389/fimmu.2022.982026.
84. Su Y, Su C, Qin L. Current landscape and perspective of oncolytic viruses and their combination therapies. Transl Oncol. 2022;25:101530. https://doi.org/10.1016/j.tranon.2022.101530.

85. Garg P, Mohanty A, Ramisetty S, Kulkarni P, Horne D, Pisick E, Salgia R, Singhal SS. Artificial intelligence and allied subsets in early detection and preclusion of gynecological cancers. Biochim Biophys Acta Rev Cancer. 2023;1878(6):189026. https://doi.org/10.1016/j.bbcan.2023.189026.
86. Xie J, Luo X, Deng X, Tang Y, Tian W, Cheng H, Zhang J, Zou Y, Guo Z, Xie X. Advances in artificial intelligence to predict cancer immunotherapy efficacy. Front Immunol. 2023;13:1076883. https://doi.org/10.3389/fimmu.2022.1076883.
87. Shahzadi M, Rafique H, Waheed A, Naz H, Waheed A, Zokirova FR, Khan H. Artificial intelligence for chimeric antigen receptor-based therapies: a comprehensive review of current applications and future perspectives. Ther Adv Vaccines Immunother. 2024;12:25151355241305856. https://doi.org/10.1177/25151355241305856.
88. Wasilewski T, Kamysz W, Gębicki J. AI-assisted detection of biomarkers by sensors and biosensors for early diagnosis and monitoring. Biosensors. 2024;14(7):356. https://doi.org/10.3390/bios14070356.
89. Garg P, Singhal G, Kulkarni P, Horne D, Salgia R, Singhal SS. Artificial intelligence-driven computational approaches in the development of anticancer drugs. Cancer. 2024;16(22):3884. https://doi.org/10.3390/cancers16223884.
90. Ventola CL. Cancer immunotherapy, part 3: challenges and future trends. P & T. 2017;42(8):514–21.
91. Medina-Olivares FJ, Gómez-De León A, Ghosh N. Obstacles to global implementation of CAR T cell therapy in myeloma and lymphoma. Front Oncol. 2024;14:1397613. https://doi.org/10.3389/fonc.2024.1397613.
92. Vidal L, Dlamini Z, Qian S, Rishi P, Karmo M, Joglekar N, Abedin S, Previs RA, Orbegoso C, Joshi C, Azim HA, Karkaria H, Harris M, Mehrotra R, Berraondo M, Werutsky G, Gupta S, Niikura N, Chico I, Saini KS. Equitable inclusion of diverse populations in oncology clinical trials: deterrents and drivers. ESMO Open. 2024;9(5):103373. https://doi.org/10.1016/j.esmoop.2024.103373.
93. Michaud-Létourneau I, Gayard M, Mathisen R, Phan LTH, Weissman A, Pelletier DL. Enhancing governance and strengthening advocacy for policy change of large collective impact initiatives. Matern Child Nutr. 2019;15(Suppl 2):e12728. https://doi.org/10.1111/mcn.12728.
94. Liu D, Wang L, Guo Y. Advances in and prospects of immunotherapy for prostate cancer. Cancer Lett. 2024;601:217155. https://doi.org/10.1016/j.canlet.2024.217155.
95. Xu Z, Wang X, Zeng S, Ren X, Yan Y, Gong Z. Applying artificial intelligence for cancer immunotherapy. Acta Pharm Sin B. 2021;11(11):3393–405. https://doi.org/10.1016/j.apsb.2021.02.007.

# Immunotherapy in Renal Cell Carcinoma 13

Miguel Zugman, Salvador Jaime-Casas, Peter D. Zang, Koral Shah, and Charles B. Nguyen

## Abbreviations

| | |
|---|---|
| CAR | chimeric antigen receptor |
| CAR-T | chimeric antigen receptor T cells |
| CBM588 | *Clostridium butyricum* MIYAIRI 588 |
| ccRCC | clear cell renal cell carcinoma |
| CLS | capillary leak syndrome |
| CR | complete response |
| DCR | disease control rate |
| HD | high dose |
| HRQOL | health-related quality of life |
| ICI | immune checkpoint inhibitor |
| IL-2 | interleukin-2 |
| IPI | ipilimumab |
| irAE | immune-related adverse event |
| KIM-1 | kidney injury molecule-1 |
| MDT | multidisciplinary team |
| NIVO | nivolumab |
| ORR | objective response rate |
| OS | overall survival |
| PFS | progression-free survival |
| RCC | renal cell carcinoma |
| TKI | tyrosine kinase inhibitor |
| VEGF | vascular endothelial growth factor |

M. Zugman · S. Jaime-Casas · P. D. Zang · K. Shah
City of Hope Comprehensive Cancer Center, Duarte, CA, USA

C. B. Nguyen (✉)
City of Hope Orange County, Irvine, CA, USA
e-mail: charnguyen@coh.org


R. Salgia, P. Kulkarni (eds.), *Immunotherapies in Solid Tumors*, Cancer Treatment and Research 129, https://doi.org/10.1007/978-3-031-97242-3_13

## 13.1 Introduction

Renal cell carcinoma (RCC) is projected to account for approximately 81,800 new cancer cases and 14,890 cancer-related deaths in the United States in 2025. This places RCC as the eighth most commonly diagnosed cancer and the tenth leading cause of cancer-related deaths among both men and women [1]. RCC is uniquely heterogeneous with a broad range of biologies and histologies. Clear cell RCC (ccRCC) is the most common subtype, representing for approximately 75% of cases. In contrast, non-clear cell RCC accounts for the remaining 25% and encompasses a varying group of histologies that include papillary, chromophobe, unclassified, and other subtypes. This chapter will mainly focus on the role of immunotherapy in clear cell RCC.

## 13.2 Early Immunotherapy Experience with High-Dose IL-2 in RCC

High-dose interleukin-2 (HD IL-2) was among the earliest immunotherapeutic approaches evaluated for metastatic RCC (mRCC), predating the advent of targeted therapies and immune checkpoint inhibitors (ICIs). Initially FDA approved in 1992, HD IL-2 was able to induce durable complete responses (CR) in a subset of patients [2]. In a pivotal study of 255 patients with mRCC, HD IL-2 led to an objective response rate (ORR) of 14%, including 5% CRs and 9% partial responses. Notably, the median duration of response among those with CRs was not reached, indicating prolonged disease control [3, 4]. Indeed, a subset of patients with mRCC treated with IL-2 remained disease-free decades later [5]. Despite the potential for durable responses, HD IL-2 therapy in mRCC has been constrained by significant toxicity, primarily due to capillary leak syndrome (CLS) which leads to increased vascular permeability, edema, and multi-organ dysfunction. While these adverse effects are typically reversible upon cessation of therapy, HD IL-2 needed to be administered in an inpatient setting equipped with experienced medical teams and intensive monitoring capabilities [6]. The broader use of HD IL-2 in mRCC was also limited by the absence of reliable predictive biomarkers [7]. Evidence suggested that patients with lower tumor burden might experience better outcomes, further restricting its use to this select subset of patients [8]. Consequently, the emergence of vascular endothelial growth factor tyrosine kinase inhibitors (VEGF-TKIs) marked a pivotal shift in the treatment paradigm for mRCC [9]. Nevertheless, the early HD-IL2 experience in RCC highlighted the potential for an immune-based approach in RCC.

## 13.3 Evolving Landscape of First-Line Treatment of mRCC

The treatment landscape for mRCC later evolved with the incorporation of VEGF-TKIs. Sunitinib was one of the first FDA-approved TKIs for first-line therapy in mRCC after it demonstrated superior efficacy compared to interferon-alfa, another cytokine therapy previously employed in RCC treatment [10]. In a randomized phase 3 trial, sunitinib achieved a median progression-free survival (PFS) of 11 months, significantly longer than the 5 months observed with interferon-alfa. Additionally, the ORR was notably higher with sunitinib at 31% compared to 6% with interferon-alfa [11].

Over the subsequent decade, significant advancements were made in the application of VEGF-TKIs for mRCC. These developments included improved toxicity management, comparative analyses of individual drug toxicity profiles, optimization of dosing strategies, implementation of treatment breaks in appropriate scenarios, and strategic sequencing of therapies in the context of emerging insights into resistance and cross-resistance [12, 13, 14, 15, 16, 17, 18, 19, 20, 21, 22]. Notably, the emergence of hypertension as a potential biomarker for TKI efficacy provided clinicians with an additional tool for monitoring treatment response [23, 24, 25]. Despite these advancements, a major paradigm shift occurred in 2018 with the FDA approval of ICI combination of ipilimumab and nivolumab (anti-PD-1 and anti-CTLA-4 inhibitors, respectively) for the treatment of mRCC, ushering in a new era of immunotherapy approaches for this disease [26]. This initial landmark shift was driven by the CheckMate-214 trial which established the efficacy of ipilimumab plus nivolumab (IPI/NIVO) in patients with intermediate and poor-risk disease [27]. This combination was notable not only for a 12% CR rate, but also for its durable long-term benefit with 22.8% of patients remaining progression-free at 90 months compared to 10.8% with sunitinib. The median duration of response was markedly longer with IPI/NIVO (76.2 months; 95% CI: 59.1–NE) versus 25.1 months (95% CI: 19.8–33.2) with sunitinib [28]. While biomarkers of ICI response (e.g., PD-L1 expression and tumor mutational burden) have not consistently shown predictive value in RCC, the presence of sarcomatoid features has been strongly associated with ICI response. Subgroup analysis of CheckMate-214 demonstrated that patients with sarcomatoid RCC had markedly higher ORR (61% versus 23%) and longer overall survival (OS) as well as PFS with IPI/NIVO compared to sunitinib [29]. Overall, many patients with mRCC treated with IPI/NIVO can achieve long-term disease control off treatment, reinforcing the concept of immunologic memory and possible cure in a subset of patients [30, 31].

In parallel, combinations of VEGF-TKIs with ICIs entered the field. However, early efforts involving specifically anti-PD-L1 inhibitors (e.g., avelumab or atezolizumab) failed to demonstrate an OS benefit compared to sunitinib, as seen in the JAVELIN Renal 101 and IMmotion151 trials, respectively [32]. These anti-PD-L1-based combinations, despite initial PFS signals, have not been widely adopted in practice. In contrast, VEGF-TKI combinations with anti-PD-1 agents have shown broader activity across risk groups and led to multiple approvals. Three combinations are currently established in the first-line setting for mRCC (Table 13.1):

- Pembrolizumab plus axitinib (KEYNOTE-426): the first to show OS and PFS benefit in all-comers, with reasonable tolerability given the shorter half-life of axitinib and widespread clinical uptake [33, 34].

**Table 13.1** Outcomes from key first-line ICI-based trials in advanced RCC

| Trial (latest update) | Regimen | ORR (%) | mPFS (months) (95% CI) | HR PFS (95% CI) | mOS (months) (95% CI) | HR OS (95% CI) | Sunitinib mOS (months) (95% CI) |
|---|---|---|---|---|---|---|---|
| CheckMate-214 *(Ann Oncol, 2024)* | Nivolumab + Ipilimumab | 39.5 | 12.4 (9.9–16.8) | 0.88 (0.75–1.03) | 52.7 (48.5–64.5) | 0.72 (0.62–0.83) | 37.8 (31.9–43.8) |
| KEYNOTE-426 *(Eur Urol 2023)* | Pembrolizumab + Axitinib | 60.6 | 15.7 (13.6–20.2) | 0.68 (0.58–0.80) | 47.2 (43.6–54.8) | 0.84 (0.70–0.99) | 40.8 (34.3–47.5) |
| CLEAR *(ASCO 23)* | Lenvatinib + Pembrolizumab | 71.3 | 23.9 (20.8–27.7) | 0.47 (0.38–0.57) | 53.7 (48.7–NE) | 0.79 (0.63–0.99) | 54.3 (40.9–NE) |
| CheckMate-9ER *(25 ASCO GU)* | Nivolumab + Cabozantinib | 55.7 | 16.4 (12.5–19.3) | 0.58 (0.49–0.70) | 46.5 (40.6–53.8) | 0.79 (0.65–0.96) | 35.5 (29.2–42.8) |

Abbreviations: *HR* hazard ratio, *mOS* median overall survival, *mPFS* median progression-free survival, *ORR* objective response rate

- Pembrolizumab plus lenvatinib (CLEAR study): demonstrated the highest ORR and CR rate among the combinations, but with increased toxicity [35, 36].
- Nivolumab plus cabozantinib (CheckMate-9ER): showed durable OS and PFS benefit, with multitarget VEGF/MET inhibition possibly contributing to its efficacy. This combination also preserved health-related quality of life (HRQOL) in several key domains [37, 38].

As long-term follow-up data have matured, all three combinations—pembrolizumab/axitinib, pembrolizumab/lenvatinib, and nivolumab/cabozantinib—continue to demonstrate OS benefits over sunitinib. However, the magnitude of benefit has diminished over time, with hazard ratios remaining below 1.0 but confidence intervals tightening toward that threshold [39, 40, 41]. These trends suggest a possible attenuation of long-term impact, highlighting the importance of interpreting these results within the context of extended follow-up and evolving treatment paradigms.

Perhaps most intriguing is the updated follow-up data from CheckMate-214, where approximately 35% of patients in the intention-to-treat population treated with IPI/NIVO remained alive at nearly 8 years with a non-significant OS trend even in favorable-risk disease patients [28]. This raises the enduring question in first-line decision-making: should clinicians prioritize the highest chance of complete and durable remission, as seen with dual ICI therapy, or opt for the highest probability of tumor response and disease control, as offered by ICI/TKI combinations? [42]. This therapeutic fork reflects not only evolving evidence but also the importance of tailoring treatment to patient-specific goals—a chance at long-term remission versus consistent disease control, durability of benefit versus speed of response in the setting of symptomatic disease, and treatment-free survival versus ongoing tolerability.

Interestingly, we may be witnessing the reemergence of strategies that combine immune checkpoint inhibitors with next-generation cytokine therapies—designed to reduce toxicity while enhancing immune activation, overcoming resistance, and potentially increasing long-term remission rates [43]. More immediately on the horizon is the integration of HIF-2α inhibitors into novel triplet ICI regimens, offering another path to deepen and extend therapeutic benefit [44]. Further advancements are undoubtedly on the way.

## 13.4 Immunotherapy Rechallenge in the Refractory Setting

When patients with mRCC experience favorable initial responses to immunotherapy but later have disease progression, oncologists naturally question if ICI rechallenge could revive previous responses. Indeed, real-world data has shown that a subset of patients initially treated with first-line ICI-based therapies later receive a different ICI combination [45]. Although theoretically promising due to previously primed and activated T-cells, there has been a lack of robust data to support the role of ICI rechallenge in this setting. However, two recent phase 3 trials provide strong data against ICI rechallenge due to limited efficacy and increased toxicity. The

CONTACT-03 trial compared atezolizumab plus cabozantinib versus cabozantinib monotherapy in 522 patients with mRCC who progressed during or shortly after a recent ICI-based line of therapy [46]. The addition of atezolizumab provided no improvement in PFS (10.6 vs. 10.8 months, HR 1.03, p = 0.78) or OS (HR 0.94, p = 0.69). Importantly, the combination therapy had an increased frequency of serious adverse events (48% vs. 33%). Similarly, the TiNivo-2 trial examined tivozanib plus nivolumab versus tivozanib alone in 343 patients with mRCC previously treated with one or two lines of therapy, including an ICI [47]. This study did not show any benefit with the addition of nivolumab to tivozanib. Interestingly, tivozanib monotherapy at 1.34 mg demonstrated superior median PFS compared to the ICI combination with tivozanib at 0.89 mg (7.4 vs. 5.7 months; HR 1.10, p = 0.49). Among patients whose immediate prior therapy was ICI, monotherapy tivozanib again outperformed combination therapy (PFS of 9.2 vs. 7.4 months). Serious adverse event rates were comparable (32% vs. 37%), further discouraging ICI rechallenge.

Despite the clear phase 3 results from CONTACT-03 and TiNivo-2, smaller studies reveal nuanced scenarios where ICI rechallenge may still be cautiously considered. The FRACTION-RCC study assessed the efficacy of IPI/NIVO in 46 patients previously treated with ICI but without prior exposure to anti-CTLA-4 therapy [48]. Although the ORR was lower (17.4%) than previously observed in CheckMate-214 of treatment-naïve patients, 43.2% of patients achieved PFS at 24 weeks, indicating potential benefit in select patients. However, the observed efficacy might primarily be attributed to the introduction of ipilimumab. Similarly, the RENIVO study included 45 patients undergoing ICI rechallenge, primarily with nivolumab monotherapy [49]. The study reported an ORR of 16%, similar with FRACTION-RCC findings. RENIVO also identified factors associated with poorer ICI rechallenge outcomes including number of metastatic sites, presence of liver metastases, performance status, poor-risk disease, and interim therapy between ICI regimens. The latter aligns with findings from the TiNivo-2 trial where patients whose last therapy was not an ICI exhibited a lower median PFS of 3.7 months in both treatment arms. Conversely, patients with longer initial IO response (PFS greater than 6 months) experienced potentially better outcomes upon rechallenge.

Overall, recent high-quality evidence discourages routine ICI rechallenge after prior ICI therapy in mRCC due to limited benefit and increased toxicity. However, smaller studies highlight possible exceptions, particularly with alternative ICI combinations or in carefully selected patients. Individualized treatment decisions and further research into biomarkers predictive of ICI rechallenge success remain essential.

## 13.5 Adjuvant Immunotherapy for RCC

Many patients with localized RCC are often cured with nephrectomy alone, but a subset will have disease recurrence. Thus, the goal of adjuvant therapy following surgery is to lower the risk of recurrence and ideally improve OS. Initial adjuvant studies in RCC explored the role of VEGF-TKIs with underwhelming results. The S-TRAC study evaluated adjuvant sunitinib in patients with RCC at high risk of disease recurrence [50]. While the study showed that sunitinib improved disease-free survival compared to placebo, there was ultimately no statistically significant difference in OS [51]. Other studies of sunitinib and other TKIs such as pazopanib, axitinib, and sorafenib failed to show an improvement in clinical outcomes [52, 53, 54, 55]. Along with notable toxicities with these agents, the role of adjuvant TKI therapy in RCC has generally been a less preferred approach.

In the immunotherapy era, several studies of ICIs have been evaluated as adjuvant treatment for RCC. Trials of adjuvant atezolizumab (IMmotion-010) and IPI/NIVO (CheckMate-914) as well as perioperative nivolumab (PROSPER) did not confer a disease-free survival benefit in patients with RCC. However, pembrolizumab was FDA-approved in 2021 for adjuvant immunotherapy in RCC based on the KEYNOTE-564 phase 3 trial [56]. In this study, patients with clear cell RCC at high risk of recurrence (pT2 with grade 4 or sarcomatoid features; any pT3–4; any node-positive disease; and oligometastatic disease rendered no evidence of disease after surgical resection) were randomized to 1 year of adjuvant pembrolizumab versus placebo. In the initial analysis, pembrolizumab led to an improvement in disease-free survival which led to the initial FDA approval [56]. Subsequent follow-up analysis showed that pembrolizumab also led to an improved OS compared to placebo [57]. Thus, adjuvant pembrolizumab should be considered for patients with RCC who are at high risk of recurrence.

An emerging challenge with adjuvant pembrolizumab is the first-line treatment selection for those who have metastatic recurrence following adjuvant immunotherapy. As discussed earlier, prospective studies of immunotherapy rechallenge in the metastatic setting have not demonstrated improvement in outcomes, but these trials enrolled a limited number of patients who had disease progression during or after adjuvant pembrolizumab. Thus, the optimal treatment approach for patients with recurrent disease following adjuvant pembrolizumab is unclear and requires additional prospective evaluation. This also underscores the need for improved patient selection for adjuvant immunotherapy. Although there are currently no established biomarkers in RCC, KIM-1 (kidney injury molecule-1) has emerged as a promising circulating biomarker that may identify patients at high risk of disease recurrence following nephrectomy [58]. However, additional prospective evaluation and validation of KIM-1 to select patients for adjuvant ICI is needed before implementation in clinical practice.

## 13.6 Emerging Novel Immunotherapeutic Strategies in RCC

While the introduction of ICIs has dramatically transformed the treatment landscape for RCC, eventual progression on these regimens is common. Given the immunogenic nature of RCC, further research in immune-based therapies for treatment in refractory disease is an area of active interest. Among these strategies, cellular therapies have gained traction in recent years and, in particular, modification of the antigen receptor on immune effector cells. These chimeric antigen receptor (CAR) immune effector cells require the extraction and culturing the patient's own immune effector cells (autologous) or can also be from other donors (allogenic). The cells are then expanded and reinfused into the patient where they can identify malignant cells through antigen binding and induce cytotoxic killing. These cellular-based therapies hold the promise of providing durable remissions after a single infusion though require intensive upfront costs including hospitalization, lymphodepleting chemotherapy, and toxicities.

Current clinical studies involving cellular therapies in RCC involve the targeting of CD70, which has been shown to be aberrantly expressed in clear cell RCC relative to normal tissues [59, 60]. Additionally, further studies also showed that CD70 expression is high in sarcomatoid and some papillary variants in RCC [61]. CD70 targeting CAR T cells (CAR-T) in RCC have recently reported promising evidence of clinical efficacy. CTX130 and ALLO-316 are two different allogenic anti-CD70 CAR-T therapies that have recently reported out encouraging results. COBALT-RCC was a phase I multicenter study that examined the safety and efficacy of CTX130. In total, 14 patients with metastatic clear cell RCC were enrolled. At the end of the study, the disease control rate (DCR) was 77% even in a patient population that had been heavily pre-treated with prior ICI and VEGF-TKI therapy. In addition, the side effect profile was manageable with 7 patients developing grade 1–2 CRS but no grade 3 or higher events [62]. The TRAVERSE study was another phase I trial that examined ALLO-316, a separate anti-CD70 CAR-T construct. 19 patients with mRCC were ultimately enrolled. Similar to CTX130, the side effect profile was manageable, and efficacy was notable with a DCR of 89%. In a sub-analysis, the DCR was 100% in those with high CD70 expression [63]. While both COBALT-RCC and TRAVERSE were early-phase studies, they showed the potential for CAR-T efficacy in heavily pre-treated mRCC with encouraging responses. In addition, the side effect profile seemed to be manageable with no rates of high-grade adverse events. Efforts are already underway to further optimize these two CAR-T products, and the results of future studies are eagerly anticipated.

## 13.7 Gut Microbiome Interventions to Improve Immunotherapy Outcomes in mRCC

A growing body of work has demonstrated the impact of the microbiome on cancer outcomes. Comprised of symbiotic microorganisms, the microbiome exerts both pro-tumorigenic and anticancer properties and has been recently integrated as a hallmark of cancer [64]. There has been emerging data on gut microbiome dysbiosis on RCC outcomes and responses to immunotherapy. In retrospective studies, concurrent antibiotic use was associated with worse outcomes in patients with RCC [65]. Stool metagenomic sequencing of patients with RCC has revealed enrichment of organisms such as *Clostridium hathewayi* and *Akkermansia muciniphila*, which correlate with ICI response [66, 67]. These data highlight the potential role of the gut microbiome composition on immunotherapy outcomes, which may represent a novel target in RCC.

Recent early-phase studies have evaluated the role of probiotic interventions in combination with ICI-based therapies to favorably modulate the gut microbiome and improve treatment responses in mRCC. In pre-clinical models, the probiotic strain *Clostridium butyricum* MIYAIRI 588 (CBM588) leads to enrichment of *Bifidobacterium* bacteria and promotes IL-17A-producing T cells [68]. In a recent phase 1 study, patients with untreated mRCC were randomized to IPI/NIVO plus CBM588 versus IPI/NIVO alone [69]. Interestingly, CBM588 supplementation led to improvements in ORR and PFS which correlated with increases in circulating cytokine levels [69]. Another phase 1 study evaluated CBM588 in combination with nivolumab and cabozantinib versus nivolumab plus cabozantinib alone in patients with untreated mRCC, which similarly showed improved ORR with CBM588 supplementation [70]. In addition to probiotic supplementation, other strategies such as fecal microbiota transplantation and dietary strategies to alter the gut microbiome in RCC are also currently under investigation.

## 13.8 Multidisciplinary Approaches in RCC

Much like the RCC treatment landscape, RCC is a heterogeneous disease with diverse histological subtypes and immuno-molecular signatures that impact the standardization of subsequent lines of care. For this reason, incorporating medical and surgical specialties in a multidisciplinary decision-making model is of utmost importance to improve patient outcomes. A multidisciplinary team (MDT) includes professionals from various departments who regularly review cancer cases to develop individualized and precise treatment plans for each patient with RCC [71, 72].

Zeng et al. performed a single-center retrospective evaluation of 269 patients with mRCC, of which 48% (n = 129) were treated with an MDT model [73]. Results showed that patients in the MDT group had improved oncologic outcomes, including OS. Patients in the MDT were also more likely to receive multi-line therapy, which resulted in longer OS for this group. The incorporation of VEGF-TKIs with ICIs in mRCC has also led to characteristic toxicity profiles including cardiovascular, dermatological, and gastrointestinal adverse events. MDT has been proposed to develop prompt recognition and management of these toxicities, consequently leading to improved treatment adherence and outcomes. Roberto et al. developed a case series showing how the incorporation of subspecialists such as endocrinologists, cardiologists, nephrologists, gastroenterologists, and dermatologists served as the cornerstone of their institutional MDT model, which led to optimized decision-making for patients with mRCC who experienced treatment-related adverse events [74]. The utility of the MDT referral has also been validated in patients with localized RCC, where the evaluation by a urologist plays critical roles in selecting patients who could potentially achieve a cure with surgery alone and forego systemic treatment. Martini et al. analyzed a prospective group of patients with RCC treated with surgery alone at a tertiary center to develop a model that incorporates age and comorbidity status, and other factors, to determine which patients benefit more from MDT referral [75]. This model suggested that patients with locally advanced disease (cT3 and T4) derive the highest benefit from MDT approach, while patients with low-stage localized disease (e.g., T1a) can be safely managed with surgery alone.

The evolving treatment landscape of RCC underscores the critical need for a multidisciplinary approach to patient care. As systemic therapies evolve, the heterogeneity of RCC necessitates individualized treatment strategies that balance oncologic efficacy with toxicity management. Evidence from retrospective and prospective studies highlights the significant survival benefits of MDT involvement, particularly in optimizing treatment sequencing and addressing complex adverse event profiles. MDT referral has demonstrated value in metastatic and non-metastatic settings, ensuring appropriate patient selection for surgery and minimizing unnecessary systemic therapy. Moving forward, integrating multidisciplinary collaboration into standard practice will be essential to refining personalized treatment approaches and ultimately improving outcomes for patients with RCC.

## 13.9 Cytoreductive Nephrectomy in the Immunotherapy Era

Cytoreductive nephrectomy was previously considered the standard of care for patients with mRCC who had good performance status. However, these studies were done in the context of nephrectomy followed by interferon-alpha therapy [76, 77]. With the evolution of systemic therapy and the introduction of newer agents, the role of cytoreductive nephrectomy in mRCC has been questioned. The CARMENA trial investigated the role of cytoreductive nephrectomy in the VEGF-TKI era by showing that sunitinib alone was not inferior to nephrectomy followed by sunitinib in patients with intermediate-risk or poor-risk mRCC [78]. However, data evaluating the role of nephrectomy in the modern ICI era are yet to be made. RCC is an immunogenic tumor, and the theoretical benefit of cytoreductive nephrectomy includes removing the primary immune-tumorigenic site while targeting key immune checkpoints with systemic therapy [79]. The PROBE (NCT04510597), NORDIC-SUN (NCT03977571), and SEVURO-CN (NCT05753839) trials are ongoing studies designed to evaluate the role of deferred cytoreductive nephrectomy versus no cytoreductive nephrectomy in the context of ICI-based therapy.

## 13.10 Managing Immune-Related Adverse Events (irAEs)

In patients with mRCC, various treatment combinations consisting of ICIs plus TKIs or dual ICI regimens are considered the standard of care in the first-line setting. Given the increasing adoption of combination regimens, characterizing the immune-related adverse event (irAE) profile is critical to optimizing patient outcomes while minimizing toxicity [80]. The overall incidence of all-grade irAEs for

ICI/TKI combinations is reported to be as high as 95–97%, with 57–72% of patients experiencing grade ≥3 irAE toxicities [35]. For dual ICI-based therapy with IPI/NIVO, all grade and grade ≥3 irAEs are reported in 94% and 48% of cases, respectively [81]. Unlike traditional chemotherapy-associated toxicities, irAEs are unique to ICIs and result from excessive immune activation against self-antigens, leading to inflammatory damage across multiple organ systems.

ICIs can induce a spectrum of inflammatory toxicities across various organ systems, with the most frequently affected being skin, liver, colon, lung, and endocrine systems. However, some irAEs may not be clinically apparent initially and are diagnosed by exclusion—specifically, diarrhea, colitis, and hepatitis. In the era of combination-based regimens, a challenging scenario can be the correct characterization of irAEs, as ICIs and TKIs share overlapping toxicities. In this scenario, it is recommended that the VEGFR-TKI be discontinued, and the ICI infusion be delayed. Improvement of toxicity relative to the drug's half-life can help characterize the offending agent [82]. A multidisciplinary collaboration between medical oncologists, dermatologists, gastroenterologists, pulmonologists, endocrinologists, and other subspecialties is crucial for the timely identification and management of irAEs. Future strategies incorporating predictive biomarkers and personalized risk stratification may further refine toxicity management, enabling a more tailored approach to immunotherapy in mRCC.

## 13.11 Conclusions and Future Directions

In summary, the treatment landscape of RCC has been revolutionized with the incorporation of immunotherapy which have improved outcomes for a majority of patients given the potential for deep and durable responses. Frontline therapies for metastatic RCC include dual ICI therapy or ICI combination therapies with TKIs. Recently, ICI therapy has moved earlier in the disease state with the recent approval of adjuvant immunotherapy. Thus, an emerging challenge is the optimal treatment decision following progression on these ICI agents given recent phase 3 data showing a lack of efficacy with ICI rechallenge. However, novel immunotherapeutic agents such as CAR-T therapies as well as gut microbiome interventions may provide a new window to harness the anti-cancer immune response in RCC. Given the treatment complexities in the ICI era, a multidisciplinary team-based approach is needed for patients with RCC.

## References

1. Siegel RL, Kratzer TB, Giaquinto AN, Sung H, Jemal A. Cancer statistics, 2025. CA Cancer J Clin. 2025;75(1):10–45.
2. McDermott DF, Atkins MB. Interleukin-2 therapy of metastatic renal cell carcinoma—predictors of response. Semin Oncol. 2006;33(5):583–7.
3. Fyfe G, Fisher RI, Rosenberg SA, Sznol M, Parkinson DR, Louie AC. Results of treatment of 255 patients with metastatic renal cell carcinoma who received high-dose recombinant interleukin-2 therapy. J Clin Oncol. 1995;13(3):688–96.

4. Fyfe GA, Fisher RI, Rosenberg SA, Sznol M, Parkinson DR, Louie AC. Long-term response data for 255 patients with metastatic renal cell carcinoma treated with high-dose recombinant interleukin-2 therapy. J Clin Oncol. 1996;14(8):2410–1.
5. Rosenberg SA. IL-2: the first effective immunotherapy for human cancer. J Immunol. 2014;192(12):5451–8.
6. McDermott DF, Atkins MB. Application of IL-2 and other cytokines in renal cancer. Expert Opin Biol Ther. 2004;4(4):455–68.
7. Klapper JA, Downey SG, Smith FO, Yang JC, Hughes MS, Kammula US, et al. High-dose interleukin-2 for the treatment of metastatic renal cell carcinoma: a retrospective analysis of response and survival in patients treated in the surgery branch at the National Cancer Institute between 1986 and 2006. Cancer. 2008;113(2):293–301.
8. Leibovich BC, Han KR, Bui MH, Pantuck AJ, Dorey FJ, Figlin RA, et al. Scoring algorithm to predict survival after nephrectomy and immunotherapy in patients with metastatic renal cell carcinoma: a stratification tool for prospective clinical trials. Cancer. 2003;98(12):2566–75.
9. Vazquez S, Leon L, Fernandez O, Lazaro M, Grande E, Aparicio L. Sunitinib: the first to arrive at first-line metastatic renal cell carcinoma. Adv Ther. 2012;29(3):202–17.
10. Schmid TA, Gore ME. Sunitinib in the treatment of metastatic renal cell carcinoma. Ther Adv Urol. 2016;8(6):348–71.
11. Motzer RJ, Hutson TE, Tomczak P, Michaelson MD, Bukowski RM, Rixe O, et al. Sunitinib versus interferon alfa in metastatic renal-cell carcinoma. N Engl J Med. 2007;356(2):115–24.
12. Schmidinger M. Understanding and managing toxicities of vascular endothelial growth factor (VEGF) inhibitors. EJC Suppl. 2013;11(2):172–91.
13. Motzer RJ, Hutson TE, Cella D, Reeves J, Hawkins R, Guo J, et al. Pazopanib versus sunitinib in metastatic renal-cell carcinoma. N Engl J Med. 2013;369(8):722–31.
14. Rini BI, Escudier B, Tomczak P, Kaprin A, Szczylik C, Hutson TE, et al. Comparative effectiveness of axitinib versus sorafenib in advanced renal cell carcinoma (AXIS): a randomised phase 3 trial. Lancet. 2011;378(9807):1931–9.
15. Rini BI, Melichar B, Ueda T, Grunwald V, Fishman MN, Arranz JA, et al. Axitinib with or without dose titration for first-line metastatic renal-cell carcinoma: a randomised double-blind phase 2 trial. Lancet Oncol. 2013;14(12):1233–42.
16. Bjarnason GA, Knox JJ, Kollmannsberger CK, Soulieres D, Ernst DS, Zalewski P, et al. The efficacy and safety of sunitinib given on an individualised schedule as first-line therapy for metastatic renal cell carcinoma: a phase 2 clinical trial. Eur J Cancer. 2019;108:69–77.
17. Brown JE, Royle KL, Gregory W, Ralph C, Maraveyas A, Din O, et al. Temporary treatment cessation versus continuation of first-line tyrosine kinase inhibitor in patients with advanced clear cell renal cell carcinoma (STAR): an open-label, non-inferiority, randomised, controlled, phase 2/3 trial. Lancet Oncol. 2023;24(3):213–27.
18. Ornstein MC, Wood LS, Elson P, Allman KD, Beach J, Martin A, et al. A phase II study of intermittent sunitinib in previously untreated patients with metastatic renal cell carcinoma. J Clin Oncol. 2017;35(16):1764–9.
19. Porta C, Tortora G, Linassier C, Papazisis K, Awada A, Berthold D, et al. Maximising the duration of disease control in metastatic renal cell carcinoma with targeted agents: an expert agreement. Med Oncol. 2012;29(3):1896–907.
20. Bergers G, Hanahan D. Modes of resistance to anti-angiogenic therapy. Nat Rev Cancer. 2008;8(8):592–603.
21. Ravaud A, Gross-Goupil M. Overcoming resistance to tyrosine kinase inhibitors in renal cell carcinoma. Cancer Treat Rev. 2012;38(8):996–1003.
22. Oudard S, Vano Y. The role of rechallenge with targeted therapies in metastatic renal-cell carcinoma. Curr Opin Urol. 2015;25(5):402–10.
23. Agarwal M, Thareja N, Benjamin M, Akhondi A, Mitchell GD. Tyrosine kinase inhibitor-induced hypertension. Curr Oncol Rep. 2018;20(8):65.
24. Rini BI, Quinn DI, Baum M, Wood LS, Tarazi J, Rosbrook B, et al. Hypertension among patients with renal cell carcinoma receiving axitinib or sorafenib: analysis from the randomized phase III AXIS trial. Target Oncol. 2015;10(1):45–53.

25. Liu Y, Zhou L, Chen Y, Liao B, Ye D, Wang K, et al. Hypertension as a prognostic factor in metastatic renal cell carcinoma treated with tyrosine kinase inhibitors: a systematic review and meta-analysis. BMC Urol. 2019;19(1):49.
26. Motzer RJ, Tannir NM, McDermott DF, Aren Frontera O, Melichar B, Choueiri TK, et al. Nivolumab plus ipilimumab versus sunitinib in advanced renal-cell carcinoma. N Engl J Med. 2018;378(14):1277–90.
27. Motzer RJ, Rini BI, McDermott DF, Aren Frontera O, Hammers HJ, Carducci MA, et al. Nivolumab plus ipilimumab versus sunitinib in first-line treatment for advanced renal cell carcinoma: extended follow-up of efficacy and safety results from a randomised, controlled, phase 3 trial. Lancet Oncol. 2019;20(10):1370–85.
28. Tannir NM, Albiges L, McDermott DF, Burotto M, Choueiri TK, Hammers HJ, et al. Nivolumab plus ipilimumab versus sunitinib for first-line treatment of advanced renal cell carcinoma: extended 8-year follow-up results of efficacy and safety from the phase III CheckMate 214 trial. Ann Oncol. 2024;35(11):1026–38.
29. Tannir NM, Signoretti S, Choueiri TK, McDermott DF, Motzer RJ, Flaifel A, et al. Efficacy and safety of nivolumab plus ipilimumab versus sunitinib in first-line treatment of patients with advanced sarcomatoid renal cell carcinoma. Clin Cancer Res. 2021;27(1):78–86.
30. Regan MM, Jegede OA, Mantia CM, Powles T, Werner L, Motzer RJ, et al. Treatment-free survival after immune checkpoint inhibitor therapy versus targeted therapy for advanced renal cell carcinoma: 42-month results of the CheckMate 214 trial. Clin Cancer Res. 2021;27(24):6687–95.
31. Choueiri TK, Penkov K, Uemura H, Campbell MT, Pal S, Kollmannsberger C, et al. Avelumab + axitinib versus sunitinib as first-line treatment for patients with advanced renal cell carcinoma: final analysis of the phase III JAVELIN renal 101 trial. Ann Oncol. 2025;36(4):387–92.
32. Motzer RJ, Powles T, Atkins MB, Escudier B, McDermott DF, Alekseev BY, et al. Final overall survival and molecular analysis in IMmotion151, a phase 3 trial comparing atezolizumab plus bevacizumab vs sunitinib in patients with previously untreated metastatic renal cell carcinoma. JAMA Oncol. 2022;8(2):275–80.
33. Rini BI, Plimack ER, Stus V, Gafanov R, Hawkins R, Nosov D, et al. Pembrolizumab plus axitinib versus sunitinib for advanced renal-cell carcinoma. N Engl J Med. 2019;380(12):1116–27.
34. Powles T, Plimack ER, Soulieres D, Waddell T, Stus V, Gafanov R, et al. Pembrolizumab plus axitinib versus sunitinib monotherapy as first-line treatment of advanced renal cell carcinoma (KEYNOTE-426): extended follow-up from a randomised, open-label, phase 3 trial. Lancet Oncol. 2020;21(12):1563–73.
35. Motzer R, Alekseev B, Rha SY, Porta C, Eto M, Powles T, et al. Lenvatinib plus pembrolizumab or everolimus for advanced renal cell carcinoma. N Engl J Med. 2021;384(14):1289–300.
36. Choueiri TK, Eto M, Motzer R, De Giorgi U, Buchler T, Basappa NS, et al. Lenvatinib plus pembrolizumab versus sunitinib as first-line treatment of patients with advanced renal cell carcinoma (CLEAR): extended follow-up from the phase 3, randomised, open-label study. Lancet Oncol. 2023;24(3):228–38.
37. Choueiri TK, Powles T, Burotto M, Escudier B, Bourlon MT, Zurawski B, et al. Nivolumab plus cabozantinib versus sunitinib for advanced renal-cell carcinoma. N Engl J Med. 2021;384(9):829–41.
38. Cella D, Motzer RJ, Suarez C, Blum SI, Ejzykowicz F, Hamilton M, et al. Patient-reported outcomes with first-line nivolumab plus cabozantinib versus sunitinib in patients with advanced renal cell carcinoma treated in CheckMate 9ER: an open-label, randomised, phase 3 trial. Lancet Oncol. 2022;23(2):292–303.
39. Motzer RJ, Escudier B, Burotto M, Powles T, Apolo AB, Bourlon MT, et al. Nivolumab plus cabozantinib (N+C) vs sunitinib (S) for previously untreated advanced renal cell carcinoma (aRCC): final follow-up results from the CheckMate 9ER trial. J Clin Oncol. 2024;43(5_suppl):102994.
40. Plimack ER, Powles T, Stus V, Gafanov R, Nosov D, Waddell T, et al. Pembrolizumab plus axitinib versus sunitinib as first-line treatment of advanced renal cell carcinoma: 43-month follow-up of the phase 3 KEYNOTE-426 study. Eur Urol. 2023;84(5):449–54.

41. Motzer RJ, Porta C, Eto M, Powles T, Grunwald V, Hutson TE, et al. Lenvatinib plus pembrolizumab versus sunitinib in first-line treatment of advanced renal cell carcinoma: final prespecified overall survival analysis of CLEAR, a phase III study. J Clin Oncol. 2024;42(11):1222–8.
42. Barragan-Carrillo R, Saad E, Saliby RM, Sun M, Albiges L, Bex A, et al. First and second-line treatments in metastatic renal cell carcinoma. Eur Urol. 2025;87(2):143–54.
43. Beebe KD, Eisner JR, Guo J, Shibata Y, Davison JM, Uronis J, et al. The immunogenomic landscape of peripheral high-dose IL-2 pharmacodynamics in patients with metastatic renal cell carcinoma: a benchmark for next-generation IL-2-based immunotherapies. J Immunol. 2024;213(1):29–39.
44. Choueiri TK, Plimack ER, Powles T, Voss MH, Gurney H, Silverman RK, et al. Phase 3 study of first-line treatment with pembrolizumab + belzutifan + lenvatinib or pembrolizumab/quavonlimab + lenvatinib versus pembrolizumab + lenvatinib for advanced renal cell carcinoma (RCC). J Clin Oncol. 2022;40(6_suppl) https://doi.org/10.1200/JCO.2022.40.6_suppl.TPS399.
45. Shah NJ, Sura SD, Shinde R, Shi J, Singhal PK, Robert NJ, et al. Real-world treatment patterns and clinical outcomes for metastatic renal cell carcinoma in the current treatment era. Eur Urol Open Sci. 2023;49:110–8.
46. Pal SK, Albiges L, Tomczak P, Suarez C, Voss MH, de Velasco G, et al. Atezolizumab plus cabozantinib versus cabozantinib monotherapy for patients with renal cell carcinoma after progression with previous immune checkpoint inhibitor treatment (CONTACT-03): a multicentre, randomised, open-label, phase 3 trial. Lancet. 2023;402(10397):185–95.
47. Choueiri TK, Albiges L, Barthelemy P, Iacovelli R, Emambux S, Molina-Cerrillo J, et al. Tivozanib plus nivolumab versus tivozanib monotherapy in patients with renal cell carcinoma following an immune checkpoint inhibitor: results of the phase 3 TiNivo-2 study. Lancet. 2024;404(10460):1309–20.
48. Choueiri TK, Kluger H, George S, Tykodi SS, Kuzel TM, Perets R, et al. FRACTION-RCC: nivolumab plus ipilimumab for advanced renal cell carcinoma after progression on immuno-oncology therapy. J Immunother Cancer. 2022;10(11):e005780.
49. Vauchier C, Auclin E, Barthelemy P, Carril-Ajuria L, Ryckewaert T, Borchiellini D, et al. REchallenge of NIVOlumab (RENIVO) or nivolumab-ipilimumab in metastatic renal cell carcinoma: an ambispective multicenter study. J Oncol. 2022;2022:3449660.
50. Ravaud A, Motzer RJ, Pandha HS, George DJ, Pantuck AJ, Patel A, et al. Adjuvant sunitinib in high-risk renal-cell carcinoma after nephrectomy. N Engl J Med. 2016;375(23):2246–54.
51. Motzer RJ, Ravaud A, Patard JJ, Pandha HS, George DJ, Patel A, et al. Adjuvant sunitinib for high-risk renal cell carcinoma after nephrectomy: subgroup analyses and updated overall survival results. Eur Urol. 2018;73(1):62–8.
52. Haas NB, Manola J, Uzzo RG, Flaherty KT, Wood CG, Kane C, et al. Adjuvant sunitinib or sorafenib for high-risk, non-metastatic renal-cell carcinoma (ECOG-ACRIN E2805): a double-blind, placebo-controlled, randomised, phase 3 trial. Lancet. 2016;387(10032):2008–16.
53. Motzer RJ, Haas NB, Donskov F, Gross-Goupil M, Varlamov S, Kopyltsov E, et al. Randomized phase III trial of adjuvant pazopanib versus placebo after nephrectomy in patients with localized or locally advanced renal cell carcinoma. J Clin Oncol. 2017;35(35):3916–23.
54. Gross-Goupil M, Kwon TG, Eto M, Ye D, Miyake H, Seo SI, et al. Axitinib versus placebo as an adjuvant treatment of renal cell carcinoma: results from the phase III, randomized ATLAS trial. Ann Oncol. 2018;29(12):2371–8.
55. Eisen T, Frangou E, Oza B, Ritchie AWS, Smith B, Kaplan R, et al. Adjuvant sorafenib for renal cell carcinoma at intermediate or high risk of relapse: results from the SORCE randomized phase III intergroup trial. J Clin Oncol. 2020;38(34):4064–75.
56. Choueiri TK, Tomczak P, Park SH, Venugopal B, Ferguson T, Chang YH, et al. Adjuvant pembrolizumab after nephrectomy in renal-cell carcinoma. N Engl J Med. 2021;385(8):683–94.
57. Choueiri TK, Tomczak P, Park SH, Venugopal B, Ferguson T, Symeonides SN, et al. Overall survival with adjuvant pembrolizumab in renal-cell carcinoma. N Engl J Med. 2024;390(15):1359–71.

58. Xu W, Puligandla M, Halbert B, Haas NB, Flaherty KT, Uzzo RG, et al. Plasma KIM-1 is associated with recurrence risk after nephrectomy for localized renal cell carcinoma: a trial of the ECOG-ACRIN research group (E2805). Clin Cancer Res. 2021;27(12):3397–403.
59. Junker K, Hindermann W, von Eggeling F, Diegmann J, Haessler K, Schubert J. CD70: a new tumor specific biomarker for renal cell carcinoma. J Urol. 2005;173(6):2150–3.
60. Diegmann J, Junker K, Gerstmayer B, Bosio A, Hindermann W, Rosenhahn J, et al. Identification of CD70 as a diagnostic biomarker for clear cell renal cell carcinoma by gene expression profiling, real-time RT-PCR and immunohistochemistry. Eur J Cancer. 2005;41(12):1794–801.
61. Jilaveanu LB, Sznol J, Aziz SA, Duchen D, Kluger HM, Camp RL. CD70 expression patterns in renal cell carcinoma. Hum Pathol. 2012;43(9):1394–9.
62. Pal SK, Tran B, Haanen J, Hurwitz ME, Sacher A, Tannir NM, et al. CD70-targeted allogeneic CAR T-cell therapy for advanced clear cell renal cell carcinoma. Cancer Discov. 2024;14(7):1176–89.
63. Srour S, Kotecha R, Curti B, Chahoud J, Drakaki A, Tang L, et al. A phase 1 multicenter study (TRAVERSE) evaluating the safety and efficacy of ALLO-316 following conditioning regimen in pts with advanced or metastatic clear cell renal cell carcinoma (ccRCC). Cancer Res. 2023;83(8_supplement):CT011.
64. Hanahan D. Hallmarks of cancer: new dimensions. Cancer Discov. 2022;12(1):31–46.
65. Derosa L, Hellmann MD, Spaziano M, Halpenny D, Fidelle M, Rizvi H, et al. Negative association of antibiotics on clinical activity of immune checkpoint inhibitors in patients with advanced renal cell and non-small-cell lung cancer. Ann Oncol. 2018;29(6):1437–44.
66. Derosa L, Routy B, Fidelle M, Iebba V, Alla L, Pasolli E, et al. Gut bacteria composition drives primary resistance to cancer immunotherapy in renal cell carcinoma patients. Eur Urol. 2020;78(2):195–206.
67. Salgia NJ, Bergerot PG, Maia MC, Dizman N, Hsu J, Gillece JD, et al. Stool microbiome profiling of patients with metastatic renal cell carcinoma receiving anti-PD-1 immune checkpoint inhibitors. Eur Urol. 2020;78(4):498–502.
68. Hagihara M, Kuroki Y, Ariyoshi T, Higashi S, Fukuda K, Yamashita R, et al. Clostridium butyricum modulates the microbiome to protect intestinal barrier function in mice with antibiotic-induced dysbiosis. iScience. 2020;23(1):100772.
69. Dizman N, Meza L, Bergerot P, Alcantara M, Dorff T, Lyou Y, et al. Nivolumab plus ipilimumab with or without live bacterial supplementation in metastatic renal cell carcinoma: a randomized phase 1 trial. Nat Med. 2022;28(4):704–12.
70. Ebrahimi H, Dizman N, Meza L, Malhotra J, Li X, Dorff T, et al. Cabozantinib and nivolumab with or without live bacterial supplementation in metastatic renal cell carcinoma: a randomized phase 1 trial. Nat Med. 2024;30(9):2576–85.
71. Koco L, Weekenstroo HHA, Lambregts DMJ, Sedelaar JPM, Prokop M, Futterer JJ, et al. The effects of multidisciplinary team meetings on clinical practice for colorectal, lung, prostate and breast cancer: a systematic review. Cancers (Basel). 2021;13(16):4159.
72. Croke JM, El-Sayed S. Multidisciplinary management of cancer patients: chasing a shadow or real value? An overview of the literature. Curr Oncol. 2012;19(4):e232–8.
73. Zeng Y, Zhu S, Wang Z, Chen J, Dai J, Liu Z, et al. Multidisciplinary team (MDT) discussion improves overall survival outcomes for metastatic renal cell carcinoma patients. J Multidiscip Healthc. 2023;16:503–13.
74. Roberto M, Panebianco M, Aschelter AM, Buccilli D, Cantisani C, Caponnetto S, et al. The value of the multidisciplinary team in metastatic renal cell carcinoma: paving the way for precision medicine in toxicities management. Front Oncol. 2022;12:1026978.
75. Martini A, Fallara G, Pellegrino AA, Nocera L, Larcher A, Raggi D, et al. Multidisciplinary team referral at diagnosis for patients with non-metastatic renal cell carcinoma. Urol Oncol. 2022;40(8):384.e9–384.e14.
76. Flanigan RC, Salmon SE, Blumenstein BA, Bearman SI, Roy V, McGrath PC, et al. Nephrectomy followed by interferon alfa-2b compared with interferon alfa-2b alone for metastatic renal-cell cancer. N Engl J Med. 2001;345(23):1655–9.

77. Mickisch GH, Garin A, van Poppel H, de Prijck L, Sylvester R, European Organisation for R, et al. Radical nephrectomy plus interferon-alfa-based immunotherapy compared with interferon alfa alone in metastatic renal-cell carcinoma: a randomised trial. Lancet. 2001;358(9286):966–70.
78. Mejean A, Ravaud A, Thezenas S, Colas S, Beauval JB, Bensalah K, et al. Sunitinib alone or after nephrectomy in metastatic renal-cell carcinoma. N Engl J Med. 2018;379(5):417–27.
79. Ingels A, Campi R, Capitanio U, Amparore D, Bertolo R, Carbonara U, et al. Complementary roles of surgery and systemic treatment in clear cell renal cell carcinoma. Nat Rev Urol. 2022;19(7):391–418.
80. Leucht K, Ali N, Foller S, Grimm MO. Management of immune-related adverse events from immune-checkpoint inhibitors in advanced or metastatic renal cell carcinoma. Cancers (Basel). 2022;14(18):4369.
81. Albiges L, Tannir NM, Burotto M, McDermott D, Plimack ER, Barthelemy P, et al. Nivolumab plus ipilimumab versus sunitinib for first-line treatment of advanced renal cell carcinoma: extended 4-year follow-up of the phase III CheckMate 214 trial. ESMO Open. 2020;5(6):e001079.
82. Qin Q, Nein E, Flaten A, Zhang T. Toxicity management of systemic kidney cancer therapies. Hematol Oncol Clin North Am. 2023;37(5):993–1003.

# Phenotypic Plasticity, Non-genetic Mechanisms, and Immune Drug Resistance in Cancer

14

Prakash Kulkarni, Sravani Ramisetty, Debora Bruno, TingTing Tan, Amartej Merla, and Ravi Salgia

## Abbreviations

| | |
|---|---|
| FDA | US Food and Drug Administration |
| TME | Tumor microenvironment |
| PD-L1 | Programmed cell death 1 ligand 1 |
| B2M | Beta-2-microglobulin |
| CTLs | Cytotoxic T lymphocytes |
| JAK1/2 | Janus kinase 1 and 2 |
| PTEN | Phosphatase and tensin homolog |
| STK11 | Serine/threonine kinase 11 |
| MHC-1 | Major histocompatibility complex, class I |

P. Kulkarni
Department of Medical Oncology and Therapeutics Research, City of Hope National Medical Center, Duarte, CA, USA

Department of Systems Biology, City of Hope National Medical Center, Duarte, CA, USA

S. Ramisetty
Department of Medical Oncology, City of Hope National Medical Center, Duarte, CA, USA

D. Bruno
Department of Medical Oncology, City of Hope, Newnan, GA, USA

T. Tan
Department of Medical Oncology, City of Hope National Medical Center, Newport Beach, CA, USA

A. Merla
Department of Medical Oncology, Lancaster, CA, USA

R. Salgia (✉)
Department of Medical Oncology and Therapeutics Research, City of Hope National Medical Center, Duarte, CA, USA
e-mail: rsalgia@coh.org



R. Salgia, P. Kulkarni (eds.), *Immunotherapies in Solid Tumors*, Cancer Treatment and Research 129, https://doi.org/10.1007/978-3-031-97242-3_14

| | |
|---|---|
| DNMT | DNA methyl transferase |
| HDAC | Histone deacetylase |
| BET | Bromodomain and extra terminal |
| FDA | United States Food and Health Administration |
| EMT | Epithelial-to-mesenchymal transition |
| MDSCs | Myeloid-derived suppressor cells |
| PI3K | Phosphoinositide 3-kinase |
| Akt | AKT serine/threonine kinase 1 |
| mTOR | Mechanistic target of rapamycin kinase |
| EMP | Epithelial-to-mesenchymal plasticity |
| IDPs | Intrinsically disordered proteins |
| IDRs | Intrinsically disordered regions |
| CAFs | Cancer-associated fibroblasts |
| EGT | Evolutionary game theory |
| TGF-b | Transforming growth factor beta |
| EGFR | Epidermal growth factor receptor |
| HER2 | Erb-B2 receptor tyrosine kinase 2 2 |
| NK | Natural killer cell |
| IFNα/IFNγ | Interferon α and γ |
| ETB | Evolutionary tumor board |
| CXCL10 | C-X-C motif chemokine ligand 10 |
| CCL5 | C-C motif chemokine ligand 5 |
| DTPs | Drug-tolerant persisters |

## 14.1 Introduction

The interactions between a patient's cancer cells and the body's immune system are dynamic and continuously evolving from disease initiation to progression to metastatic disease. Obviously, these events are dependent on the cancer cell's ability to evade the body's immune system. With the advent of cancer immunotherapy, there has been a significant impact on disease treatment in cancer patients. Immunotherapy, which includes several different types, such as T-cell therapy, immune checkpoint inhibitors, monoclonal antibodies, cancer vaccines, and many others, can result in sustainable response in patients with a wide range of metastatic disease [1] (Fig. 14.1).

Cancer immunotherapy leverages the power of the patient's immune system and specifically targets cancer cells compared to traditional chemotherapeutic approaches [2]. However, not all tumors are responsive to immunotherapy. Cancers that respond well to immunotherapy can be characterized by an active immune profile and are referred to as "hot" (immune-inflamed) tumors. "Hot" tumors are defined as those tumors that show accumulation of proinflammatory cytokines and T cell infiltration. In contrast, some cancers are non-responsive and referred to as

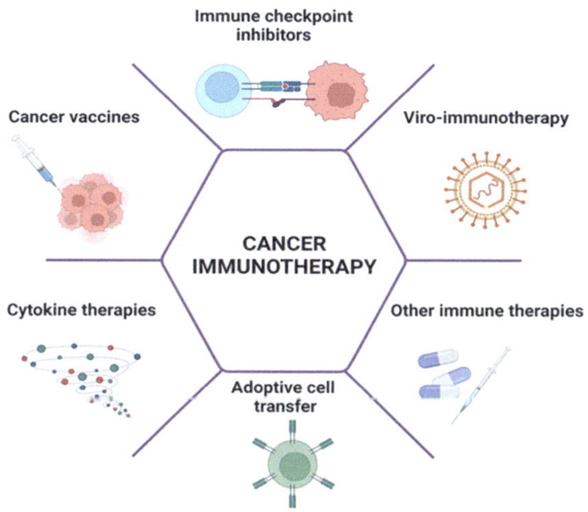


**Fig. 14.1** Cancer immunotherapy types include the use of immune-checkpoint inhibitors, cancer vaccines, cytokines, viruses, and adoptive cell transfer. (Created with BioRender.com, accessed on 23 April 2023 [1]. Taken from Kciuk et al. [1] with permission)

"cold" (immune-desert) tumors [3, 4]. Although turning nonresponsive "cold" tumors into responsive "hot" ones could accelerate therapeutic outcomes, the diversity of mechanisms underlying immune evasion presents a formidable impediment [5]. Therefore, understanding the mechanisms that control these transitions, as well as tumor immunotyping can provide much needed insights into designing effective immunotherapeutic strategies against cancer.

Several immunotherapies are now approved by the US Food and Drug Administration (FDA) and have shown remarkable clinical success against many cancer types. Unfortunately, despite the promise and potential, only a fraction of cancer patients who are eligible for immunotherapy, actually benefit from this treatment, depending on tumor grade/stage and other host factors. As is the case with most therapeutic treatments, cancer cells develop resistance to immunotherapy. As a result, patients either fail to respond or rapidly develop resistance, and hyper- and pseudo-progression can also occur in certain patient populations [6–9].

Resistance to immunotherapy can be either due to cell intrinsic or cell extrinsic factors such as other cells within the tumor microenvironment (TME). Further, while some patients may have primary or innate resistance, meaning they fail to respond to treatment from the start, others can develop secondary resistance [10]. Thus, a deeper understanding of the mechanisms that limit the use of cancer immunotherapy is imperative if we were to overcome treatment resistance and have increased positive clinical outcomes for patients [6].

In this chapter, we summarize the mechanisms underlying cancer immunotherapy resistance, especially the contributions of phenotypic plasticity and the underlying non-genetic mechanisms. Furthermore, recent developments in preventing relapses following treatment to increase the efficacy of immunotherapy for cancer patients are also briefly discussed [11, 12].

## 14.2 Genetic and Non-genetic Resistance in Cancer Immunotherapy

Contrary to the prevailing wisdom, it is now unequivocal that cancer cells can develop drug resistance including resistance to immunotherapy through genetic as well as non-genetic mechanisms. In fact, the ability of cancer cells to exploit both genetic and non-genetic mechanisms to acquire therapeutic resistance highlights cancer's remarkable resilience. Notably, these events are frequently linked underscoring the genetic/non-genetic duality of drug resistance in cancer [13], and while some oncogenic mutations enable cancer cells to rapidly adapt their transcriptional and/or metabolic programs to evade the therapeutic pressure, others promote phenotypic plasticity enabling cancer cells to evade the body's immunosurveillance mechanisms [13, 14]. Furthermore, drug resistance in cancer appears to develop through cell-state transition trajectories together with progressive increase in cell fitness, the so-called "resistance continuum", highlighting the dynamic nature of cellular adaptation [15].

Genetic mechanisms include pre-existing mutations in cancer cells that make them resistant to certain therapies. For example, mutations in genes that affect programmed cell death ligand 1 (PD-L1) expression can lead to immunotherapy resistance. Alterations in PD-L1 expression can preclude immune cells from effectively attacking cancer cells, rendering immunotherapy less effective [16–18]. Similarly, mutations in Beta-2-microglobulin (B2M) can lead to a lack of CD8 T cell [also known as cytotoxic T lymphocytes (CTLs)] recognition [19], and mutations in Janus Kinase 1 and 2 (JAK1/2) can permit cancer cells to escape the effects of interferon gamma [20, 21]. Likewise, mutations in the tumor suppressors phosphatase and tensin homolog (PTEN) [22–24] and serine/threonine kinase 11 (STK11) [25–27] genes are also known to contribute to immunotherapy resistance. Lastly, while it is well known that mutations in the oncogene KRAS can promote cancer cell growth and anti-apoptosis, emerging evidence indicates that mutant KRAS also mediates autocrine and paracrine effects and crosstalk with other constituents of the TME. For example, exosomes derived from KRAS mutant lung cancer cells or lung cancer patients carrying a KRAS mutation could induce CD4+ T cells to switch their phenotype to FOXP3+ Treg-like cells that are immune-suppressive [28]. These results underscore a novel paracrine role for KRAS in T cell phenotypic switching in lung cancer. Thus, tumor-promoting inflammation and immune modulation due to mutant KRAS can cause immune escape in the TME [29, 30], and in colorectal cancer, it was observed that the therapeutic efficacy of cetuximab-mediated antibody-dependent cellular cytotoxicity is impaired by KRAS mutation [31].

While some mutations that drive drug resistance can pre-exist, the so-called innate resistance, cancer cells can also acquire mutations (also known as acquired resistance) during drug treatment. Furthermore, in many instances, while cancer cells initially respond well to a given therapy, they can develop a so-called "drug

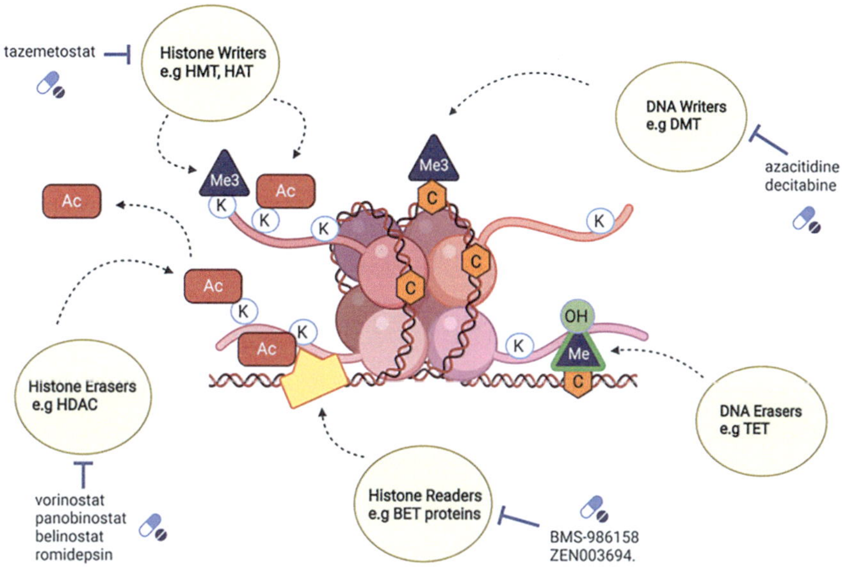


**Fig. 14.2** Conceptual diagram describing key epigenetic modifiers, their mode of action, and their select inhibitors. Histone writers add methyl groups (Me3) or acetyl groups (Ac) can be inhibited by approved drug tazemetostat. DNA writers, such as DMT (DNA methyltransferases) remove methyl groups (Me3) and can be inhibited by approved drugs; azacitidine and decitabine. Histone erasers such as HDAC (histone deacetylases) remove acetyl groups (Ac) and can be inhibited by approved drugs; vorinostat, panobinostat, belinostat, and romidepsin, while DNA erasers such as TET (ten-eleven translocation) oxidize 5-methyl cytosine into 5 hydroxymethyl cytosine. Histone readers such as the BET proteins can recognize acetylated lysine residues on histone tails, and they can be inhibited by BMS-986158 and ZEN003694. (Created with BioRender.com. Taken from Kumar et al. [32] with permission)

tolerant" state which is reversible if the treatment is withdrawn, underscoring the non-genetic nature of reversible drug tolerance but can progress to a bona fide resistant state that is irreversible and is caused by genetic mutations.

Among the different non-genetic mechanisms, epigenetic changes that include DNA methylation, histone modifications, and RNA-associated silencing are widely recognized and can contribute to immunotherapy resistance via multiple ways [32] (Fig. 14.2). For example, they can affect the plasticity of tumor cells, their DNA repair capability, and their susceptibility to cell death pathways [32, 33]. Several drugs that target various epigenetic modulators such as DNA methyl transferase (DNMT), histone deacetylase (HDAC), bromodomain and extra terminal (BET), and some non-coding RNAs, are either FDA-approved or in various stages of clinical development [32, 33]. Additionally, epigenetic changes can regulate reprogramming of cancer cells into cancer stem cell-like cells or epithelial-to-mesenchymal transition (EMT) [34–36].

Other non-genetic mechanisms include abnormalities in antigen presentation such as loss of major histocompatibility complex, Class I (MHC-1) expression that can lead to abnormalities in antigen presentation [37, 38], alternative signaling pathways that can dampen the immune response such as the phosphoinositide 3-kinase (PI3K)/AKT serine/threonine kinase 1(Akt)/mechanistic target of rapamycin kinase (mTOR) pathway that can suppress immune responses by inhibiting T cell function and promoting immune exhaustion, the Notch signaling pathway which can lead to immune suppression by promoting the development of myeloid-derived suppressor cells (MDSCs), which in turn suppress T cell activity, and the Wnt signaling pathway. Aberrant activation of Wnt signaling results in increased programmed cell death ligand 1 (PD-L1) expression facilitating the cancer cells to evade the body's immune surveillance [39, 40]. Some other non-genetic mechanisms also include changes in the TME to limit the effectiveness of antibodies, and chronic inflammation which can promote an immunosuppressive niche and consequently, impair immune surveillance [41, 42]. Finally, certain microRNAs have been reported to contribute to cancer immunotherapy resistance [43–45].

## 14.3 Phenotypic Plasticity, an Emerging Factor in Resistance to Cancer Immunotherapy

Phenotypic plasticity, that is the ability of an organism to change its phenotype in response to perturbations in the environment, is yet another non-genetic mechanism contributing to cancer immunotherapy resistance. In fact, phenotypic plasticity is now emerging as a major factor in cancer [46]. Indeed, phenotypic plasticity and non-genetic mechanisms are the more recently recognized hallmarks of cancer [47] that enable cancer cells to adapt to stressful environments. For example, inflammation which is augmented by drug treatment, can tip transitions between the various T cell phenotypes such as functional cytotoxic cells, reversibly exhausted cells that have minimal cytotoxicity, and cells that are terminally exhausted, resulting in resistance to immune checkpoint inhibitors via a non-genetic mechanism [48]. Thus, phenotypic plasticity can contribute to cancer progression, metastasis, and drug resistance including cancer immunotherapy [49–53].

Phenotypic plasticity in cancer cells can also facilitate dynamically switching between different cell states, for example from an epithelial to a mesenchymal phenotype, also referred to as epithelial-to-mesenchymal plasticity (EMP) [54], allowing them to evade immune detection. Cancer cells can evade the body's immune system by several mechanisms such as altering their surface markers, expressing immunosuppressive molecules, and adapting to the tumor microenvironment [55–59]. Furthermore, different cancer cell populations within a tumor can exhibit varying degrees of plasticity [60, 61]. This tumor heterogeneity presents additional challenges to target all resistant cells with a single immunotherapy strategy. It can also give rise to drug-tolerant persisters (DTPs) in the population. DTPs serve as a bet-hedging strategy by ensuring that, in the case of an unanticipated adverse event, at least some individuals in a population can survive. DTPs can revert to being drug-sensitive in the absence of the drug treatment, they can eventually give rise to irreversible drug resistance.

## 14.4 IDPs and Phenotypic Plasticity

Intrinsically disordered proteins (IDPs) are proteins or regions of intrinsic disorder (IDRs) within ordered proteins that lack unique 3D structure. Instead, IDPs/IDRs exist as interconverting conformational ensembles. Because of their structural plasticity, IDPs can interact with different protein partners in the cell. Cellular protein interactions create a network (protein interaction networks or PINs) that form the main conduit of information flow in the cell. Because of their high degree of malleability, IDPs typically occupy hub positions in PINs. Therefore, dysregulation of IDPs in response to specific perturbation such as stress due to drug treatment contributes to increased stochastic and "promiscuous" interactions between the IDPs and partner proteins. Consequently, latent pathways are uncovered which is defined as PIN rewiring. The latter can lead to altered pathological states such as cancer [62] and phenotypes such as an immunotherapy-tolerant phenotype underscoring the critical role of IDPs in regulating phenotypic plasticity of the cancer cell [63]. Indeed, about 80% of all cancer-associated proteins are predicted to be IDPs [64].

However, if the stress (immunotherapy treatment) persists chronically, the PIN is frustrated. As a result, mutations occur in specific locations (mutational hot spots) in key proteins including IDPs to relieve frustration, and eventually lead to irreversible drug resistance [65, 66]. Such a two-step mechanism, that is a reversible drug-tolerant state leading to a permanent (irreversible) drug-resistant state, has also been observed in bacteria [67]. Furthermore, theoretical studies modeling stochastic bacterial phenotypic switching [68] revealed that switching to a different phenotype that has increased fitness allows the population enough time to acquire compensatory mutations, highlighting how phenotypic switching can serve as a robust strategy to decrease the adaptation time by orders of magnitude [69] (Fig. 14.3). Taken together, these observations underscore not only the role of IDPs but also that of phenotypic plasticity in developing immunity to therapy while speeding up the evolution of therapy-resistant clones [70].

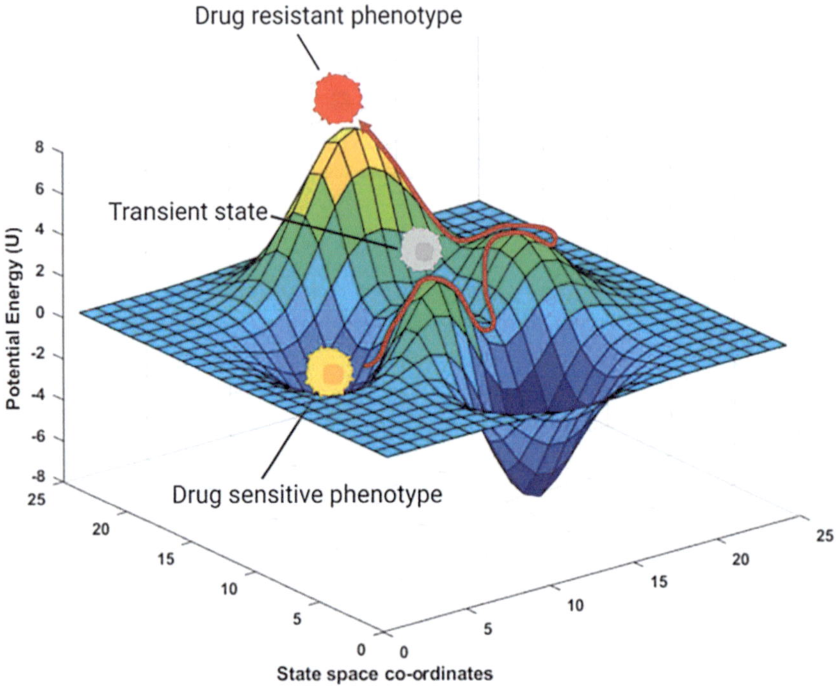


**Fig. 14.3** Cancer network state space as an energy landscape. The energy landscape shows cancer cell states over time with drug exposure. The x–y plane represents state space coordinates, and the z-axis represents potential energy *U*, indicating cell fate stability. Initially, stable drug-naïve cancer cells occupy fixed points and low-energy attractors. Upon drug treatment, cancer cells transition from the stable phenotype (yellow cell) towards other high-energy yet less stable attractors to increase their fitness (red cell). During this transition, cancer cells may traverse transient states (gray cells). (Taken from Ramisetty et al. [69] with permission)

## 14.5 Group Behavior and Therapy Resistance

In addition to the non-genetic mechanism described above, it is now well recognized that resistance to therapy is also due to intricate group behavior of groups of cells within the tumor that is highly heterogeneous and the surrounding TME [65].

Group behavior of cancer cells such as competition and cooperation between distinct phenotypes, is mediated via cell–cell communication. Further, the TME embodies several other types of supporting cells such as cancer-associated fibroblasts (CAFs), various types of immune cells, as well as the endothelial cells, in addition to cancer cells. A major function of these supporting cells is to promote tumor cell growth by producing growth factors and proinflammatory cytokines that promote angiogenesis [71]. Furthermore, group behavior can enable cancer cells to sustain a heterogeneous cell population of cells which can switch phenotypes to give rise to a temporary drug tolerant phenotype while facilitating eventual permanent drug resistance [72].

Group behavior is associated with costs and benefits to the participating cancer cells which can be captured in the form of a game pay-off matrix. Thus, the cancer cell dynamics and tumor progression can be modeled using evolutionary game theory (EGT) which provides a conceptual framework to account for the frequency-dependent nature of ecosystem dynamics. EGT can also be leveraged to discern the games cancer cells play in the presence of selective pressure (stress, such as drug treatment) [69]. Therefore, treatment strategies designed with the strategies cancer cells adopt to deal with therapies could potentially delay or preclude the development of drug tolerance and eventually, the drug resistance phenotype [73, 74].

## 14.6 Potential Therapies to Target Phenotypic Plasticity

Several strategies have been explored to overcome the problems posed by phenotypic plasticity. For example, inhibitors that target EMT-inducing master regulators, transcription factors, or signaling pathways such as the transforming growth factor beta (TGF-b) pathway, could prevent cancer cells from switching to a mesenchymal phenotype, which typically promotes metastasis and therapy resistance [51, 52, 75]. Alternatively, checkpoint therapy could be combined with TGF-β blockade [76].

Additional strategies include targeting the TME and state-gating therapies. Manipulating the TME to downregulate immunosuppressive factors while enhancing immune cell infiltration could also improve response to immunotherapy [77]. State-gating therapies target phenotypic plasticity to limit the spread of cancer as well as its resistance to therapy [78].

## 14.7 Intermittent Therapy

Yet another strategy to address the inevitable resistance to immunotherapy is intermittent therapy. There is now emerging evidence that the classical treatment protocols that call for administering a therapeutic drug continuously at the maximum tolerated dose for the entire treatment cycle can actually encourage the selection of resistant clones. Instead, adopting an intermittent therapy strategy whereby, interventions are administered in on/off cycles meaning, alternating between periods of treatment and rest [79] (Fig. 14.4), can attenuate onset of drug resistance, resulting in improved progression-free survival [80, 81].

Indeed, recent reports also indicate that intermittent therapy can improve efficacy and circumvent resistance to targeted antibody therapies as well, especially to antibody-dependent cellular cytotoxicity [82]. The authors investigated the resistance against cetuximab in colorectal cancer cells. They found that resistant clones showed decreased epidermal growth factor receptor (EGFR)/Erb-B2 Receptor Tyrosine Kinase 2 2 (HER2) expression, upregulation of interferon-related pathways, and downregulation of natural killer (NK) cell activation. More importantly however, the resistant clones reverted to becoming sensitive upon the withdrawal of therapeutic pressure, underscoring the involvement of phenotypic plasticity and

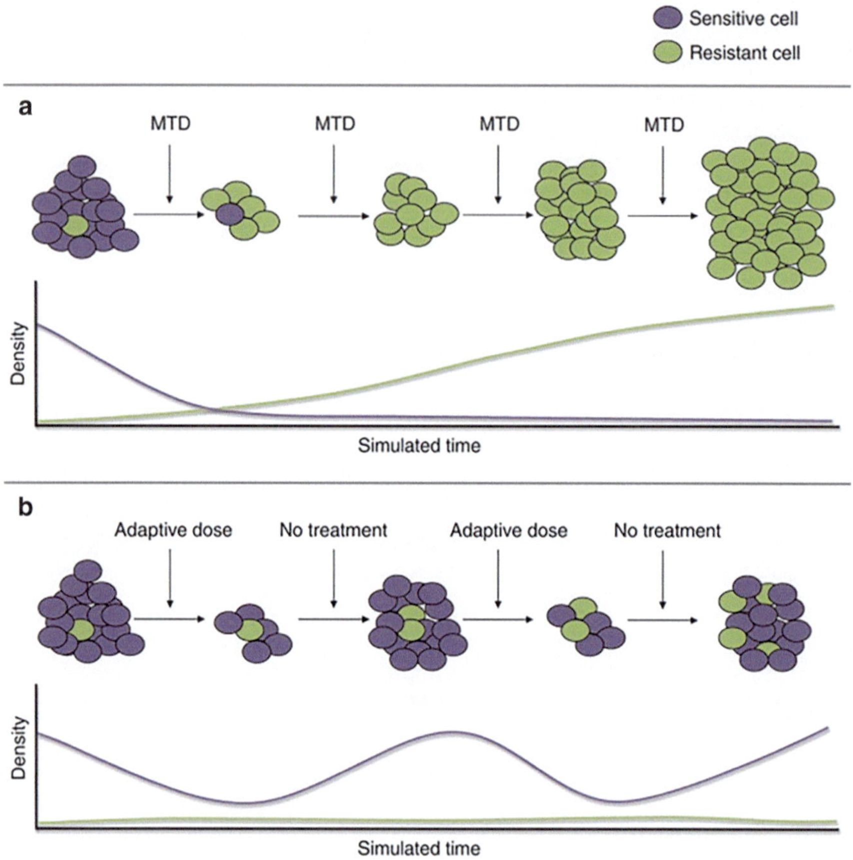


**Fig. 14.4** Illustration of the designed evolutionary dynamics in adaptive therapy. (**a**, **b**) The purple cells are sensitive to the treatment and the green cells are resistant. The graphs represent the simulated density of each population over time during treatment. The top row represents standard therapy in which the maximum tolerated dose is given continuously after initiation. The cells sensitive to treatment are eliminated quickly. This intensely selects for cells that are resistant to the treatment, in this case T− cells, and eliminates the competition effects of the T+ population, resulting in competitive release with rapid treatment failure and tumor progression. The bottom row represents an evolution-based strategy in which therapy is halted before all of the sensitive cells are eliminated. In the absence of therapy, the sensitive cells out-compete the resistant cells due to their fitness advantage. This "steers" the tumor back to the pretreatment so that it remains sensitive to treatment. The resistant cells, or T− population, will increase slightly with each cycle so that this treatment eventually fails. However, mathematical models demonstrate control may be durably maintained for up to 20 cycles—significantly longer than continuous therapy. (Taken from Zhang et al. [79] with permission)

non-genetic mechanisms. Furthermore, a mathematical model predicted that a strategy that administers intermittent dosing is superior to that calling for a continuous regimen in delaying treatment resistance [82].

Likewise, [83] Qi et al. (2022) found that combining an immune checkpoint inhibitor with a targeted therapy, namely BAY1082439, an anti-PI3Kα/β/δ inhibitor, could result in overcoming immunotherapy resistance in PTEN-null mouse prostate cancer models. Importantly, however, the authors observed that intermittent but continuous therapeutic administration could overcome immune checkpoint inhibitor resistance and promote $CD8^+$ T cell-dependent anti-tumor immunity in this mouse model. Mechanistically, BAY1082439 converted the cell-intrinsic immune-suppression to immune-stimulation in the cancer cells by stimulating the interferon α and γ (IFNα/IFNγ) pathway activation, β2-microglubin expression and C-X-C motif chemokine ligand 10 (CXCL10)/C-C motif chemokine ligand 5 (CCL5) secretion. These preclinical data suggest that combination therapy given intermittently but not continuously turn "cold" tumors into "hot" T cell-inflamed tumors, underscoring intermittent therapy as a potential strategy to overcome resistance to immunotherapy [83].

Consistent with the above observations in preclinical studies, a phase II clinical trial that included intermittent ipilimumab/nivolumab treatment with reinduction at progression was conducted (NCT03126331). The main aim of this study was to determine (i) duration of therapy and (ii) determine the safety/efficacy of reinduction at progression in patients who had treatment-naïve renal cell carcinoma [84]. The results were very encouraging and showed that in patients who have a radiographic response to ipilimumab/nivolumab, it is possible to have prolonged treatment-free intervals. Although additional studies designed with de-escalation strategies are clearly warranted, the study by [84] Ornstein et al. (2024) lends further credence to intermittent therapy.

Considered together, these studies on intermittent therapy and several others conducted over the last 20 years have clearly illustrated the virtues of this treatment strategy for several cancer types, especially in light of high and ever-increasing costs [85, 86].

## 14.8 Conclusions and Future Directions

From the foregoing, it is evident that understanding phenotypic plasticity and non-genetic mechanisms is imperative to developing therapeutic strategies to overcome immunotherapy resistance. Targeting mechanisms that underlie phenotypic switching and intermittent therapy are obviously imminent as are some others discussed above. The latter include but are not limited to targeting specific signaling pathways associated with EMT or other phenotypic transitions.

In addition to addressing immunotherapy resistance, research in the future is expected to focus on how to improve treatment durability. State-of-the-art technologies including next-generation antibodies, personalized cancer vaccines, and advanced CAR-T cell therapies hold the promise to address this limitation. For example, bispecific antibodies and antibody-drug conjugates offer new opportunities to target aggressive tumors more effectively. Similarly, incorporating mRNA technology appears to have tremendous potential to advance the field further by facilitating the rapid and precise vaccine development personalized to each patient [87].

With the advent of these new and exciting technologies and the rapid advances in the field, a Team Medicine approach that involves an interdisciplinary team of clinicians and basic research scientists would be ideal in order to leverage the benefits of cancer immunotherapy to the maximum extent [69]. Adopting such non-conventional strategies such as "Evolutionary Tumor Board" (ETB) into clinical protocols is likely to enhance patient outcomes with regard to progression-free and overall survival rates [88]. Besides, in light of the amazing plasticity of cancer, a more dynamic and personalized approach to treating cancer seems imminent. Thus, the eco-evolutionary ETB approach which integrates knowledge and information from preclinical and clinical observations and mathematical models to predict how a patient would respond to different therapies, is well suited for this purpose [89]. Hence, an interdisciplinary Team Medicine approach that is personalized to each patient, is a logical next step in treating and managing patients with this debilitating disease.

## References

1. Kciuk M, et al. Recent advances in molecular mechanisms of cancer immunotherapy. Cancer. 2023;15(10):2721.
2. Ling SP, et al. Role of immunotherapy in the treatment of cancer: a systematic review. Cancer. 2022;14(21):5205.
3. Duan Q, Zhang H, Zheng J, Zhang L. Turning cold into hot: firing up the tumor microenvironment. Trends Cancer. 2020;6(7):605–18.
4. Kuleshov MV, et al. Enrichr: a comprehensive gene set enrichment analysis web server 2016 update. Nucleic Acids Res. 2016;44(W1):W90–7.
5. Zhang J, Huang D, Saw PE, Song E. Turning cold tumors hot: from molecular mechanisms to clinical applications. Trends Immunol. 2022;43(7):523–45.
6. Sharma P, Hu-Lieskovan S, Wargo JA, Ribas A. Primary, adaptive, and acquired resistance to cancer immunotherapy. Cell. 2017;168(4):707–23.
7. Jenkins RW, Barbie DA, Flaherty KT. Mechanisms of resistance to immune checkpoint inhibitors. Br J Cancer. 2018;118(1):9–16.
8. Fares CM, Van Allen EM, Drake CG, Allison JP, Hu-Lieskovan S. Mechanisms of resistance to immune checkpoint blockade: why does checkpoint inhibitor immunotherapy not work for all patients? Am Soc Clin Oncol Educ Book. 2019;39:147–64.
9. Bell HN, Zou W. Beyond the barrier: unraveling the mechanisms of immunotherapy resistance. Annu Rev Immunol. 2024;42(1):521–50.
10. Said SS, Ibrahim WN. Cancer resistance to immunotherapy: comprehensive insights with future perspectives. Pharmaceutics. 2023;15(4):1143.
11. Santiago-Sánchez GS, Fabian KP, Hodge JW. A landscape of checkpoint blockade resistance in cancer: underlying mechanisms and current strategies to overcome resistance. Cancer Biol Ther. 2024;25(1):2308097.

12. Emens LA, et al. Challenges and opportunities in cancer immunotherapy: a Society for Immunotherapy of Cancer (SITC) strategic vision. J Immunother Cancer. 2024;12(6):e009063.
13. Salgia R, Kulkarni P. The genetic/non-genetic duality of drug 'resistance' in cancer. Trends Cancer. 2018;4(2):110–8.
14. Marine JC, Dawson SJ, Dawson MA. Non-genetic mechanisms of therapeutic resistance in cancer. Nat Rev Cancer. 2020;20(12):743–56.
15. França GS, et al. Cellular adaptation to cancer therapy along a resistance continuum. Nature. 2024;631(8022):876–83.
16. Zaretsky JM, et al. Mutations associated with acquired resistance to PD-1 blockade in melanoma. N Engl J Med. 2016;375(9):819–29.
17. Ljunggren HG, Jonsson R, Höglund P. Seminal immunologic discoveries with direct clinical implications: the 2018 Nobel Prize in Physiology or Medicine honours discoveries in cancer immunotherapy. Scand J Immunol. 2018;88(6):e12731.
18. Han Y, Liu D, Li L. PD-1/PD-L1 pathway: current researches in cancer. Am J Cancer Res. 2020;10(3):727–42.
19. Wang H, Liu B, Wei J. Beta2-microglobulin(B2M) in cancer immunotherapies: biological function, resistance and remedy. Cancer Lett. 2021;517:96–104.
20. Shin DS, et al. Primary resistance to PD-1 blockade mediated by JAK1/2 mutations. Cancer Discov. 2017;7(2):188–201.
21. Xue C, et al. Evolving cognition of the JAK-STAT signaling pathway: autoimmune disorders and cancer. Signal Transduct Target Ther. 2023;8(1):204.
22. Peng W, et al. Loss of PTEN promotes resistance to T cell-mediated immunotherapy. Cancer Discov. 2016;6(2):202–16.
23. Cheng F, Eng C. PTEN mutations trigger resistance to immunotherapy. Trends Mol Med. 2019;25(6):461–3.
24. Vidotto T, et al. Emerging role of PTEN loss in evasion of the immune response to tumours. Br J Cancer. 2020;122(12):1732–43.
25. Skoulidis F, et al. STK11/LKB1 mutations and PD-1 inhibitor resistance in KRAS-mutant lung adenocarcinoma. Cancer Discov. 2018;8(7):822–35.
26. Bai R, et al. Mechanisms of cancer resistance to immunotherapy. Front Oncol. 2020;10:1290.
27. Xu K, Lu W, Yu A, Wu H, He J. Effect of the STK11 mutation on therapeutic efficacy and prognosis in patients with non-small cell lung cancer: a comprehensive study based on meta-analyses and bioinformatics analyses. BMC Cancer. 2024;24(1):491.
28. Kalvala A, et al. Phenotypic switching of naïve T cells to immune-suppressive Treg-like cells by mutant KRAS. J Clin Med. 2019;8(10):1726.
29. Hamarsheh S, Groß O, Brummer T, Zeiser R. Immune modulatory effects of oncogenic KRAS in cancer. Nat Commun. 2020;11(1):5439.
30. Pereira F, et al. KRAS as a modulator of the inflammatory tumor microenvironment: therapeutic implications. Cells. 2022;11(3):398.
31. Nakadate Y, et al. KRAS mutation confers resistance to antibody-dependent cellular cytotoxicity of cetuximab against human colorectal cancer cells. Int J Cancer. 2014;134(9):2146–55.
32. Kumar VE, et al. Targeting epigenetic modifiers of tumor plasticity and cancer stem cell behavior. Cells. 2022;11(9):1403.
33. Lu Y, et al. Epigenetic regulation in human cancer: the potential role of epi-drug in cancer therapy. Mol Cancer. 2020;19(1):79.
34. O'Brien-Ball C, Biddle A. Reprogramming to developmental plasticity in cancer stem cells. Dev Biol. 2017;430(2):266–74.
35. Wainwright EN, Scaffidi P. Epigenetics and cancer stem cells: unleashing, hijacking, and restricting cellular plasticity. Trends Cancer. 2017;3(5):372–86.
36. Verona F, et al. Targeting epigenetic alterations in cancer stem cells. Front Mol Med. 2022;2:1011882.

37. Taylor BC, Balko JM. Mechanisms of MHC-I downregulation and role in immunotherapy response. Front Immunol. 2022;13:844866.
38. Sari G, Rock KL. Tumor immune evasion through loss of MHC class-I antigen presentation. Curr Opin Immunol. 2023;83:102329.
39. Yang L, Li A, Lei Q, Zhang Y. Tumor-intrinsic signaling pathways: key roles in the regulation of the immunosuppressive tumor microenvironment. J Hematol Oncol. 2019;12(1):125.
40. Zhao H, et al. Inflammation and tumor progression: signaling pathways and targeted intervention. Signal Transduct Target Ther. 2021;6(1):263.
41. Labani-Motlagh A, Ashja-Mahdavi M, Loskog A. The tumor microenvironment: a milieu hindering and obstructing antitumor immune responses. Front Immunol. 2020;11:940.
42. Jiménez-Morales S, Aranda-Uribe IS, Pérez-Amado CJ, Ramírez-Bello J, Hidalgo-Miranda A. Mechanisms of immunosuppressive tumor evasion: focus on acute lymphoblastic leukemia. Front Immunol. 2021;12:737340.
43. Daveri E, et al. microRNAs shape myeloid cell-mediated resistance to cancer immunotherapy. Front Immunol. 2020;11:1214.
44. Nguyen MT, et al. miRNA as a modulator of immunotherapy and immune response in melanoma. Biomol Ther. 2021;11(11):1648.
45. Nam DY, Rhee JK. Identifying microRNAs associated with tumor immunotherapy response using an interpretable machine learning model. Sci Rep. 2024;14(1):6172.
46. Bell CC, Gilan O. Principles and mechanisms of non-genetic resistance in cancer. Br J Cancer. 2020;122(4):465–72.
47. Hanahan D. Hallmarks of cancer: new dimensions. Cancer Discov. 2022;12(1):31–46.
48. Kareva I, Gevertz JL. Mitigating non-genetic resistance to checkpoint inhibition based on multiple states of immune exhaustion. NPJ Syst Biol Appl. 2024;10(1):14.
49. Horn LA, Fousek K, Palena C. Tumor plasticity and resistance to immunotherapy. Trends Cancer. 2020;6(5):432–41.
50. Benboubker V, Boivin F, Dalle S, Caramel J. Cancer cell phenotype plasticity as a driver of immune escape in melanoma. Front Immunol. 2022;13:873116.
51. Shah S, et al. Understanding and leveraging phenotypic plasticity during metastasis formation. NPJ Syst Biol Appl. 2023;9(1):48.
52. Tímár J, Honn KV, Hendrix MJC, Marko-Varga G, Jalkanen S. Newly identified form of phenotypic plasticity of cancer: immunogenic mimicry. Cancer Metastasis Rev. 2023;42(1):323–34.
53. Sievers C, et al. Phenotypic plasticity and reduced tissue retention of exhausted tumor-infiltrating T cells following neoadjuvant immunotherapy in head and neck cancer. Cancer Cell. 2023;41(5):887–902.e885.
54. Gu Y, Zhang Z, Ten Dijke P. Harnessing epithelial-mesenchymal plasticity to boost cancer immunotherapy. Cell Mol Immunol. 2023;20(4):318–40.
55. Sahoo S, et al. Immunosuppressive traits of the hybrid epithelial/mesenchymal phenotype. Front Immunol. 2021;12:797261.
56. Taki M, et al. Tumor immune microenvironment during epithelial-mesenchymal transition. Clin Cancer Res. 2021;27(17):4669–79.
57. Wang G, et al. The pan-cancer landscape of crosstalk between epithelial-mesenchymal transition and immune evasion relevant to prognosis and immunotherapy response. NPJ Precis Oncol. 2021;5(1):56.
58. Jeong H, et al. Epithelial-mesenchymal transition induced by tumor cell-intrinsic PD-L1 signaling predicts a poor response to immune checkpoint inhibitors in PD-L1-high lung cancer. Br J Cancer. 2024;131(1):23–36.
59. Singh D, Siddique HR. Epithelial-to-mesenchymal transition in cancer progression: unraveling the immunosuppressive module driving therapy resistance. Cancer Metastasis Rev. 2024;43(1):155–73.
60. Tripathi S, Chakraborty P, Levine H, Jolly MK. A mechanism for epithelial-mesenchymal heterogeneity in a population of cancer cells. PLoS Comput Biol. 2020;16(2):e1007619.

61. Subbalakshmi AR, et al. Phenotypic plasticity and cancer: a system biology perspective. J Clin Med. 2024;13(15):4302.
62. Kulkarni V, Kulkarni P. Intrinsically disordered proteins and phenotypic switching: implications in cancer. Prog Mol Biol Transl Sci. 2019;166:63–84.
63. Kulkarni P, et al. Protein conformational dynamics and phenotypic switching. Biophys Rev. 2021;13(6):1127–38.
64. Uversky VN, Oldfield CJ, Dunker AK. Intrinsically disordered proteins in human diseases: introducing the D2 concept. Annu Rev Biophys. 2008;37:215–46.
65. Bhattacharya S, et al. Group behavior and emergence of cancer drug resistance. Trends Cancer. 2021;7(4):323–34.
66. Kulkarni P, et al. A nexus between genetic and non-genetic mechanisms guides KRAS inhibitor resistance in lung cancer. Biomol Ther. 2023;13(11):1587.
67. Hug SM, Gaut BS. The phenotypic signature of adaptation to thermal stress in Escherichia coli. BMC Evol Biol. 2015;15:177.
68. Tadrowski AC, Evans MR, Waclaw B. Phenotypic switching can speed up microbial evolution. Sci Rep. 2018;8(1):8941.
69. Ramisetty S, et al. Leveraging cancer phenotypic plasticity for novel treatment strategies. J Clin Med. 2024;13(11):3337.
70. Kulkarni P, Salgia R. Comprehending phenotypic plasticity in cancer and evolution. iScience. 2024;27(3):109308.
71. Yoshida GJ, Azuma A, Miura Y, Orimo A. Activated fibroblast program orchestrates tumor initiation and progression; molecular mechanisms and the associated therapeutic strategies. Int J Mol Sci. 2019;20(9):2256.
72. Kulkarni P, et al. Addressing drug resistance in cancer: a team medicine approach. J Clin Med. 2022;11(19) https://doi.org/10.3390/jcm11195701.
73. Stanková K, Brown JS, Dalton WS, Gatenby RA. Optimizing cancer treatment using game theory: a review. JAMA Oncol. 2019;5(1):96–103.
74. Stein A, et al. Stackelberg evolutionary game theory: how to manage evolving systems. Philos Trans R Soc Lond Ser B Biol Sci. 2023;378(1876):20210495.
75. Gupta PB, Pastushenko I, Skibinski A, Blanpain C, Kuperwasser C. Phenotypic plasticity: driver of cancer initiation, progression, and therapy resistance. Cell Stem Cell. 2019;24(1):65–78.
76. Shrestha R, Prithviraj P, Bridle KR, Crawford DHG, Jayachandran A. Combined inhibition of TGF-β1-induced EMT and PD-L1 silencing re-sensitizes hepatocellular carcinoma to sorafenib treatment. J Clin Med. 2021;10(9):1889.
77. Pellegrino M, et al. Manipulating the tumor immune microenvironment to improve cancer immunotherapy: IGF1R, a promising target. Front Immunol. 2024;15:1356321.
78. Burkhardt DB, San Juan BP, Lock JG, Krishnaswamy S, Chaffer CL. Mapping phenotypic plasticity upon the cancer cell state landscape using manifold learning. Cancer Discov. 2022;12(8):1847–59.
79. Zhang J, Cunningham JJ, Brown JS, Gatenby RA. Integrating evolutionary dynamics into treatment of metastatic castrate-resistant prostate cancer. Nat Commun. 2017;8(1):1816.
80. Bayer P, et al. Coordination games in cancer. PLoS One. 2022;17(1):e0261578.
81. Chahoud J, Anderson ARA, Zhang J, Brown J, Gatenby RA. Evolutionary dynamics and intermittent therapy for metastatic cancers. J Clin Oncol. 2023;41(28):4469–71.
82. Zhou J, Liu C, Tang Y, Li Z, Cao Y. Phenotypic switching as a non-genetic mechanism of resistance predicts antibody therapy regimens. iScience. 2024;27(4):109450.
83. Qi Z, et al. Overcoming resistance to immune checkpoint therapy in PTEN-null prostate cancer by intermittent anti-PI3Kα/β/δ treatment. Nat Commun. 2022;13(1):182.
84. Ornstein MC, et al. Phase II trial of intermittent therapy in patients with metastatic renal cell carcinoma treated with front-line ipilimumab and nivolumab. Clin Genitourin Cancer. 2024;22(6):102181.

85. Danson S, et al. Are we over-treating with checkpoint inhibitors? Br J Cancer. 2019;121(8):629–30.
86. Henderson RH, et al. Spend less to achieve more: economic analysis of intermittent versus continuous cetuximab in KRAS wild-type patients with metastatic colorectal cancer. J Cancer Policy. 2022;33:100342.
87. Ghemrawi R, et al. Revolutionizing cancer treatment: recent advances in immunotherapy. Biomedicine. 2024;12(9):2158.
88. Robertson-Tessi M, et al. Feasibility of an evolutionary tumor board for generating novel personalized therapeutic strategies. medRxiv:20232001201823284628. 2023
89. Strobl MAR, Gallaher J, Robertson-Tessi M, West J, Anderson ARA. Treatment of evolving cancers will require dynamic decision support. Ann Oncol. 2023;34(10):867–84.

# Index




R. Salgia, P. Kulkarni (eds.), *Immunotherapies in Solid Tumors*, Cancer Treatment and Research 129, https://doi.org/10.1007/978-3-031-97242-3

**D**



**E**



**G**

MIX
Papier aus verantwortungsvollen Quellen
Paper from responsible sources
FSC® C105338

FSC
www.fsc.org

If you have any concerns about our products,
you can contact us on
**ProductSafety@springernature.com**

In case Publisher is established outside the EU,
the EU authorized representative is:
**Springer Nature Customer Service Center GmbH**
**Europaplatz 3, 69115 Heidelberg, Germany**

Printed by Libri Plureos GmbH
in Hamburg, Germany